T0263385

Gender Affirming Surgery

Editors

LEE C. ZHAO
RACHEL BLUEBOND-LANGNER

UROLOGIC CLINICS OF NORTH AMERICA

www.urologic.theclinics.com

Consulting Editor
SAMIR S. TANEJA

November 2019 • Volume 46 • Number 4

ELSEVIER

1600 John F. Kennedy Boulevard • Suite 1800 • Philadelphia, Pennsylvania, 19103-2899

http://www.theclinics.com

UROLOGIC CLINICS OF NORTH AMERICA Volume 46, Number 4
November 2019 ISSN 0094-0143, ISBN-13: 978-0-323-71049-7

Editor: Kerry Holland
Developmental Editor: Laura Kavanaugh

© **2019 Elsevier Inc. All rights reserved.**

This periodical and the individual contributions contained in it are protected under copyright by Elsevier, and the following terms and conditions apply to their use:

Photocopying
Single photocopies of single articles may be made for personal use as allowed by national copyright laws. Permission of the Publisher and payment of a fee is required for all other photocopying, including multiple or systematic copying, copying for advertising or promotional purposes, resale, and all forms of document delivery. Special rates are available for educational institutions that wish to make photocopies for non-profit educational classroom use. For information on how to seek permission visit www.elsevier.com/permissions or call: (+44) 1865 843830 (UK)/(+1) 215 239 3804 (USA).

Derivative Works
Subscribers may reproduce tables of contents or prepare lists of articles including abstracts for internal circulation within their institutions. Permission of the Publisher is required for resale or distribution outside the institution. Permission of the Publisher is required for all other derivative works, including compilations and translations (please consult www.elsevier.com/permissions).

Electronic Storage or Usage
Permission of the Publisher is required to store or use electronically any material contained in this periodical, including any article or part of an article (please consult www.elsevier.com/permissions). Except as outlined above, no part of this publication may be reproduced, stored in a retrieval system or transmitted in any form or by any means, electronic, mechanical, photocopying, recording or otherwise, without prior written permission of the Publisher.

Notice
No responsibility is assumed by the Publisher for any injury and/or damage to persons or property as a matter of products liability, negligence or otherwise, or from any use or operation of any methods, products, instructions or ideas contained in the material herein. Because of rapid advances in the medical sciences, in particular, independent verification of diagnoses and drug dosages should be made.

Although all advertising material is expected to conform to ethical (medical) standards, inclusion in this publication does not constitute a guarantee or endorsement of the quality or value of such product or of the claims made of it by its manufacturer.

Urologic Clinics of North America (ISSN 0094-0143) is published quarterly by Elsevier Inc., 360 Park Avenue South, New York, NY 10010-1710. Months of issue are February, May, August, and November. Business and Editorial Offices: 1600 John F. Kennedy Blvd., Suite 1800, Philadelphia, PA 19103-2899. Periodicals postage paid at New York, NY and additional mailing offices. Subscription prices are $387.00 per year (US individuals), $757.00 per year (US institutions), $100.00 per year (US students and residents), $450.00 per year (Canadian individuals), $946.00 per year (Canadian institutions), $520.00 per year (foreign individuals), $946.00 per year (foreign institutions), and $240.00 per year (Canadian and foreign students/residents). Foreign air speed delivery is included in all *Clinics* subscription prices. All prices are subject to change without notice. **POSTMASTER:** Send address changes to *Urologic Clinics of North America*, Elsevier Health Sciences Division, Subscription Customer Service, 3251 Riverport Lane, Maryland Heights, MO 63043. **Customer Service: 1-800-654-2452 (US). From outside the United States, call 1-314-447-8871. Fax: 1-314-447-8029. E-mail: JournalsCustomerServiceusa@elsevier.com (for print support)** and **JournalsOnlineSupport-usa@elsevier.com (for online support)**.

Reprints. For copies of 100 or more, of articles in this publication, please contact the Commercial Reprints Department, Elsevier Inc., 360 Park Avenue South, New York, New York 10010-1710. Tel.: 212-633-3874; Fax: 212-633-3820; E-mail: reprints@ elsevier.com.

Urologic Clinics of North America is covered in MEDLINE/PubMed (*Index Medicus*), *Excerpta Medica, Current Contents/Clinical Medicine, Science Citation Index,* and *ISI/BIOMED.*

Contributors

CONSULTING EDITOR

SAMIR S. TANEJA, MD
The James M. Neissa and Janet Riha Neissa
Professor of Urologic Oncology, Professor of
Urology, Radiology, and Biomedical
Engineering, GU Program Leader, Perlmutter
Cancer Center, Director, Division of Urologic
Oncology, Department of Urology, NYU
Langone Health, New York, New York, USA

EDITORS

LEE C. ZHAO, MD, MS
Assistant Professor, Department of Urology,
NYU Langone Health, New York, New York,
USA

RACHEL BLUEBOND-LANGNER, MD
Associate Professor, Department of Plastic
Surgery, NYU Langone Health, New York,
New York, USA

AUTHORS

JOSEPH P. ALUKAL, MD
Associate Professor, Department of Urology,
New York Presbyterian Hospital, Columbia
University Medical Center, New York,
New York, USA

JENS URS BERLI, MD
Division of Plastic and Reconstructive Surgery,
Assistant Professor, Residency Program
Director, PLS Gender Surgery Fellowship
Director, Oregon Health &
Science University, Portland, Oregon,
USA

MARTA R. BIZIC, MD, PhD
Belgrade Center for Genitourinary
Reconstructive Surgery, Department of
Urology, Faculty of Medicine, University of
Belgrade, Belgrade, Serbia

JENNIFER K. BLAKEMORE, MD
NYU Langone Fertility Center, New York, New
York, USA

GIDEON A. BLECHER, MBBS, FRACS (Urol)
Consultant Urologist, The Alfred Hospital,
Melbourne, Australia; Consultant Urologist,
Monash Health, Bentleigh East,
Australia

MARK-BRAM BOUMAN, MD, PhD
Department of Plastic, Reconstructive and
Hand Surgery, Center of Expertise on Gender
Dysphoria, Amsterdam University Medical
Center, Amsterdam, The Netherlands

SAMANTHA BUSA, PsyD
Clinical Assistant Professor, Department of
Child and Adolescent Psychiatry, Hassenfeld
Children's Hospital at NYU Langone, New
York, New York, USA

MANG L. CHEN, MD
GU Recon, San Francisco, California, USA

NIM CHRISTOPHER, MPhil, FRCS (Urol)
Consultant Urologist, University College
London Hospitals & St Peter's Andrology,
London, United Kingdom

SARA DANKER, MD
Division of Plastic and Reconstructive Surgery, Oregon Health & Science University, Portland, Oregon, USA

MIROSLAV L. DJORDJEVIC, MD, PhD
Professor, Belgrade Center for Genitourinary Reconstructive Surgery, Faculty of Medicine, University of Belgrade, Belgrade, Serbia

DANIEL DUGI III, MD, FACS
Associate Professor, Department of Urology, Co-founder and Director of Surgical Services, Transgender Health Program, Oregon Health & Science University, Portland, Oregon, USA

GEOLANI W. DY, MD
Department of Urology, New York University School of Medicine, New York, New York, USA

NICK ESMONDE, MD, MPH
Division of Plastic and Reconstructive Surgery, Oregon Health & Science University, Portland, Oregon, USA

M. ELIZABETH FINO, MD
New York University Langone Fertility Center, New York, New York, USA

MARAH C. HEHEMANN, MD
Division of Urology, NorthShore University HealthSystem, Glenview, Illinois, USA

ARON JANSSEN, MD
Vice Chair, Department of Child and Adolescent Psychiatry, Hassenfeld Children's Hospital at NYU Langone, New York, New York, USA

IVANA JOKSIC, MD, PhD
Belgrade Center for Genitourinary Reconstructive Surgery, Clinic for Gynecology and Obstetrics "Narodni Front," Belgrade, Serbia

NATHAN LEVITT, FNP-BC
Hansjörg Wyss Department of Plastic Surgery, New York University School of Medicine, New York University Rory Meyers College of Nursing, New York, New York, USA

WEN LIU, MD, MPH
Resident, Department of Urology, NYU Langone Medical Center, New York University School of Medicine, New York, New York, USA

KAREEN MATOUK, MA
Department of Child and Adolescent Psychiatry, Hassenfeld Children's Hospital at NYU Langone, New York, New York, USA

WILHELMUS J.H.J. MEIJERINK, MD, PhD
Professor, Department of Surgery, Center of Expertise on Gender Dysphoria, Amsterdam University Medical Center, Amsterdam University Medical Center, Amsterdam, The Netherlands; Department of Operation Rooms, Radboud University Medical Centre, Nijmegen, The Netherlands

BOBBY B. NAJARI, MD, MSc
Assistant Professor, Departments of Urology and Population Health, NYU Langone Medical Center, New York University School of Medicine, New York, New York, USA

JOEY NICHOLSON, MLIS, MPH
NYU Langone, Health Sciences Library, New York, New York, USA

DMITRIY NIKOLAVSKY, MD
Physician, Department of Urology, SUNY Upstate Medical University, Syracuse, New York, USA

IAN T. NOLAN, BM
New York University School of Medicine, New York, New York, USA

GWENDOLYN P. QUINN, PhD
Department of Obstetrics and Gynecology, New York University Langone Health, New York, New York, USA

ASA RADIX, MD, MPH, MPhil, FACP
Senior Director of Research and Education, Callen-Lorde Community Health Center, Clinical Associate Professor of Medicine, Department of Medicine, NYU School of Medicine, New York, New York, USA

DAVID J. RALPH, BSc, MS, FRCS (Urol)
Professor of Urology, Department Head, University College London Hospitals & St Peter's Andrology, London, United Kingdom

BAUBACK SAFA, MD
The Buncke Clinic, San Francisco, California, USA

JESSICA N. SCHARDEIN, MS, MD
Resident Physician, Department of Urology,
SUNY Upstate Medical University, Syracuse,
New York, USA

MICHAEL L. SCHULSTER, MD
Resident, Department of Urology, NYU
Langone Medical Center, New York University
School of Medicine, New York, New York, USA

POONE SHOURESHI, MD
Department of Urology, Oregon Health &
Science University, Portland, Oregon,
USA

BORKO STOJANOVIC, MD
Belgrade Center for Genitourinary
Reconstructive Surgery, Faculty of Medicine,
University of Belgrade, Belgrade, Serbia

JURRIAAN B. TUYNMAN, MD, PhD
Department of Surgery, Center of Expertise
on Gender Dysphoria, Amsterdam University
Medical Center, Amsterdam, The Netherlands

WOUTER B. VAN DER SLUIS, MD, PhD
Department of Plastic, Reconstructive and
Hand Surgery, Center of Expertise on Gender
Dysphoria, Amsterdam University Medical
Center, Amsterdam, The Netherlands

THOMAS J. WALSH, MD, MS
Department of Urology, University of
Washington, Seattle, Washington, USA

SUPORN WATANYUSAKUL, MD
Suporn Clinic, Muang District, Chonburi,
Thailand

JEREMY A. WERNICK, LMSW
Clinical Assistant Professor, Department of
Child and Adolescent Psychiatry, Hassenfeld
Children's Hospital at NYU Langone, New
York, New York, USA

LEE C. ZHAO, MD, MS
Assistant Professor, Department of Urology,
NYU Langone Health, New York, New York,
USA

JESSICA N. SCHARDEIN, MS, MD
Attending Physician, Department of Urology, SUNY Upstate Medical University, Syracuse, New York, USA

MICHAEL L. SCHULSTER, MD
Resident, Department of Urology, NYU Langone Medical Center, New York University School of Medicine, New York, New York, USA

POONE SHOUERESHI, MD
Department of Urology, Oregon Health & Science University, Portland, Oregon, USA

BORKO STOJANOVIC, MD
Belgrade Center for Genital Reconstructive Surgery, Faculty of Medicine, University of Belgrade, Belgrade, Serbia

LUQRAAN B. TUYIMAN, MD, PhD
Department of Surgery, Center of Expertise on Gender Dysphoria, Amsterdam University Medical Center, Amsterdam, The Netherlands

WOUTER B. VAN DER SLUIS, MD, PhD
Department of Plastic, Reconstructive and Hand Surgery, Center of Expertise on Gender Dysphoria, Amsterdam University Medical Center, Amsterdam, The Netherlands

THOMAS J. WALSH, MD, MS
Department of Urology, University of Washington, Seattle, Washington, USA

SUPORN WATANYUSAKUL, MD
Suporn Clinic, Muang District, Chonburi, Thailand

JEREMY A. WERNICK, LMSW
Clinical Assistant Professor, Department of Child and Adolescent Psychiatry, Hassenfeld Children's Hospital at NYU Langone, New York, New York, USA

LEE C. ZHAO, MD, MS
Associate Professor, Department of Urology, NYU Langone Health, New York, New York, USA

Contents

> The transgender and nonbinary (TGNB) population is a significant minority, comprising at least 0.6% of the population. Visibility is growing rapidly, especially in younger generations. Gender affirming health care must adapt to this population's needs. Demographic data regarding TGNB health care are limited, but several disparities are clear, stemming from sociopolitical factors, such as external discrimination and insensitive and/or uninformed care. Most self-identifying TGNB patients receive some type of nonsurgical care, including hormonal and/or mental health. Gender-affirming surgery is highly prevalent as well, with at least one-quarter of TGNB people having had some combination of the procedures in this category.

> Transgender people have a gender identity that differs from their sex assigned at birth. For many transgender individuals accessing gender affirming hormone therapy (GAHT) is an important and medically necessary step in their gender transition. Both feminizing and masculinizing regimens are safe when used within established hormone protocols and are associated with significant improvements in mental health outcomes, including reduction in depression, anxiety and gender dysphoria. Clinicians should be aware of the current best practice guidelines for initiating and maintaining patients on GAHT.

> For individuals with gender dysphoria, gender-affirming surgeries (GAS) are one means of reducing the significant distress associated with primary and secondary sex characteristics misaligned with their gender identity. This article uses a systematic review to examine the existing literature on the psychological benefits of GAS. Findings from this review indicate that GAS can lead to multiple, significant improvements in psychological functioning. Methodological differences in the literature demonstrate the need for additional research to draw more definitive conclusions about the psychological benefits of GAS.

> Gender dysphoria, or the incongruence between gender identification and sex assigned at birth with associated discomfort or distress, manifests in transgender

patients, whose multifaceted care includes puberty suppression, cross-sex hormonal therapy, and gender-affirming surgery. Discussion of fertility preservation (FP) is paramount because many treatments compromise future fertility, and although transgender patients demonstrate desire for children, use of FP remains low for a plethora of reasons. In transgender women, established FP options include ejaculated sperm cryopreservation, electroejaculation, or testicular sperm extraction. Further research is needed regarding reproductive health and FP in transgender patients.

The process of gender affirmation may have an impact on fertility. Counseling on the impact of affirmation and opportunities for fertility, future family building, and reproductive health is an important first step in the affirmation process. This article discusses the options for fertility preservation for transmen. The barriers and outcomes in this unique population are also considered. In addition, insights are provided on the future of fertility preservation and suggestions are made for how to build a comprehensive team for male transgender patients.

Simple orchiectomy for gender affirmation is a low-risk, minimally invasive, generalizable procedure that eliminates circulating endogenous testosterone, allowing reduced hormonal supplementation. This article describes a technique that serves as a step in definitive phenotypic transition while maximally preserving healthy tissue for future sex reassignment surgery. Orchiectomy should be offered routinely as a bridge or alternative to vaginoplasty, particularly in the setting of limited access to specialized centers for transgender surgery.

Penile inversion vaginoplasty is a technique of gender-affirming genital surgery that uses primarily genital skin to construct the vulva and neovagina for patients assigned male sex at birth. This article presents present the authors' techniques and other contemporary techniques for this surgery, with particular attention to neovaginal canal construction, neoclitoral construction, and urethroplasty.

Surgical (re)construction of a vagina (vaginoplasty) is performed in biological women with congenital or postablative vaginal absence and in transgender women. Penile inversion vaginoplasty is the gold surgical standard for genital Gender Affirmation Surgery in transgender women. In absence of sufficient penoscrotal skin, due to penoscrotal hypoplasia, circumcision, penile trauma with loss of penile skin quantity and/or quality, or when primary vaginoplasty has failed, intestinal vaginoplasty can be performed. This article provides an update on surgical indications of intestinal vaginoplasty, operative technique, perioperative care, and short- and long-term postoperative issues. A review of recent literature is performed.

Vaginoplasty Modifications to Improve Vulvar Aesthetics   541

Suporn Watanyusakul

Penile inversion vaginoplasty leaves limited penile tissue to reconstruct a realistic vulvar aesthetic appearance. The author introduces a non-penile inversion modification technique for vulvar aesthetics improvement without compromising sexual sensation or vaginal depth by using dorsal neurovascular whole glans penis preputial island flap for sensate clitoris, clitoral hood and frenulum, and inner surface of labia minora reconstruction. It offers two different techniques (type A using preputial flap and penile skin flap, type B using penile and scrotal skin flap) for the double surface of labia minora reconstruction. Simple full-thickness genital skin-mucosal graft vaginoplasty is used for the neovaginal wall lining.

Metoidioplasty   555

Marta R. Bizic, Borko Stojanovic, Ivana Joksic, and Miroslav L. Djordjevic

Gender affirmation surgery for transmale patients is still challenging, as creation of the neophallus is one of the most demanding steps in surgical treatment. Metoidioplasty, as a one-stage procedure, can be considered in patients who desire gender affirmation surgery without undergoing a complex, multistage procedure with creation of an adult-sized neophallus. Metoidioplasty presents one of the variants of phalloplasty for patients in whom the clitoris is large enough under testosterone treatment. Advanced urethral reconstruction provides low complication rates with satisfying results of standing micturition.

Single-Stage Phalloplasty   567

Mang L. Chen and Bauback Safa

Single-stage phalloplasty may be accomplished by having both the microsurgical and the reconstructive urology team operate simultaneously. Phalloplasty with pars pendulans urethroplasty is completed by the microsurgeons, and pars fixa urethroplasty, vaginectomy, scrotoplasty, and perineal reconstruction are performed by the reconstructive urologist. Some surgeons prefer separating phalloplasty from the urologic portions of the procedure. The single-staged approach is favored in patients whose ultimate goal is to have an aesthetic, sensate, and functional phallus and scrotum. Complications remain high but are predictably lower in higher-volume centers. Reconstructive urologists manage the urethral complications that develop.

"Staging" in Phalloplasty   581

Sara Danker, Nick Esmonde, and Jens Urs Berli

The treatment of gender dysphoria related to genitourinary anatomy can be effectively treated with phalloplasty. A phalloplasty may include some or all of the following: penile shaft, glans, shaft urethra, perineal urethra, scrotoplasty, vaginectomy, testicular implants, and erectile devices. The literature does not currently support a gold standard for how best to stage these procedures. This article reviews current techniques for phalloplasty staging and proposes that a staged urethral reconstruction is a reliable technique that allows for potential complications to be managed individually, while minimizing the severity of complications and their impact on the outcome of the final reconstruction.

Gideon A. Blecher, Nim Christopher, and David J. Ralph

Significant developments have enabled the transformation of phalloplasty to a functional organ. Differences exist in the surgical placement of a prosthesis when within a phallus, such as the lack of corpora, pubic fixation requirement, distal sock placement, and the consideration of a vascular pedicle. Increased complications compared with nonphalloplasty cohorts remain one of the biggest challenges, including rates of infection, erosion, mechanical malfunction, and malposition. Nonetheless, the placement of penile prosthesis within a phalloplasty enables trans men to achieve a once near-impossible goal of penetrative sexual intercourse without an external device.

Jessica N. Scahrdein, Lee C. Zhao, and Dmitriy Nikolavsky

As more transgender patients undergo gender-affirming genital reconstructive surgery, such as vaginoplasty and phalloplasty, it is imperative for health care providers, including urologists, to understand the new anatomy and most common complications to diagnose and treat patients effectively. Although there have been several modifications to prior techniques as well as development of new techniques over the years, complications are still common after vaginoplasty and phalloplasty. This article focuses on the most common complications as well as the evaluation and management of those complications.

UROLOGIC CLINICS OF NORTH AMERICA

Foreword

Gender Reassignment Surgery: A New Frontier for Urologists

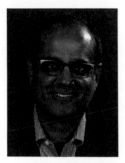

Samir S. Taneja, MD
Consulting Editor

Throughout the history of this specialty, urologists have continued to expand the scope and magnitude of their work. As we learn of new approaches to urologic disease, we often seek out new applications for such approaches, thereby broadening the umbrella of our care. Similarly, we have learned that surgical techniques developed to address one problem may be very applicable in approaching new challenges, allowing us to participate in the advancement of surgery, both within confines of conventional urologic disease and in new areas not previously considered to be urologic in nature.

The field of gender reassignment surgery is not new, but the expanding role of urologists into the area is a response for the increasing patient demand, social acceptance of the need for gender affirmation, and allocation of health care resources to the area. Intuitively, techniques used in male and female genitourinary reconstruction are highly valuable in genitourinary construction at the time of gender reassignment. At the core of the procedures, establishing urinary tract continuity at the time of neophallus construction, continence at the time of neovagina construction, and maintaining potency and genital sensitivity are all highly specialized surgical goals, unique to the urologist.

In this issue of the *Urologic Clinics*, Drs Lee Zhao and Rachel Bluebond-Langner have assembled a series of articles highlighting the spectrum of surgical procedures used within gender reassignment. The range of procedures demonstrates the complexity of the caring for the whole patient, and the critical decisions that must be made on an individual basis, depending upon the patient's goals and care priorities. For most practicing urologists, this issue will serve as an introduction to a new subspecialization within Urology. For some, it will serve as a motivation to enter this new field with their own patients, while for others, it may serve as a nidus for innovation. After all, if genitourinary reconstructive principles have shaped genitourinary construction, refinements in genitourinary construction may allow us to further improve genitourinary reconstruction. We are indebted to Drs Zhao and Bluebond-Langner, and the many authors who have shared their experience, in the creation of this very unique resource for practicing urologists and urologists in training.

Samir S. Taneja, MD
Perlmutter Cancer Center
Division of Urologic Oncology
Department of Urology
NYU Langone Health
222 East 41st Street, 12th Floor
New York, NY 10017, USA

E-mail address:
samir.taneja@nyumc.org

urologic.theclinics.com

Foreword
Gender Reassignment Surgery: A New Frontier for Urologists

Serge S. Ginzburg, MD
Einstein Cancer Center
Division of Urologic Oncology
Department of Urology
NYU Langone Health
222 East 41st Street, 12th Floor
New York, NY 10017, USA

E-mail address:
serge.ginzburg@nyu.org

Urol Clin N Am 46 (2019) xiii
https://doi.org/10.1016/j.ucl.2019.08.001
0094-0143/19/© 2019 Published by Elsevier Inc.

Preface

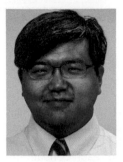
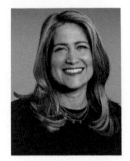

Lee C. Zhao, MD, MS   Rachel Bluebond-Langner, MD

Editors

Due to changing social mores and insurance coverage, gender-affirming surgery for transgender patients is becoming more common worldwide. In this issue of *Urologic Clinics*, we have assembled authors from around the world to review the current status of gender-affirming surgery pertinent to Urologic practice.

We start with demographic trends in treating gender dysphoria. Hormonal therapy is a prerequisite for surgery. Next, the psychological benefit of gender-affirming surgery is discussed. Given that both hormonal therapy and surgery can affect reproduction, fertility preservation for both transmasculine and transfeminine individuals is reviewed.

Next, we delve into feminizing procedures for transfeminine individuals. Orchiectomy is a viable option to reduce testosterone suppression and can be performed prior to or instead of vaginoplasty. For patients undergoing vaginoplasty, the penile inversion vaginoplasty is most prevalent. Intestinal vaginoplasty is a viable technique in patients who do not have sufficient penile and scrotal skin. Regardless of the lining of the vaginal canal, the external appearance of the vulva plays an important role in patient satisfaction.

For masculinizing procedures, genital operations include metoidioplasty and phalloplasty. Phalloplasty can be performed in stages, although authors vary in the process of staging. The placement of penile prosthesis in the neophallus is challenging due to the absence of corpora cavernosa.

Due to many patients traveling to distant centers for gender-affirming surgery, urologists who were not involved in the original surgery may be presented with the challenge of managing complications of gender-affirming surgery. These complications are reviewed to conclude this issue of *Urologic Clinics*.

We are especially grateful for the experts who took time from their families and practices to contribute these articles.

Lee C. Zhao, MD, MS
Department of Urology
NYU Langone Health
222 41st St, 11th Floor
New York, NY 10017, USA

Rachel Bluebond-Langner, MD
Department of Plastic Surgery
NYU Langone Health
222 41st St, 7th Floor
New York, NY 10017, USA

E-mail addresses:
Lee.zhao@nyumc.org (L.C. Zhao)
rachel.bluebond-langner@nyumc.org
(R. Bluebond-Langner)

Urol Clin N Am 46 (2019) xv
https://doi.org/10.1016/j.ucl.2019.09.001
0094-0143/19/© 2019 Published by Elsevier Inc.

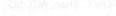

Considerations in Gender-Affirming Surgery
Demographic Trends

Ian T. Nolan, BM[a], Geolani W. Dy, MD[b], Nathan Levitt, FNP-BC[c,d],*

KEYWORDS

- Transgender • Gender-affirming surgery • Demographic • Prevalence • Disparities • Top surgery
- Bottom surgery • Phalloplasty

KEY POINTS

- The transgender and nonbinary (TGNB) population is a significant minority, likely comprising at least 0.6% of the general population. It also is growing rapidly, especially in younger generations.
- Gender-affirming surgery is highly prevalent, with at least one-quarter of TGNB people having had some combination of the many procedures in this category.
- For transgender men, chest surgery is highly prevalent whereas phalloplasty and metoidioplasty are relatively rare.
- For transgender women, surgery is less prevalent than for transgender men, but breast and genital surgery is still relatively common.

DEMOGRAPHIC TRENDS OF TRANSGENDER AND NONBINARY IDENTITY

Specialized care for transgender and nonbinary (TGNB) patients needs to meet the growing needs of a TGNB population whose visibility and access to health care is rapidly expanding. Several data sources from online surveys, explorations of health care databases, and smaller-scale clinic-based surveys provide data regarding trends in TGNB demographics. Several significant trends emerge in the literature, including that TGNB identities are a significant minority, they are identified more commonly in relatively young cohorts, and they are rapidly expanding in visibility. All demographic trends regarding TGNB populations should be understood in the context that TGNB communities exist in all ages and subgroups of society, and research methods should be evaluated for all studies to avoid false conclusions.

The true prevalence of TGNB identities in the United States and worldwide is as yet unknown. Within the United States, the likely best estimate of prevalence is 0.6%, from an analysis of the Centers for Disease Control and Prevention Behavioral Risk Factor Surveillance System in 19 States.[1] Upper estimates of the prevalence of TGNB identities in Western countries are as high as 2.7%, with more conservative numbers estimating it at approximately 0.3% (**Table 1**).[2–6] A few meta-analyses have explored the topic of TGNB prevalence but have been unable to definitively do so due to several limitations in the available literature. A summary of the literature's description of the prevalence of TGNB identity as well as gender-affirming surgery (GAS) overall

Disclosure Statement: None.
[a] New York University School of Medicine, 550 1st Avenue, New York, NY 10016, USA; [b] Department of Urology, New York University School of Medicine, 550 1st Avenue, New York, NY 10016, USA; [c] Hansjörg Wyss Department of Plastic Surgery, New York University School of Medicine, 222 East 41st Street, New York, NY 10017, USA; [d] New York University Rory Meyers College of Nursing, 433 1st Avenue, New York, NY 10010, USA
* Corresponding author. Hansjörg Wyss Department of Plastic Surgery, New York University School of Medicine, 222 East 41st Street, New York, NY 10017, USA
E-mail address: Nathan.levitt@nyumc.org

0094-0143/19/© 2019 Elsevier Inc. All rights reserved.

urologic.theclinics.com

Table 1
Demographic trends of gender-affirming surgery

Parameter	Range of Estimated Prevalence Among Transgender People in the United States (%)
TGNB identity[a]	0.39–2.7[a] [1–4,6,7,9,45]
GAS overall	25–35[10,22]
• GAS in trans men	42–54[10,22]
• GAS is trans women	28[10]
• GAS in nonbinary	9[10]
Genital surgery	4–13[22,26]
• Trans men	25–50[10,25,26]
Hysterectomy	14[10]
Phalloplasty	3[10]
Metoidioplasty	2[10]
• Trans women	5–13[10,22,25,26]
• Nonbinary assigned male at birth	1[10]
• Nonbinary assigned female at birth	<1[10]
• Hysterectomy	2[10]
• Chest/breast surgery	8–25[22,26]

[a] Estimated percent of total US population.

and specific procedures in specific populations is given in **Table 1**.

A few trends are clear. Almost all available data show that TGNB-identified populations are growing in visibility over time. Flores and colleagues[1] note that their estimated prevalence of transgender identity in the United States was twice as high in 2016 as in 2011. Arcelus and colleagues[9] describe an increase in TGNB prevalence in Europe from 1960 to 2014. One recent national survey of more than 50,000 Swedish people in 2014 reported rates of noncisgender identity as high as 2.1% (2100/100,000) and an 8-fold increase in prevalence of transsexualism diagnoses from 2005 to 2015.[6] These trends likely are due to several factors, including greater visibility and acceptance of TGNB individuals, greater willingness to self-identify as TGNB and seek transition, increased quality and availability of gender-affirming care, and better recording of TGNB identities by medical records.[7]

Another consensus among available data is that TGNB identification seems more common among younger age groups. By Williams Institute estimates, TGNB prevalence among adults is highest in the 18-year-old to 24-year-old age group: 0.7% (700/100,000)—higher than 0.6% prevalence in

ages 25 years to 64 years and 0.5% in ages 65 yeras and older. Similarly, approximately half U.S. Transgender Survey (USTS) respondents were between the ages of 18 years and 24 years, although the survey's online nature likely skewed results. The USTS is the largest available data source, from an online cohort of 27,715 subjects enrolled by the National Center for Transgender Equality. A 2016 study of 9th graders and 11th graders by the Minnesota Department of Education reported exceptionally high rates of TGNB identities, as high as 2.7%.[2] This study, which targeted young Minnesotans, is the highest available estimate of TGNB prevalence.

Evidence supports that the apparent increase in TGNB identities and the high prevalence of these identities in younger people come not from an actual increase in the prevalence of transgender identities but rather from an increased acceptance and awareness. Most TGNB people start to identify that they are not cisgender at a fairly young age. According to the USTS, 94% of respondents began to feel that their gender was different from the sex assigned at birth by age 20, regardless of their age at the time of survey.[8] This suggests that older TGNB people were not unaware of their gender identity before coming out but were perhaps not familiar or comfortable with the concept of coming out or of affirming their gender publicly, which may be due to a variety of factors including discrimination, fear, and issues around safety.

Two main patterns emerge in the literature regarding demographic trends of specific TGNB subgroups. The first is that transgender women (females assigned male at birth) are consistently identified at higher rates than are transgender men (males assigned female at birth). This trend is consistent and significant, with some studies reporting transgender women at prevalences twice that of transgender men.[2,9] These proportions are likely skewed, however, by several factors, including those factors that limit all TGNB demographic research, which are discussed later.

Another notable trend is the high prevalence of nonbinary identities. Nonbinary gender identities are those that fall outside the traditional male-female dichotomy. Many nonbinary patients are not cisgender; that is, they do not identify wholly with the sex that was assigned them at birth but also do not identify entirely with the opposite gender. The USTS reported approximately a one-third prevalence of nonbinary respondents, and a large survey of high-school age students reported approximately half.[2,10]

Some studies also suggest that nonwhite groups are more likely to endorse nonbinary identities.

Flores and colleagues[11] estimate that TGNB identity in non-Hispanic whites was 0.48%, whereas it was 0.77% in non-Hispanic blacks, 0.84% for Hispanic/Latino Americans, and 0.64% for other non-Hispanic groups. This could be due to several factors, including variations of gender interpretation between cultures and other societal influences.

NON–TRANSITION-RELATED TRANSGENDER AND NONBINARY HEALTH CARE

TGNB health care involves managing both TGNB-specific health concerns as well as health maintenance that is common to all patients regardless of gender identity. Urologists and plastic surgeons performing GAS should be familiar with both transition-related (gender-affirming) care and as TGNB-specific care that is not directly related to transitioning.

As for all patients, comprehensive urologic care for TGNB people involves management of common health issues unrelated to gender or sex. Other health concerns related to TGNB patients' sex but are not directly related to being TGNB. For example, TGNB patients are likely at different risk for several cancers than their cisgender counterparts, such as prostate cancer in transgender women or breast cancer in transgender men. Increased risk comes not from TGNB identity but from lower screening rates, largely because of insensitive or misinformed practices that are slowly changing to accommodate TGNB patients.[12] Data regarding breast, cervical, and prostate cancer in TGNB patients, however, and evidence-based consensus regarding recommended screening for these diseases are remarkably limited.[13–15]

TGNB health care also should be informed by a several significant health disparities that exist for groups within this population. The term, TGNB, is an umbrella term for patients with several distinct gender identities and who also have intersectional identities that are associated with differing risks for various health concerns. Thus, discussions of TGNB health issues often are oversimplifications. Epidemiologic trends concerning TGNB populations also should be discussed in a nonpathologizing way and should be informed by the various sociopolitical factors that contribute to existing health disparities. The health disparities that affect TGNB populations often are attributed to factors, such as limited access to health care, discrimination in health care settings, poor physician training around TGNB issues, and higher rates of unemployment and poverty.

One significant disparity that is directly actionable by health care providers is the limited scope and poor quality of training around TGNB health concerns. Most medical professionals report lack of comfort managing TGNB patients, and TGNB patients often are turned away because of provider discomfort.[10,16,17] Denying patients care because of their TGNB status is discriminatory and likely contributes to existing health care and health access disparities for TGNB populations.

High rates of HIV and psychiatric concerns create further disparity and seem relatively consistent worldwide.[18–20] HIV affected 1.3% of USTS respondents, notably 19% of black USTS respondents. These rates are especially concerning compared with the 0.4% overall prevalence rate in the United States. Significant to urologists, TGNB populations also are associated with higher rates of other sexually transmitted diseases, which often stem from lower rates of screening due to providers using gendered or insensitive language.

TGNB patients also are more likely to carry various psychiatric diagnoses, such as depression and anxiety. According to the USTS, 39% of respondents "currently experienced serious psychological distress" compared with 5% of the general population; 7% of respondents had attempted suicide in the past year alone.[10] Psychiatric concerns typically arise from issues unrelated to gender, from external discrimination, or from gender dysphoria.

TRANSITION-RELATED TRANSGENDER AND NONBINARY HEALTH CARE

Gender-affirming health care can help lessen mental health concerns affecting TGNB patients. It is effective and medically necessary for those who seek it.[21] Psychological care, hormonal care, and surgical care for TGNB patients with gender dysphoria have all been unambiguously associated with improvements in gender dysphoria, anxiety, and depression. Nonsurgical care, including counseling, hormones, and/or puberty blockers, is the most commonly sought gender-affirming care, with 91% of TGNB reporting desire for these interventions.[10] Estrogen use among transgender women may carry significant thrombotic implications for GAS, and many providers recommend cessation of hormones perioperatively, although this is largely provider dependent.

Utilization of GAS is high in TGNB populations, with most studies reporting at least a 25% prevalence.[10,22] Rates of GAS are rapidly expanding as well. According to the American Society of Plastic Surgeons, GAS is among the most rapidly increasing surgical domains, with a 289% increase for transgender men and a 41% increase for transgender women between 2016 and 2017 (no data available for 2018).[23] Increased rates of GAS are likely due to increases in awareness, demand, surgeon familiarity with the procedures, or insurance coverage.[24]

Subsets of TGNB populations have different rates of GAS utilization. Important modifiers are age, income, and race. Older TGNB patients are more likely to have had GAS.[25] One study found a 4% increased likelihood of having had GAS for each additional year of age.[26] Not surprisingly, more affluent TGNB patients also are more likely to have had GAS. Specifically, those with income below $35,000 to $50,000 are much less likely to have had GAS. Those with income below $10,000 have a 15% GAS prevalence, whereas those with income over $50,000 have 43% prevalence. (Those with much higher income were not much more likely to have had GAS than those with average incomes, consistent with interpretation of GAS as a necessity rather than a luxury.) Nonwhite race is also negatively associated with GAS prevalence, although the effect is small.[27]

Effect of financial status on GAS utilization is critical to TGNB health. According to one survey, cost was the most prohibitive factor to obtaining GAS for approximately 25% of respondents.[26] Lack of insurance coverage is a major barrier. As recently as 2015, more than half of USTS respondents were denied coverage for GAS.[10] Even after interpretation of Section 1557 of the Affordable Care Act as forbidding insurance coverage discrimination on the basis of sex or gender identity, coverage of GAS is still limited for many by slow adoption or persistent discriminatory exclusion policies from private providers not directly affected by the Affordable Care Act.[28–30] Even when coverage is offered, preoperative requirements often are more stringent than for similar procedures for cisgender patients.[31] For example, a transgender man seeking chest (top) surgery may be required to provide letters from psychiatric providers attesting to the appropriateness for surgery, to legally change his name, and/or to live as a member of his identified gender for an extended period of time before GAS can be offered. These requirements are not typical for a cisgender man seeking a similar procedure for gynecomastia.[31] Even when coverage is fully attained, many patients still face significant financial barriers to obtaining surgery, due in part to high rates of poverty, unemployment, and social support compared with the general population.[10,32]

Rates of GAS likely will expand dramatically if insurance coverage for these procedures continues to expand. There is evidence that expanding coverage of GAS is likely to be financially feasible and beneficial for public health, due to decreased health toll and treatment cost from comorbid conditions like HIV, depression, and suicide.[33,34] It is also the authors' opinion that coverage is defensible from multiple ethical and moral standpoints.[34]

GAS utilization is highly variable between subsets of the TGNB population. The specific procedures comprising a given patient's GAS are dependent on patient preferences, which often are influenced by their identified gender, existing anatomy, and degree of gender dysphoria associated with the chest/breast, genitals, face, and other body parts. In general, transgender men seek and have GAS more commonly than do transgender women or nonbinary patients. The best available data suggest 42% to 54% prevalence in transgender men versus 28% and 9% in transgender women and nonbinary patients, respectively.[10,22,26]

For TGNB patients generally, chest surgery is more common than genital (bottom) surgery. As an aggregate, chest surgery is reported at rates of 8% to 25%.[22,26] In transgender men, it is more common than in transgender women (36% vs 11% according to the USTS). The popularity of chest surgery may be due its high saliency regarding outward gender expression for many individuals, because the presence or absence of breast tissue is a highly visible external indicator of gender and sex. Chest surgery also is more accessible, because all plastic surgeons are trained in similar breast augmentation and mastectomy procedures for non–gender-affirming implications like macromastia or gynecomastia.[35] Furthermore, chest surgery typically costs much less than genital surgery and is less morbid.

In contrast, genital surgery is less common. As an aggregate, prevalence of genital surgery among TGNB patients is estimated at 4% to 13%.[22,26] Surgical options for genital surgery are more diverse than for chest surgery, and the prevalences of each type differ greatly.

Feminizing genital surgery options include vaginoplasty (most commonly intestinal or penile inversion) with labiaplasty and/or clitoroplasty, penectomy, and orchiectomy.[36] Prevalence of these procedures is estimated at 5% to 10%, with desire for these procedures at approximately 50%.[10,22,25,26] Among nonbinary people assigned male at birth, 1% have had feminizing genital surgery, and 11% desire it in the future.[10] Most revision vaginoplasties are intended to correct vaginal stenosis resulting from lack of dilation.

Masculinizing genital surgery is less prevalent, estimated at less than 5%.[10,22,25,26] Phalloplasty, metoidioplasty, and hysterectomy are the most common surgical options, based on patient desires to create a neophallus and/or remove internal female reproductive organs.[36] Lower prevalence of genital surgery in transgender men and transmasculine individuals is most likely due to inferior urologic, sexual, and cosmetic outcomes compared with vaginoplasty. Patient priorities may vary greatly with regard to masculinizing genital surgery outcomes, so a detailed description of each procedure's strengths and weaknesses is crucial to understanding its popularity and prevalence.[36–38]

Phalloplasty involves neophallus creation via free or pedicled tissue transfer to the mons pubis, most commonly from the forearm or thigh. It is slightly more common than metoidioplasty, with prevalence of 3% and reported future interest in the procedure at 19%.[10] Phalloplasty is often sought because it potentially results in a sizable phallus that can be used for standing micturition and penetrative sex after urethral lengthening and erectile prosthesis placement, respectively. The procedure is associated, however, with significant donor site morbidity (which often also is stigmatizing in the case of a forearm scar), high rates of urologic complications like fistula and urethral stricture, somewhat limited cosmesis due to flap bulk and skin texture, and need for additional procedures to achieve urinary and sexual function.[39]

Metoidioplasty involves creation of a neophallus via mobilization of a hormonally hypertrophied clitoris with manipulation of surrounding soft tissue. The USTS reports a 2% prevalence and 25% future interest in the procedure.[9] It can be performed with or without urethral lengthening to achieve standing micturition. Metoidioplasty is often aesthetically satisfactory to patients, can be performed in a single stage, allows for standing micturition, and sometimes allows for penetrative sex.[40] Urethral lengthening is associated with high rates of urologic complications, however, and the neophallus is much smaller than one created via phalloplasty.

Additional genital surgery options for transgender men include procedures to remove female genitalia. Hysterectomy is significantly more common than either metoidioplasty or phalloplasty. Prevalence is approximately 14% and future interest is reported by more than half of those who have not yet had this procedure.[10] Unlike neophallus creation, hysterectomy is also relatively common in nonbinary people assigned female at birth: 2% have had it and another 30% express future interest.[9]

Other surgical options, beyond chest surgery and genital surgery, also are available to address additional body parts associated with significant gender dysphoria. Procedures altering the face, body contour, body hair, and voice constitute approximately 10% of all transgender inpatient hospital visits and are much more common in transgender women than in transgender men.[10,22,25,41,42] Prevalences are approximately 50% for hair removal, 17% for silicone injections, 3% to 8% for facial feminization, and 1% for feminizing phonosurgery. Silicone injections are of particular health relevance, because they may have serious or fatal health consequences.[43,44]

LIMITATIONS OF TRANSGENDER AND NONBINARY DEMOGRAPHIC DATA

Although the available literature clearly demonstrates the trends discussed previously, there are considerable limitations to the available data regarding TGNB demographics and health concerns that warrant discussion. Direct study of TGNB patients risks outing publicly, which can lead to discrimination and physical harm. As a result, many studies are performed at TGNB-specific clinics; however, this introduces response bias and limits external validity. Online surveys also preserve anonymity but preclude correlation of responses with actual chart data.

Inadequate sexual orientation and gender identity (SOGI) data reporting continues to be a major limitation. Current United States federal census surveys, which normally provide a wealth of demographic information, do not include SOGI data.[1,45] Physician discomfort with SOGI data also is common and has been well documented.[16,46] SOGI data historically have not been consistently recorded in electronic medical records, frequently precluding accurate coding of transition-related care.[47,48] SOGI data that are collected, especially less recent data, often are limited by inaccurate or obsolete terminology surrounding gender and sex.[49] Studies that utilize coding data, such as *International Classification of Diseases* (*ICD*) codes, are further limited by the relatively poor ability of ICD-10 codes to effectively identify TGNB patients.[7] The overall low quality of available data limits any high-level meta-analytic comparisons.

One effort that may improve the quality of data regarding TGNB demographics is taking a standardized, 2-step approach to SOGI data collection. This approach, which involves asking patients to first state their current gender and then their sex assigned at birth, aids in accurate identification of TGNB people, especially in nonbinary people, in a nonpathologizing way.[50,51] Doing so is beneficial for patient care and demographic data and also is a US Centers for Medicare & Medicaid Services mandate for electronic medical records.[47,48]

SUMMARY

The TGNB population is a significant minority, comprising up to 0.6% of the US population. It also is growing rapidly, especially in younger generations. Therefore, gender-affirming health care, which historically has been limited both in scope and quality, must adapt to this population's needs. Demographic data regarding TGNB health care is still limited, but several disparities are clear, including high rates of HIV and psychiatric concerns. Almost all self-identifying TGNB patients receive some type of nonsurgical care, including hormonal and/or mental health treatments. GAS is highly prevalent as well. At least one-quarter of TGNB people have had some combination of the many procedures in this category, with higher prevalence among older, affluent, white patients. GAS is most common in transgender men, with approximately one-third of them having undergone chest surgery and much fewer having undergone genital surgery in the form of neophallus creation. Both chest surgery and genital surgery are completed by only a minority of transgender women. Nonbinary patients are relatively unlikely to seek GAS.

REFERENCES

1. Flores AR, Herman JL, Gates GJ, et al. How many adults identify as transgender in the United States? Los Angeles (CA): The Williams Institute; 2016.
2. Rider GN, McMorris BJ, Gower AL, et al. Health and care utilization of transgender and gender nonconforming youth: a population-based study. Pediatrics 2018;141(3) [pii:e20171683].
3. Conron KJ, Scott G, Stowell GS, et al. Transgender health in Massachusetts: results from a household probability sample of adults. Am J Public Health 2012;102(1):118–22.
4. Deutsch MB. Making it count: improving estimates of the size of transgender and gender nonconforming populations. LGBT Health 2016;3(3):181–5.
5. American Psychological Association. Report of the task force on gender identity and gender variance. Washington, DC: Author; 2009.
6. Ahs JW, Dhejne C, Magnusson C, et al. Proportion of adults in the general population of Stockholm County who want gender-affirming medical treatment. PLoS One 2018;13(10):e0204606.
7. Ewald ER, Guerino P, Dragon C, et al. Identifying medicare beneficiaries accessing transgender-related care in the era of ICD-10. LGBT Health 2019;6(4):166–73.
8. Herman JL, Flores AR, Brown TNT, et al. Age of individuals who identify as transgender in the United States. Los Angeles (CA): The Williams Institute; 2017.
9. Arcelus J, Bouman WP, Van Den Noortgate W, et al. Systematic review and meta-analysis of prevalence studies in transsexualism. Eur Psychiatry 2015; 30(6):807–15.
10. James SE, Herman JL, Rankin S, et al. The report of the 2015 U.S. Transgender survey. Washington, DC: National Center for Transgender Equality; 2016.
11. Flores AR, Brown TNT, Herman JL. Race and ethnicity of adults who identify as transgender in the United States. Los Angeles (CA): The Williams Institute; 2016.
12. Kiran T, Davie S, Singh D, et al. Cancer screening rates among transgender adults: cross-sectional analysis of primary care data. Can Fam Physician 2019;65(1):e30–7.
13. Stone JP, Hartley RL, Temple-Oberle C. Breast cancer in transgender patients: a systematic review. Part 2: female to male. Eur J Surg Oncol 2018; 44(10):1463–8.
14. Hartley RL, Stone JP, Temple-Oberle C. Breast cancer in transgender patients: a systematic review. Part 1: male to female. Eur J Surg Oncol 2018; 44(10):1455–62.
15. Ingham MD, Lee RJ, MacDermed D, et al. Prostate cancer in transgender women. Urol Oncol 2018; 36(12):518–25.
16. Dubin SN, Nolan IT, Streed CG Jr, et al. Transgender health care: improving medical students' and residents' training and awareness. Adv Med Educ Pract 2018;9:377–91.
17. Ben-Asher B. The necessity of sex change: a struggle for intersex and transsex liberties. Harvard Journal of Law and Gender 2006;51.
18. Cheung AS, Ooi O, Leemaqz S, et al. Sociodemographic and clinical characteristics of transgender adults in Australia. Transgend Health 2018;3(1): 229–38.
19. Chen R, Zhu X, Wright L, et al. Suicidal ideation and attempted suicide amongst Chinese transgender persons: national population study. J Affect Disord 2019;245:1126–34.
20. Jellestad L, Jaggi T, Corbisiero S, et al. Quality of life in transitioned trans persons: a retrospective cross-sectional cohort study. Biomed Res Int 2018;2018: 8684625.
21. Coleman E, Bockting W, Botzer M, et al. Standards of care for the health of transsexual, transgender, and gender-nonconforming people, version 7. Int J Transgend 2012;13(4):165–232.
22. Kailas M, Lu HMS, Rothman EF, et al. Prevalence and Types of gender-affirming surgery among a sample of transgender endocrinology patients prior to state expansion of insurance coverage. Endocr Pract 2017;23(7):780–6.
23. Surgeons, American Society of Plastic. Plastic Surgery Statistics Report. 2017.
24. Shen JK, Seebacher NA, Morrison SD. Global interest in gender affirmation surgery: a google trends analysis. Plast Reconstr Surg 2018;143(1): 254e–6e.

25. Beckwith N, Reisner SL, Zaslow S, et al. Factors associated with gender-affirming surgery and age of hormone therapy initiation among transgender adults. Transgend Health 2017;2(1):156–64.

26. Sineath RC, Woodyatt C, Sanchez T, et al. Determinants of and barriers to hormonal and surgical treatment receipt among transgender people. Transgend Health 2016;1(1):129–36.

27. Wilson EC, Chen YH, Arayasirikul S, et al. Connecting the dots: examining transgender women's utilization of transition-related medical care and associations with mental health, substance use, and HIV. J Urban Health 2015;92(1):182–92.

28. Gage SE. The transgender eligibility gap: how the ACA fails to cover medically necessary treatment for transgender individuals and how HHS can fix it. New Engl Law Rev 2015;49(3):42.

29. Services, Department of Health and Human. Access to healthcare: nondiscrimination. 2017.

30. Gelfer MP, Van Dong BR. A preliminary study on the use of vocal function exercises to improve voice in male-to-female transgender clients. J Voice 2013; 27(3):321–34.

31. Almazan AN, Boskey ER, Labow B, et al. Insurance policy trends for breast surgery in cisgender women, cisgender men, and transgender men. Plast Reconstr Surg 2019;144(2):334e–6e.

32. Nolan I, et al. Continued barriers to top surgery among transgender men. PRS viewpoints, in press.

33. Padula WV, Heru S, Campbell JD. Societal implications of health insurance coverage for medically necessary services in the U.S. transgender population: a cost-effectiveness analysis. J Gen Intern Med 2016;31(4):394–401.

34. Go JJ. Should gender reassignment surgery be publicly funded? J Bioeth Inq 2018;15(4):527–34.

35. Dy GW, Osbun NC, Morrison SD, et al. Exposure to and attitudes regarding transgender education among urology residents. J Sex Med 2016;13(10): 1466–72.

36. van de Grift TC, Pigot GLS, Boudhan S, et al. A longitudinal study of motivations before and psychosexual outcomes after genital gender-confirming surgery in transmen. J Sex Med 2017; 14(12):1621–8.

37. Beek TF, Kreukels BP, Cohen-Kettenis PT, et al. Partial treatment requests and underlying motives of applicants for gender affirming interventions. J Sex Med 2015;12(11):2201–5.

38. Jacobsson J, Andreasson M, Kolby L, et al. Patients' priorities regarding female-to-male gender affirmation surgery of the genitalia-a pilot study of 47 patients in Sweden. J Sex Med 2017;14(6):857–64.

39. Rooker SA, Vyas KS, DiFilippo EC, et al. The rise of the neophallus: a systematic review of penile prosthetic outcomes and complications in gender-affirming surgery. J Sex Med 2019;16(5):661–72.

40. Frey JD, Poudrier G, Chiodo MV, et al. A systematic review of metoidioplasty and radial forearm flap phalloplasty in female-to-male transgender genital reconstruction: is the "ideal" neophallus an achievable goal? Plast Reconstr Surg Glob open 2016; 4(12):e1131.

41. Canner JK, Harfouch O, Kodadek LM, et al. Temporal trends in gender-affirming surgery among transgender patients in the united states. JAMA Surg 2018;153(7):609–16.

42. Morrison SD, Vyas KS, Motakef S, et al. Facial feminization: systematic review of the literature. Plast Reconstr Surg 2016;137(6):1759–70.

43. Wilson E, Rapues J, Jin H, et al. The use and correlates of illicit silicone or "fillers" in a population-based sample of transwomen, San Francisco, 2013. J Sex Med 2014;11(7):1717–24.

44. Leonardi NR, Compoginis JM, Luce EA. Illicit cosmetic silicone injection: a recent reiteration of history. Ann Plast Surg 2016;77(4):485–90.

45. Meerwijk EL, Sevelius JM. Transgender population size in the United States: a meta-regression of population-based probability samples. Am J Public Health 2017;107(2):e1–8.

46. Kodadek LM, Peterson S, Shields RY, et al. Collecting sexual orientation and gender identity information in the emergency department : the divide between patient and provider perspectives. Emerg Med J 2019;36(3):136–41.

47. Alper JF, MN, Sanders JQ. Collecting sexual orientation and gender identity data in electronic health records: workshop summary. Washington, DC: Institute of Medicine; 2013.

48. Centers for Medicare and Medicaid Services (CMS), HHS. Medicare and Medicaid Programs; Electronic Health Record Incentive Program–Stage 3 and Modifications to Meaningful Use in 2015 Through 2017. Final rules with comment period. Fed Regist. 2015; 80(200):62761–955.

49. Rachlin K, Green J, Lombardi E. Utilization of health care among female-to-male transgender individuals in the United States. J Homosex 2008;54(3):243–58.

50. Deutsch MB, Buchholz D. Electronic health records and transgender patients–practical recommendations for the collection of gender identity data. J Gen Intern Med 2015;30(6):843–7.

51. Tate CC, Ledbetter JN, Youssef CP. A two-question method for assessing gender categories in the social and medical sciences. J Sex Res 2013;50(8):767–76.

Hormone Therapy for Transgender Adults

Asa Radix, MD, MPH, MPhil[a,b],*

KEYWORDS

- Transgender • Hormones • Gender-affirming care • Clinical guidelines • Transmasculine
- Transfeminine • Endocrine treatment • Cross-gender hormones

KEY POINTS

- Transgender people have a gender identity that differs from their sex assigned at birth and may seek medical interventions to better align their gender identity.
- Regimens for transgender women usually include estrogen therapy in combination with antiandrogens, whereas those for transgender men include testosterone treatment.
- Gender-affirming hormone therapy is safe when used following established guidelines and results in improved psychological outcomes, including reduced anxiety and depression.
- Feminizing regimens may be associated with elevated risk of venous thromboembolism, cardiovascular risk, and dyslipidemias, requiring optimal control of modifiable risk factors.

INTRODUCTION

Transgender people have a gender identity that differs from their sex assigned at birth.[1,2] Some transgender individuals experience distress from this gender incongruence, or gender dysphoria, and may seek medical interventions, in part to better align their outward appearance with their gender identity. For many transgender individuals accessing hormone therapy is an important and medically necessary step in their gender transition.

Compared with cisgender (ie, not transgender) people, transgender individuals experience higher rates of mental health issues (anxiety, depression) and substance use disorders as well as a wide range of medical issues, including lower rates of health utilization, higher rates of tobacco use, sexually transmitted infections, and human immunodeficiency virus infection.[3–7] More than 40% of transgender people have attempted suicide in their lives.[3] These health disparities are thought to be explained by the *minority stress model* that proposes that exposure to stressors, including high rates of enacted stigma (discrimination, rejection, and victimization), internalized stigma, and concealment of identity, adversely influences physical and mental health outcomes.[8–12] Provision of gender-affirming hormone therapy (GAHT) has been shown to improve quality of life and reduces mood disorders, such as anxiety and depression.[13–15] This paper summarizes models of care for hormone provision, describes established hormone protocols, and discusses primary care considerations for transgender people receiving GAHT.

HISTORICAL PERSPECTIVE

It was not until estrogens and testosterone were chemically synthesized and became commercially available in the 1930s and 1940s[16,17] that transgender people were able to access effective hormonal interventions. In 1967 Harry Benjamin published his highly acclaimed book "The Transsexual Phenomenon" where he outlined his experiences providing hormone therapy to transgender people.[18] It was not until 1979, however, that the first standards of care for transgender people were developed by the Harry Benjamin International Gender Dysphoria Association, later

[a] Callen-Lorde Community Health Center, 356 West 18th Street, New York, NY 10011, USA; [b] Department of Medicine, NYU School of Medicine, New York, NY, USA
* 356 West 18th Street, New York, NY 10011.
E-mail address: aradix@callen-lorde.org

Urol Clin N Am 46 (2019) 467–473
https://doi.org/10.1016/j.ucl.2019.07.001
0094-0143/19/© 2019 Elsevier Inc. All rights reserved.

renamed The World Professional Association of Transgender Health (WPATH). WPATH is an international organization of multidisciplinary health professionals and researchers dedicated to transgender medicine. The most recent edition of the standards of care (Version 7) was published in 2011[1] and version 8 is currently underway. Additional guidelines for hormonal treatment have been published by the Endocrine Society[19] as well as by institutions such as the UCSF Center of Excellence for Transgender Health and several international organizations, including the World Health Organization[20–24] (Table 1).

The early standards of care for transgender health required a specified period of psychological and/or psychiatric evaluation and a confirmed psychiatric diagnosis of gender identity disorder (GID) before individuals were eligible for hormonal interventions, which were usually prescribed by an endocrinologist. Over time there has been improved understanding of gender identity development resulting in a more flexible and patient-centered approach to GAHT provision. This has occurred alongside important changes in diagnostic tools such as the Diagnostic and Scientific Manual (DSM-5) and the International Classification of Diseases (ICD-11), which removed GID diagnoses in favor of gender dysphoria and gender incongruence (GI) respectively and removed GI from the list of mental health disorders.[25–27]

GOALS OF HORMONE THERAPY

The key principle for hormonal treatment of transgender adults is to replicate as closely as possible the hormone environment that is concordant with the person's gender identity. This includes suppressing endogenous hormones and replacing them with the hormones consistent with the affirmed gender.[1,19] The current guidelines for hormone treatment predominately focus on transgender people with binary identities (eg, transgender man or transgender woman) and not those who identify as another gender, between genders, or who do not identify with any gender, including gender nonbinary, gender-nonconforming/genderqueer, or agender people. Similar principles of hormonal therapy apply to people with nonbinary gender identities, which is to prescribe hormones that achieve the goal of the individual patient and that are within usual safety parameters. Although some people may wish to achieve full masculinization or feminization possible from hormonal interventions, others may only want sufficient hormones to achieve an androgenous appearance or to relieve symptoms of gender dysphoria.

Table 1
Clinical guidelines in transgender medicine

Agency	Year	Guideline
The Endocrine Society, USA	2017	Endocrine Treatment of Gender-Dysphoric/ Gender-Incongruent Persons: An Endocrine Society Clinical Practice Guideline
Center of Excellence for Transgender Health, University of California, San Francisco	2016	Guidelines for the Primary Care of Transgender, Gender Nonconforming, and Gender Nonbinary People.
Health Policy Project, Asia Pacific Transgender Network, United Nations Development Programme[21]	2015	Blueprint for the provision of comprehensive care for transpeople and trans communities in Asia and the Pacific
Pan American Health Organization[22]	2014	Blueprint for the provision of comprehensive care for transpersons and their communities in the Caribbean and other anglophone countries
Royal College of Psychiatrists, London, UK[23]	2013	Good practice guidelines for the assessment and treatment of adults with gender dysphoria, 2013
Transgender Health Research Lab, University of Waikato[24]	2018	Guidelines for gender affirming healthcare for gender diverse and transgender children, young people and adults in Aotearoa, New Zealand
The World Professional Association of Transgender Health (WPATH)[1]	2011	Standards of care for the health of transsexual, transgender, and gender-nonconforming people, Version 7

MEDICAL ASSESSMENT BEFORE HORMONE INITIATION

Although some centers use a multidisciplinary team model that includes mental health and medical providers to assess adults before initiating GAHT, it is also acceptable to use a single practitioner model whereby medical providers who are knowledgeable in transgender medicine evaluate patients for coexisting medical or mental health concerns and provide the initial prescriptions and ongoing hormone management. Institutions and providers that care for transgender adolescents younger than 18 years usually follow specific adolescent protocols for hormone initiation due to important considerations including the need for parental consent, stage of pubertal development, and eligibility for puberty suppression.[28]

The medical assessment should start with a detailed medical and psychosocial history that details the individual's sex assigned at birth, gender identity, name and pronoun use, and all medical, social, and legal steps taken to affirm their gender identity, including use of hormones obtained outside of traditional medical settings and interventions such as silicone and soft tissue fillers. Past medical history should focus on issues that may increase the risks associated with or that may be exacerbated by hormonal therapy (**Table 2**). Patients should also be asked about mental health diagnoses,

suicidal ideation, past psychiatric hospitalizations, and childhood trauma. Patients need to be able to make an informed decision about GAHT, so an assessment of capacity to provide informed consent is necessary. Patients should be counseled about smoking cessation because tobacco is associated with higher risk of complications, especially thromboembolic and cardiovascular disease.[29] Because patients may previously have avoided medical care due to experiences of discrimination,[3] they may be unaware of existing health issues and a complete physical examination should be done on all patients with attention to signs of cardiovascular compromise. Genital examinations are not mandated before initiation of GAHT but should be done after rapport is built and the patient is willing. Medical providers can offer preventive health screenings and update immunizations at this time.

FEMINIZING HORMONE REGIMENS

The optimal medical treatment offered to transgender women includes an estrogen in combination with an androgen blocker (the latter can be stopped after gonadectomy) to reduce endogenous testosterone levels. Estrogen therapy usually consists of 17-beta estradiol, which can be administered by oral, transdermal, or parenteral routes. Previously other estrogens were used, including ethinyl estradiol and conjugated estrogens; however, these are no longer recommended due to the high rates of venous thromboembolism.[29–31]

The usual dosing of oral estradiol is 2 mg daily, which can be titrated up to 6 mg if tolerated. If using injectable estradiol this is given biweekly. Transdermal estradiol patches are associated with lower risk of thromboembolism and may be preferred in certain circumstances where age is greater than 45 years and there is history of venous thromboembolic disease, cardiovascular disease risk factors, or tobacco use.[31–33]

The androgen blocker used most frequently in the United States is spironolactone, an oral mineralocorticoid-receptor antagonist with antiandrogen properties.[19,34] Spironolactone is dosed 100 mg to 300 mg daily. Cyproterone acetate and gonadotropin-releasing hormone (GnRH) agonists are the androgen blockers most frequently used in Europe.[23,35] Five alpha-reductase inhibitors such as finasteride have also been used for GAHT. (**Table 3**) summarizes available GAHT regimens. Feminizing hormonal regimens result in breast growth, softening of the skin, slowing of androgenetic hair loss, fat redistribution from the abdomen to the hips, and reduced prostate and testicular size but have no effect on facial

Table 2
Medical risks and hormone therapy

Testosterone	Estrogen
Erythrocytosis	Thromboembolic disease
Coronary artery disease	Coronary artery disease
Cerebrovascular disease	Cerebrovascular disease
Hypertension	Dyslipidemia (high triglycerides)
Breast/uterine cancer	Breast cancer
Fertility decreased	Gall bladder disease
Dyslipidemia (low HDL, high LDL)	Prolactinoma
	Fertility decreased

Abbreviations: HDL, high-density lipoprotein; LDL, low-density lipoprotein.

Data from Hembree WC, Cohen-Kettenis PT, Gooren L, et al. Endocrine Treatment of Gender-Dysphoric/Gender-Incongruent Persons: An Endocrine Society* Clinical Practice Guideline. *The Journal of Clinical Endocrinology & Metabolism.* 2017;102(11) and Abramowitz J, Tangpricha V. Hormonal Management for Transfeminine Individuals. *Clinics in plastic surgery.* 2018;45(3):313-317.

Table 3 Gender-affirming hormone regimens		
Feminizing Hormone Regimens	**Route**	**Dose**
Estradiol oral	Oral or sublingual	2–6 mg daily
Estradiol valerate	Intramuscular (IM)	5–20 mg every 2 wk
Estradiol patch transdermal	Transdermal	25–200 mcg daily
Antiandrogen	**Route**	**Dose**
Spironolactone	Oral	25–300 mg daily
Finasteride	Oral	1–5 mg daily
Cyproterone acetate	Oral	25–50 mg daily
Leuprolide acetate	Subcutaneous/IM	3.75 mg/mo or 11.25 mg/3 mo
Masculinizing Hormone Regimens	**Route**	**Dose**
Testosterone cypionate/enanthate	Subcutaneous/IM	20–100 mg/wk
Testosterone topical gel 1%	Transdermal	12.5–100 mg daily
Testosterone topical gel 1.62%	Transdermal	20.25–103.25 mg daily
Testosterone nasal gel 5.5 mg/0.122 gm	Nasal	5.5 mg each nostril, 3 times daily
Testosterone undecanoate	IM	750 mg IM at 10 wk intervals

Data from Hembree WC, Cohen-Kettenis PT, Gooren L, et al. Endocrine Treatment of Gender-Dysphoric/Gender-Incongruent Persons: An Endocrine Society* Clinical Practice Guideline. *The Journal of Clinical Endocrinology & Metabolism.* 2017;102(11) and Center of Excellence for Transgender Health, Department of Family and Community Medicine, University of California San Francisco,. Guidelines for the Primary and Gender-Affirming Care of Transgender and Gender Nonbinary People. In: Deutsch M, ed. 2nd ed. San Francisco, CA: University of California San Francisco; 2016. Available at: www.transhealth.ucsf.edu/ Accessed 12/20/2018.

beard hair, for which permanent hair removal, for example, electrolysis, is recommended. Feminizing regimens do not change the voice.[1,34] These regimens will usually decrease libido and cause erectile dysfunction and poor ejaculation. This may or may not be consistent with an individual's goals. When this is a problem options include reducing the androgen blocker dose or initiating phosphodiesterase type 5 inhibitor agents.

After initiating hormonal treatment, patients are usually seen at 1 month and then every 3 months for 1 year. If there are no complications and hormone levels are stable, subsequent follow-up can occur every 6 to 12 months. Laboratory testing should include complete blood count, lipid profile, serum glucose, electrolytes, and hepatic profile before and after initiating hormones and thereafter based on clinical necessity and whenever regimen doses change. Close attention should be paid to potassium levels for patients receiving spironolactone. Hormone levels (estradiol and total testosterone) should be done at each visit, with the goal to achieve an estradiol level of approximately 200 pg/mL.[19] Testosterone levels vary according to the blocker used. With GnRH analogues it is possible to achieve levels less than 50 ng/dL; however, the decrease in testosterone levels is not predictable with spironolactone, and testosterone level will increase if using 5-alpha reductase inhibitors.

MASCULINIZING HORMONE REGIMENS

Testosterone treatment is the mainstay of GAHT for transgender men and nonbinary identified people wanting to achieve masculinizing effects. Testosterone can be administered by injection, transdermal (patch or gel), and nasal routes. An oral formulation of testosterone undecanoate was recently approved by the Food and Drug Administration; however, there is insufficient experience to recommend its use in transgender regimens. There are no studies to recommend a particular route and so this decision is made with the patient, taking into account issues such as cost, comfort with self-injection, possibility of testosterone gel transferring to others, and understanding that low-dose gel may not adequately suppress menses. The usual dose of testosterone cypionate is 50 to 100 mg subcutaneous injection (or 100–200 mg intramuscularly every 2 weeks). The benefit to subcutaneous injection is a smaller gauge needle that most patients prefer.[36] The effects of testosterone include changes in fat redistribution (more fat in the abdominal area), facial hair, deepening of the voice, clitoromegaly, oily skin, acne, vaginal dryness, increase in muscle mass/strength, increased sex drive, and cessation of menses. Some patients may experience androgenetic hair loss.[19] Although testosterone frequently causes amenorrhea, it is not an effective method of contraception; therefore, patients should be counseled about the need for options such as depot medroxyprogesterone, intrauterine devices, and other long-acting reversal contraception.[37,38]

It is important to discuss fertility preservation with all patients before initiating GAHT and any surgeries that can result in sterility. Both feminizing and masculinizing regimens can reduce fertility while people are actively taking hormones; however little is known about long-term effects. Options for patients who want genetic offspring include oocyte/embryo cryopreservation and semen cryopreservation.[39] Although these procedures are best done before initiation of GAHT, patients can also discontinue hormones later on in order to attempt pregnancy or gamete cryopreservation.[1,39,40]

After initiating hormonal treatment patients are usually seen at 1 month and then every 3 months for 1 year. If there are no complications and hormone levels are stable, subsequent follow-up can occur every 6 to 12 months. Laboratory testing should include complete blood count, lipid profile, serum glucose, and hepatic profile before and after initiating hormones and thereafter based on clinical necessity. Hormone levels (total testosterone) and hematocrit should be done at each visit, with the goal to achieve a testosterone level in the usual male range of 400 to 700 ng/dL.[19]

PRIMARY CARE ISSUES

Transgender women require ongoing preventive health care with attention to medical conditions that may be exacerbated by GAHT. Estrogen therapy is associated with higher rates of venous thromboembolism and possible higher risk for cerebrovascular disease.[41] Research indicates that before starting hormones bone mineral density is lower than cisgender men; however initiation of GAHT seems to mitigate this risk.[42,43] Screening by dual-energy x-ray absorptiometry should occur at age 65 years and earlier in the setting of known risk factors.[42] Transgender women retain their prostate even after genital surgery, so recommendations for discussing prostate cancer risk and evaluation should be followed. Current guidelines recommend following breast cancer screening guidelines for transgender women on hormones.[19,44] Medical providers should seek to optimize cardiovascular and bone health for transgender patients by encouraging healthy eating and exercise and adequate vitamin D intake and treating hypertension, diabetes, dyslipidemias, and tobacco use.

Transgender men should continue to receive cervical and breast cancer screening according to guidelines for cisgender women. If they have had chest masculinization surgery (mastectomy), chest wall examinations as well as breast cancer screening should be discussed, as complete removal of breast tissue during surgery does not usually occur.[19,44] Screening for osteoporosis follows the same guidelines as for cisgender women.[42]

SUMMARY

Transgender patients often seek GAHT to align with their gender identity and reduce gender dysphoria. Both feminizing and masculinizing regimens are safe when used within established hormone protocols. Access to GAHT is associated with significant improvements in mental health outcomes, including reduction in depression and anxiety. Clinicians need to be aware of the current guidelines for initiating and maintaining patients on GAHT and be familiar with potential adverse effects to be monitored. They should be able to counsel transgender individuals about risks and benefits to hormonal therapy, including the impact on fertility. Medical providers should offer preventive care interventions to patients according to best clinical practice recommendations.

REFERENCES

1. Coleman E, Bockting W, Botzer M, et al. Standards of care for the health of transsexual, transgender, and gender-nonconforming people, version 7. Int J Transgend 2011;13:165.
2. Winter S, Diamond M, Green J, et al. Transgender people: health at the margins of society. Lancet 2016;388(10042):390–400.
3. James SE, Herman JL, Rankin S, et al. The report of the 2015 U.S. transgender survey. Washington, DC: National Center for Transgender Equality; 2016.
4. Herbst JH, Jacobs ED, Finlayson TJ, et al. Estimating HIV prevalence and risk behaviors of transgender persons in the United States: a systematic review. AIDS Behav 2008;12(1):1–17.
5. Bye L, Gruskin E, Greenwood G, et al. California lesbians, gays, bisexuals, and transgender tobacco use survey - 2004. Sacramento (CA): Califrnia Department of Health Services; 2005.
6. Becasen JS, Denard CL, Mullins MM, et al. Estimating the prevalence of HIV and sexual behaviors among the US transgender population: a systematic

review and meta-analysis, 2006-2017. Am J PublicHealth 2019;109(1):e1–8.

7. Grant JM, Mottet LA, Tanis J. National transgender discrimination survey report on health and health care. Washington, DC: National Center for Transgender Equality and the National Gay and Lesbian Task Force; 2010.

8. Carmel TC, Erickson-Schroth L. Mental health and the transgender population. J PsychosocNursMent Health Serv 2016;54(12):44–8.

9. Nuttbrock L, Bockting W, Rosenblum A, et al. Gender abuse and major depression among transgender women: a prospective study of vulnerability and resilience. Am J PublicHealth 2014;104(11): 2191–8.

10. Bockting WO, Miner MH, Swinburne Romine RE, et al. Stigma, mental health, and resilience in an online sample of the US transgender population. Am J PublicHealth 2013;103(5):943–51.

11. Meyer IH. Prejudice, social stress, and mental health in lesbian, gay, and bisexual populations: conceptual issues and research evidence. Psychol Bull 2003;129(5):674–97.

12. Gonzalez CA, Gallego JD, Bockting WO. Demographic characteristics, components of sexuality and gender, and minority stress and their associations to excessive alcohol, cannabis, and illicit (non-cannabis) drug use among a large sample of transgender people in the United States. J Prim Prev 2017;38(4):419–45.

13. Nguyen HB, Chavez AM, Lipner E, et al. Gender-affirming hormone use in transgender individuals: impact on behavioral health and cognition. Curr Psychiatry Rep 2018;20(12):110.

14. Dhejne C, Van Vlerken R, Heylens G, et al. Mental health and gender dysphoria: a review of the literature. Int Rev Psychiatry 2016;28(1):44–57.

15. Witcomb GL, Bouman WP, Claes L, et al. Levels of depression in transgender people and its predictors: results of a large matched control study with transgender people accessing clinical services. J Affect Disord 2018;235:308–15.

16. Stefanick ML. Estrogens and progestins: background and history, trends in use, and guidelines and regimens approved by the US Food and Drug Administration. Am J Med 2005;118(Suppl12B):64–73.

17. Nieschlag E, Nieschlag S. ENDOCRINE HISTORY: the history of discovery, synthesis and development of testosterone for clinical use. Eur J Endocrinol 2019;180(6):R201–r212.

18. Benjamin H. The transsexual phenomenon. New York: Julian; 1966.

19. Hembree WC, Cohen-Kettenis PT, Gooren L, et al. Endocrine treatment of gender-dysphoric/gender-incongruent persons: an endocrine society* clinical practice guideline. J ClinEndocrinolMetab 2017; 102(11):3869–903.

20. UCSF Transgender Care, Department of Family and Community Medicine, University of California San Francisco. Guidelines for the Primary and Gender-Affirming Care of Transgender and Gender Nonbinary People. In: Deutsch MB, editor. 2nd edition 2016. Available at: transcare.ucsf.edu/. Accessed December 20, 2018.

21. Health Policy Project APTN, United Nations Development Programme. Blueprint for the provision of comprehensive care for trans people and trans communities. Washington, DC: Futures Group, Health Policy Project.; 2015.

22. Pan American Health Organization [PAHO] JS, Inc, World Professional Association for Transgender, Health ea. Blueprint for the provision of comprehensive care for trans persons and their communities in the Caribbean and other Anglophone countries. Arlington (VA): John Snow Inc; 2014.

23. Wylie K, Barrett J, Besser M, et al. Good practice guidelines for the assessment and treatment of adults with Gender Dysphoria. Sexual and Relationship Therapy 2014;29:154–214.

24. Oliphant J, Veale J, Macdonald J, et al. Guidelines for gender affirming healthcare for gender diverse and transgender children, young people and adults in Aotearoa, New Zealand. Transgender Health Research Lab, University of Waikato, 2018. Available at: https://researchcommons.waikato.ac.nz/handle/10289/12160%20. Accessed August 8, 2019.

25. American Psychiatric Association. Diagnostic and statistical manual of mental disorders. 5th Edition. Arlington (VA): American Psychiatric Association; 2013.

26. Beek TF, Cohen-Kettenis PT, Kreukels BP. Gender incongruence/gender dysphoria and its classification history. Int Rev Psychiatry 2016;28(1):5–12.

27. World Health Organization. International classification of diseases ICD-11: classifying disease to map the way we live and die. Coding disease and death 2018. Available at: https://www.who.int/health-topics/international-classification-of-diseases. Accessed May 27, 2019.

28. Radix A, Silva M. Beyond the guidelines: challenges, controversies, and unanswered questions. Pediatr Ann 2014;43(6):e145–50.

29. Streed CG Jr, Harfouch O, Marvel F, et al. Cardiovascular disease among transgender adults receiving hormone therapy: a narrative review. Ann Intern Med 2017;167(4):256–67.

30. Defreyne J, Van de Bruaene LDL, Rietzschel E, et al. Effects of gender-affirming hormones on lipid, metabolic, and cardiac surrogate blood markers in transgender persons. Clin Chem 2019;65(1):119–34.

31. Gooren LJ, T'Sjoen G. Endocrine treatment of aging transgender people. Rev EndocrMetabDisord 2018; 19(3):253–62.

32. Vehkavaara S, Silveira A, Hakala-Ala-Pietila T, et al. Effects of oral and transdermal estrogen replacement therapy on markers of coagulation, fibrinolysis, inflammation and serum lipids and lipoproteins in postmenopausal women. ThrombHaemost 2001; 85(4):619–25.

33. Canonico M, Oger E, Plu-Bureau G, et al. Hormone therapy and venous thromboembolism among postmenopausal women: impact of the route of estrogen administration and progestogens: the ESTHER study. Circulation 2007;115(7):840–5.

34. Hembree WC, Cohen-Kettenis P, Delemarre-van de Waal HA, et al. Endocrine treatment of transsexual persons: an Endocrine Society clinical practice guideline. J ClinEndocrinolMetab 2009; 94(9):3132–54.

35. Asscheman H, Giltay EJ, Megens JA, et al. A long-term follow-up study of mortality in transsexuals receiving treatment with cross-sex hormones. Eur J Endocrinol 2011;164(4):635–42.

36. Spratt DI, Stewart II, Savage C, et al. Subcutaneous injection of testosterone is an effective and preferred alternative to intramuscular injection: demonstration in female-to-male transgender patients. J ClinEndocrinolMetab 2017;102(7):2349–55.

37. Light AD, Obedin-Maliver J, Sevelius JM, et al. Transgender men who experienced pregnancy after female-to-male gender transitioning. Obstet Gynecol 2014;124(6):1120–7.

38. Light A, Wang LF, Zeymo A, et al. Family planning and contraception use in transgender men. Contraception 2018;98(4):266–9.

39. Mattawanon N, Spencer JB, Schirmer DA 3rd, et al. Fertility preservation options in transgender people: A review. Rev EndocrMetabDisord 2018;19(3): 231–42.

40. T'Sjoen G, Van Caenegem E, Wierckx K. Transgenderism and reproduction. CurrOpinEndocrinol Diabetes Obes 2013;20(6):575–9.

41. Getahun D, Nash R, Flanders WD, et al. Cross-sex hormones and acute cardiovascular events in transgender persons: a cohort study. Ann Intern Med 2018;169(4):205–13.

42. Stevenson MO, Tangpricha V. Osteoporosis and bone health in transgender persons. EndocrinolMetabClin North Am 2019;48(2):421–7.

43. Van Caenegem E, Taes Y, Wierckx K, et al. Low bone mass is prevalent in male-to-female transsexual persons before the start of cross-sex hormonal therapy and gonadectomy. Bone 2013;54(1):92–7.

44. Deutsch MB, Radix A, Wesp L. Breast cancer screening, management, and a review of case study literature in transgender populations. SeminReprod Med 2017;35(5):434–41.

A Systematic Review of the Psychological Benefits of Gender-Affirming Surgery

Jeremy A. Wernick, LMSW[a],*, Samantha Busa, PsyD[a], Kareen Matouk, MA[a], Joey Nicholson, MLIS, MPH[b], Aron Janssen, MD[c]

KEYWORDS

- Gender-affirming surgery • Gender dysphoria • Transgender health • Mental health • Well-being

KEY POINTS

- There is limited research examining how gender-affirming surgeries (GAS) specifically affect the mental health of individuals with gender dysphoria.
- This article uses a systematic review to evaluate the existing literature on the psychological benefits of GAS.
- Most of the studies included in this review indicate that GAS lead to multiple, significant psychological benefits among individuals with gender dysphoria.
- Future research on this topic should focus on gathering more prospective data and standardizing the assessment of psychological well-being post-GAS.

INTRODUCTION

Transgender is an umbrella term that can be defined as identifying with a gender that differs from one's sex assigned at birth. This incongruence between one's gender identity and sex assigned at birth can lead to distress across settings. Many transgender individuals may meet criteria for gender dysphoria, which is a term used to characterize the aforementioned distress.[1] Gender dysphoria is used by the American Psychiatric Association in the Diagnostic and Statistical Manual of Mental Disorder, Fifth Edition (DSM-5) to replace the diagnosis previously known as "gender identity disorder." With the addition of gender dysphoria, it is now necessary for children, adolescents, and adults to experience significant distress and an incongruence between their gender identity and sex assigned at birth to meet criteria for the diagnosis. This shift in understanding the experience of transgender individuals affirms that transgender identities are not pathologic and refocuses transgender care to the reduction of distress and functional impairments.

The distress and impairment associated with gender dysphoria can negatively affect psychological functioning. Research continues to demonstrate that individuals with gender dysphoria have a higher prevalence of co-occurring mental health disorders compared with those without gender dysphoria.[2,3] Several epidemiologic studies have found that the lifetime prevalence of depression among those who identify themselves as "transgender" or "gender nonconforming" may be between 50% and 67%, significantly higher than the lifetime prevalence for the general population.[3] Transgender youth have increased rates of self-injurious behaviors, and studies continue to demonstrate the increased rate of suicidal ideation (SI) and suicide attempts among

---

Disclosure Statement: No disclosures to report.
[a] Department of Child and Adolescent Psychiatry, Hassenfeld Children's Hospital at NYU Langone, 1 Park Avenue, 7th Floor, New York, NY 10016, USA; [b] NYU Langone, Health Sciences Library, New York, NY, USA; [c] Ann and Robert H. Lurie Children's Hospital of Chicago, Department of Psychiatry, 225 E Chicago Avenue, Chicago, IL 60611, USA
* Corresponding author.
E-mail address: jeremy.wernick@nyulangone.org

Urol Clin N Am 46 (2019) 475–486
https://doi.org/10.1016/j.ucl.2019.07.002
0094-0143/19/© 2019 Elsevier Inc. All rights reserved.

the transgender population.[2] Compared with the general population, transgender and gender nonconforming individuals are also more likely to be diagnosed with a substance use disorder.[2-5] Minority stress theory suggests that the aforementioned mental health disparities are the result of identity-based discrimination and chronic social stressors that affect psychological functioning. Furthermore, the transgender community experiences disproportionate rates of bullying; harassment; verbal, physical, and sexual violence; and institutional discrimination.[6] Despite the evident need for gender-affirming interventions that improve the mental health of those experiencing gender dysphoria, little research has been conducted on the impact of gender-affirming interventions on psychological well-being.

For many individuals experiencing gender dysphoria, gender-affirming care may involve both social and medical interventions. Social interventions may include changing the pronouns or name used to describe a person, consistently expressing one's gender identity through clothing or hair style, legally changing identity documents to reflect one's preferred gender marker, and other reversible interventions that affirm a person's gender identity and expression. Collectively, these social changes makeup what is referred to as "social transition." Although a growing body of research has demonstrated the functional improvements and mental health benefits associated with social transition and familial support,[7] there is limited research examining how gender-affirming medical interventions specifically affect the mental health of individuals with gender dysphoria.

Seeking out gender-affirming medical interventions is one way that individuals with gender dysphoria can reduce the significant distress associated with primary and secondary sex characteristics misaligned with their gender identity. Although not all individuals experiencing gender dysphoria pursue gender-affirming medical interventions, gender-affirming health care has expanded rapidly in recent years and access to these interventions has increased across the lifespan. Gender-affirming medical interventions may include puberty suppression, gender-affirming hormones, and surgical interventions to alter the primary or secondary sex characteristics. Currently, epidemiologic data suggest that approximately 0.6% of all adults in the United States identify as transgender, and in 2015, a survey of 27,000 transgender adults showed that 25% had already undergone a gender-affirming surgery (GAS).[8,9] GASs include surgical procedures that feminize or masculinize physical characteristics to help alleviate anatomic dysphoria by aligning several physical characteristics with a person's gender identity. Individuals with gender dysphoria who pursue feminizing GAS may undergo procedures to raise their vocal pitch or feminize their facial features, as well as breast augmentation, orchiectomy, and vaginoplasty.[10] For individuals pursuing masculinizing surgeries, these interventions may also include procedures for creating more masculine facial features, removing breast tissue, as well as metoidioplasty, phalloplasty, and salpingo-oophorectomy.[11]

In order to provide individuals with gender dysphoria, safe and effective means for accessing gender-affirming medical interventions, the World Professional Association for Transgender Health (WPATH) publishes Standards of Care (SOC) for providers offering gender-affirming services. One of the many stated goals of the SOC is to improve the "health, psychological well-being, and self-fulfillment" of individuals with gender dysphoria by giving health care professionals guidelines for improving access to gender-affirming care. In recognition of the previously discussed disproportionate rate of co-occurring mental health disorders, Version 7 of the Standards of Care for the Health of Transsexual, Transgender, and Gender Nonconforming People (2012) highlights the importance of mental health professionals in the treatment of gender dysphoria and in the process of consent for and recovery from GAS.[12] However, psychotherapeutic treatment with a mental health professional is not an absolute requirement for GAS but access to GAS may improve psychological distress.

Despite the disproportionate mental health risks among individuals with gender dysphoria and the recent increase in access to GAS, there is a paucity of research examining how psychological functioning is affected by these surgical interventions. In order to understand the impact of GAS on the psychological well-being of individuals with gender dysphoria, this article aims to assess the existing literature on the potential psychological benefits of GAS using a systematic review.

METHODS
Search Strategy

Systematic searches were conducted by an experienced medical librarian across 7 databases: PubMed/MEDLINE, EMBASE via Ovid, Cochrane CENTRAL via Ovid, PsyINFO via Ovid, CINAHL via Ebsco, LGBT Life via Ebsco, and Web of Science Complete. Searches included a comprehensive list of subject headings and keywords for 3 concepts of quality of life, gender-confirmation surgical procedures, and transgender persons.

No date or language limits were applied in the searches; each search was run from database inception to January 25, 2019. A complete list of search strategies in each database is available in Appendix 1.

Study Selection

Results were exported from each database into EndNote for initial management, then study selection was completed using Covidence. Study selection followed a typical 2-stage screening process. One screener initially reviewed all titles/abstracts for relevance to the research question, then the first and a second screener reviewed all remaining articles in full text and assessed for eligibility using a prior inclusion and exclusion criteria. Eligible studies included both surgical outcomes and psychiatric well-being outcomes, were observational studies that included more than just a single case, were available in English, and were not conference abstracts.

Data Extraction/Synthesis

Data extraction focused primarily on validated measurements of psychological well-being and details about experiences with gender-affirming surgical intervention among the sampled populations. For each study, 2 reviewers extracted data related to study design, demographic information

about the sample population, surgical procedures performed, psychological constructs measured, as well as measurement tools used to assess possible psychological benefit. The reviewers have expertise in gender diversity and transgender health.

A total of 2792 abstracts were initially retrieved for study selection; following computer deduplication, 2093 titles/abstracts were screened for relevance. Of these, 129 full-text articles were assessed for eligibility, with 33 meeting the inclusion criteria. A PRISMA flow outlines the study selection process in **Fig. 1**.

RESULTS

In order to better draw conclusions about the psychological benefits of GAS, the results of this review were evaluated by separating studies with pre- and postoperative data for the identified sample and studies that examined between-group differences for individuals with and without GAS. **Table 1** shows studies with pre- and postoperative data and **Table 2** shows studies that examined between-group differences for those without and with GAS.

Pre- and Postoperative Data

Our search yielded 16 studies comparing pre- and postoperative data (see **Table 1**). Of the 16

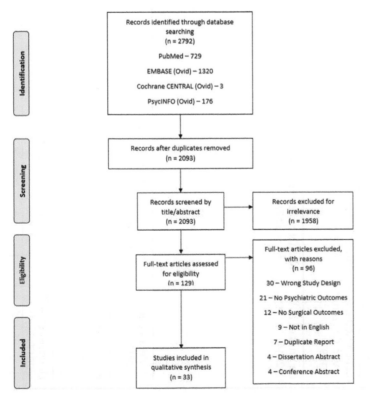

Fig. 1. Graphical depiction of search strategy and study selection. (*Adapted from* Moher D, Liberati A, Tetzlaff J, Altman DG, The PRISMA Group (2009). Preferred Reporting Items for Systematic Reviews and Meta-Analyses: The PRISMA Statement. PLoS Med 6(7): e1000097. https://doi.org/10.1371/journal.pmed1000097; with permission.)

Table 1
Studies comparing pre- and postoperative data

Authors, Year	Sample Population (Sample Size, Mean Age)	GAS	Measures	Constructs Measured
Agarwal et al,[13] 2018	FtM (N = 41, M = 27.7)	Top surgery[a]	Body Uneasiness Test (BUT-A), Modified BREAST-Q	Quality of life, body image
Becker et al,[21] 2018	FtM (N = 62), MtF (N = 20, M = 17)	GRS[b]	Body Image Assessment Questionnaire (FBeK)	Body image
Cardoso da Silva et al,[14] 2016	MtF (N = 47, M = 31.23)	Bottom surgery[c]	World Health Organization Quality of Life Assessment (WHOQOL-100)	Quality of life
Cohen-Kettenis & Van Goozen,[22] 1997	MtF (N = 5), FtM (N = 14, M = 22)	GRS[b]	Adapted Body Image Scale, Dutch Personality Questionnaire, Social Reactions Questionnaire, Utrecht Gender Dysphoria Scale	Gender dysphoria, body image, personality, social reactions
de Vries et al,[15] 2014	MtF (N = 22), FtM (N = 33, M = 20.7)	GRS[b]	Beck Depression Inventory (BDI), Child Behavior Checklist (CBCL), Children's Global Assessment Scale (CGAS), Satisfaction With Life Scale (SWLS), Spielberger's Trait Anger Scale (TPI), Spielberger's Trait Anxiety Scale (STAI), Subjective Happiness Scale (SHS), Youth Self-Report (YSR), Abbreviated World Health Organization Quality of Life Assessment (WHOQOL-BREF)	Gender dysphoria, body image, global functioning, depression, anger, anxiety, personality, behavioral/emotional problems, subjective well-being/quality of life
Heylens et al,[25] 2014	MtF (N = 46), FtM (N = 11); age range not specified	GRS[b]	Symptom Checklist-90 (SCL-90), modified questions on psychosocial functioning	Overall psychopathology
Isung et al,[16] 2017	MtF (N = 10, M = 44)	Craniofacial reconstructive surgery	Body Image Scale, Hospital Anxiety and Depression Scale (HADS), Sheehan Disability Scale (SDS), Transgender Congruence Scale (TCS)	Body image, depression, anxiety, transgender congruence, quality of life
Lindqvist et al,[19] 2017	MtF (N = 190, M = 36)	GRS[b]	Short Form-36 Health Survey (SF-36)	Quality of life

Study	Population	Surgery type	Measures	Outcomes
Mora et al,[17] 2018	MtF (N = 53, M = 35)	Surgical voice feminization	Voice Handicap Index	Voice quality of life
Mueller et al,[26] 2016	MtF (N = 39, M = 30)	Top surgery[a]	Rumination scale from Response Styles Questionnaire (RSQ), MINI	Rumination
Papadopulos et al,[18] 2017	MtF (N = 39, M = 38.6)	GRS[b]	Freiburg Personality Inventory (FPI), Patient Health Questionnaire-4 (PHQ-4), Rosenberg Self-Esteem Scale (RSES), Questions on Life Satisfaction (FLZM)	Quality of life, depression
Smith et al,[27] 2002	MtF (N = 6), FtM (N = 13, M = 22.5)	GRS[b]	Rorschach	General psychological functioning
Udeze et al,[28] 2008	MtF (N = 40, M = 47.33)	GRS[b]	Symptom Checklist-90R (SCL-90R)	General psychological functioning
van de Grift et al,[23] 2016	FtM (N = 33, M = 26.1)	Top surgery[a]	Appearance Schemas Inventory (ASI), Body Image Scale for Transsexuals (BIS), Body Image Quality of Life Inventory (BIQLI), Multidimensional Body Self Relations Questionnaire (MBSRQ), Rosenberg Self-Esteem Scale (RSES), Situational Inventory of Body Image Dysphoria (SIBID)	Body image and self-esteem
van de Grift et al,[20] 2017	FtM (N = 21, M = 40)	GRS[b]	Body Image Scale (BIS), Cantril Ladder of Life Scale (CL), Hospital Anxiety and Depression Scale (HADS), Rosenberg Self-Esteem Scale (RSES), Satisfaction With Life Scale (SWLS), Subjective Happiness Scale (SHS)	Body image, psychosocial outcomes, quality of life, self-esteem, sexuality, depression and anxiety
Weigert et al,[24] 2013	MtF (N = 35, M = 42.2)	Top surgery[a]	BREAST-Q	Psychosocial well-being, satisfaction with breasts, sexual well-being

Abbreviations: FtM, female-to-male; GRS, gender/sex reassignment surgery; MtF, male-to-female; Post-op, postoperative; Pre-op, preoperative.

[a] Mastectomy or breast construction.

[b] Mastectomy or breast construction, facial surgery, or genital surgery.

[c] Any genital surgery.

Table 2
Studies comparing between group differences of individuals with versus without GAS

Authors, Year	Sample Population (Sample Size, Mean Age)	GAS	Measures	Constructs Measured
Ainsworth & Spiegel,[44] 2010	MtF with FFS only (N = 28, M = 51); MtF with GS only (N = 25, M = 50); MtF with both FFS and GS (N = 47, M = 59); MtF with no FFS/GS (N = 147, M = 46)	FFS and/or GS[a]	San Francisco Short Form Health Questionnaire (SF-36v2)	Quality of life
Barrett,[45] 1998	FtM, pre-op: (N = 23, M = 35), post-op: (N = 31, M = 40)	GS[a]	BEM Sex Role Inventory, General Health Questionnaire (GHQ), Symptoms Checklist 90 (SCL-90), Social Roles Performance Schedule (SRPS), Modified questions about life and sexual/body satisfaction	Psychological and social functioning
Butler et al,[29] 2019	MtF (N = 291); FtM (N = 424); (M = 33.99)	GRS[b]	Mini-Social Phobia Inventory (MiniSPIN)	Social anxiety
Davis & Meier,[41] 2014	FtM (N = 208, M = 31.5); HT (N = 118), CRS (N = 84), No HT or CRS (N = 78)	CRS	Beck Anxiety Index (BAI), Beck Depression Inventory (BDI), Snell Clinical Anger Scale (CAS), custom scale for body dissatisfaction, qualitative questions about mood and sexuality	Anxiety, depression, anger, body dissatisfaction
Fleming et al,[30] 1982	FtM (N = 22, M = 31.8) Cisgender men (N = 22), matched in age to FtM group	GRS[b]	Body-Cathexis Scale (BCS), Janis- Field-Eagly Self-Esteem Measure	Body image
Jellestad et al,[31] 2018	MtF (N = 77, M = 51); FtM (N = 41, M = 36); Nonbinary (N = 25, M = 42)	GRS[b]	Short Form-36 Health Survey (SF-36), Short Form of the Center for Epidemiologic Studies-Depression Scale (ADS-K)	Quality of life, depression
Kraemer et al,[32] 2008	Pre-op: MtF (N = 12), FtM (N = 3), (M = 33); Post-op: MtF (N = 14), FtM (N = 8), (M = 38.2)	GRS[b]	Body Image Measure (FBeK)	Quality of life
Motmans et al,[33] 2012	MtF (N = 148, M = 42); FtM (N = 107, M = 37)	GRS[b]	Short Form-36 Health Survey (SF-36)	Health-related quality of life
Olson-Kennedy et al,[42] 2018	FtM, Surgical (N = 68, M = 19), nonsurgical (N = 68, M = 17)	CRS	Chest Dysphoria Scale	Chest dysphoria
Owen-Smith et al,[34] 2018	FtM (N = 347); MtF (N = 350); 18+ y old	GRS[b]	Beck Anxiety Index (BAI), Body Attractiveness Subscale of Revised Physical Self-Perception Profile, Center for Epidemiologic Studies Depression Scale (CES-D-10), Transgender Congruence Scale (TCS)	Body congruence, body image satisfaction, depression, anxiety

Study	Sample	Surgery	Measures	Outcomes
Ozata Yildizhan et al,[35] 2018	GRS Group: FtM (N = 9), MtF (N = 11), (M = 33); no GRS Group: FtM (N = 30), MtF (N = 20), (M = 27)	GRS[b]	Abbreviated World Health Organization Quality of Life Assessment (WHOQOL-BREF), Family Assessment Device (FAD), Multidimensional Scale for Perceived Social Support (MSPSS), Structured Clinical Interview for DSM-IV-TR Axis I Disorders (SCID-I)	Psychological diagnoses, family functioning, perceived social support, quality of life
Simbar et al,[36] 2018	FtM (N = 27), MtF (N = 60); (15–44 y old)	GRS[b]	Fisher's Body Image Questionnaire, Abbreviated World Health Organization Quality of Life Assessment (WHOQOL-BREF)	Quality of life, body image
Smith et al,[37] 2001	GRS Group: MtF (N = 7), FtM (N = 13), (M = 21); nonsurgical group: MtF (N = 9), FtM (N = 5), (M = 21)	GRS[b]	Appraisal of Appearance Inventory (AAI), Body Image Scale (BIS), Minnesota Multiphasic Personality Inventory (MMPI), Symptom Checklist-90 (SCL-90)	Gender dysphoria, body dissatisfaction, psychological functioning
Testa et al,[38] 2017	MtF (N = 154, M = 36.8); FtM (N = 288, M = 30.2)	GRS[b]	Body Areas Satisfaction Scale (BASS) of the Multidimensional Body-Self Relations Questionnaire- Appearance Scales, Eating Attitudes Test (EAT-26), questions on gender identity nonaffirmation and desire for and utilization of gender-confirming medical interventions	Body satisfaction, eating disorder symptoms
Tucker et al,[39] 2018	MtF (N = 178); FtM (N = 28); GRS on both chest and genitalia (N = 28), GRS on genitalia only (N = 20), GRS on chest only (N = 17), HT only (N = 105), no medical interventions (N = 36); (M = 48.5)	GRS[b]	Patient Health Questionnaire-9 (PHQ-9), Suicidal Behaviors Questionnaire - Revised (SBQ-R)	Suicidal ideation, depression
van de Grift et al,[40] 2017	MtF (N = 135, M = 39.2); FtM (N = 66, M = 30.6); HT and GRS (N = 136); HT only (N = 36); no medical interventions (N = 29)	GRS[b]	Body Image Scale (BIS), Cantril Ladder of Life Scale (CL), Multidimensional Sexuality Questionnaire (MSQ), Symptom Checklist-90 (SCL-90), Satisfaction With Life Scale (SWLS), Subjective Happiness Scale (SHS), Utrecht Gender Dysphoria Scale	Psychological functioning, gender dysphoria, body image, subjective well-being, social support
van de Grift et al,[43] 2018	FtM, pre-op: (N = 50, (M = 24.5); post-op: (N = 51, M = 26.4)	CRS	BODY-Q, Single-item screening question on depression and anxiety	Body image and psychosocial function

Abbreviations: CRS, chest reconstruction surgery; FFS, facial feminization surgery; FtM, female-to-male; GRS, gender/sex reassignment surgery; GS, genital surgery; HT, hormone therapy; MtF, male-to-female.
 [a] Any genital surgery.
 [b] Mastectomy or breast construction, facial surgery, vocal surgery, or genital surgery.

studies, 9 measured the psychological impact of "gender/sex reassignment surgeries (GRS)," generally. These 9 studies included individuals who had undergone breast augmentation, mastectomy, chest reconstruction, surgical voice feminization, craniofacial reconstructive surgery, vaginoplasty, or phalloplasty. Seven of the 16 studies with pre- and postoperative data assessed the psychological impact of specific surgical procedures. Overall, most of the studies demonstrated significant improvements in the psychological constructs measured pre- and post-GAS. Three studies did not produce any significant results. Common constructs that were assessed included quality of life, body image, gender dysphoria, general psychological functioning, depression, anxiety, and psychosocial outcomes.

Eight of the 16 studies assessed for quality of life and 10 different measurements of quality of life were used across studies. The most common measurement tools used to assess quality of life were the BREAST-Q, Satisfaction with Life Scale (SWLS), and the World Health Organization Quality of Life Assessment (WHOQOL-100). Six studies yielded statistically significant results.[13–18] Two studies that measured quality of life pre- and post-GAS did not yield statistically significant results.[19,20] Lindqvist and colleagues[19] found that in a sample of transgender women, quality of life and overall well-being improved initially post-GAS and gradually declined in comparison to the general population over a 5-year period. In a study of transgender men who underwent genital surgeries specifically, no statistically significant improvements in quality of life were found post-GAS.[14] With regard to the 6 studies that demonstrated improvements in quality of life post-GAS, findings suggest that transgender men and transgender women who access breast augmentation, chest reconstruction, surgical voice feminization, craniofacial reconstructive surgery, vaginoplasty, or phalloplasty may experience significant improvements in quality of life.[13–18]

Eight of the 16 studies with pre- and post-GAS data measured body image/satisfaction related to gender dysphoria and 6 different measurement tools were used across studies. The most common measurements tools used were the Body Image Scale (BIS) and the BREAST-Q. All 8 studies demonstrated statistically significant improvements post-GAS.[14,15,17,18,21–24] A study including 21 transgender men who underwent genital surgeries showed that gender dysphoria and body dissatisfaction were significantly lower following GAS in comparison to the time of admission. While satisfaction with specific body characteristics improved, high dissatisfaction at admission and lower psychological functioning at follow-up were associated with persistent body dissatisfaction.[14] Another study that looked specifically at transgender men who underwent mastectomy showed significant improvements in overall body image post-GAS, with body satisfaction having the most significant improvements.[23] de Vries and colleagues[15] also found that significant improvements in body image/satisfaction were correlated with improvements in gender dysphoria and overall psychological functioning for both transgender men and women.

Nine of the 16 studies measured several aspects of general psychological functioning and well-being among individuals with gender dysphoria pre- and post-GAS and more than 15 measurements were used across studies. The most common measurement tools were the Rosenberg Self-Esteem Scale (RSES), Hospital Anxiety and Depression Scale (HADS), and the Symptom Checklist-90 (SCL-90). All 9 studies identified demonstrated statistically significant improvements.[14,17,18,22,24–28] In a study including transgender women who had undergone genital surgeries, multiple measures demonstrated statistically significant improvements in subjective emotional stability, self-esteem, as well as fewer symptoms of depression and anxiety.[20] Another study, including both transgender men and women who had a range of GAS, found significant decreases in anxiety, depression, interpersonal sensitivity, and hostility post-GAS. Of note, most of the participants in this study reported the most significant improvements in the measured constructs of psychological functioning after initiation of hormone therapy compared with post-GAS.[25] One study measured rumination as an indicator of psychological well-being among transgender women undergoing multiple GAS. Rumination and associated distress decreased significantly after surgical procedures on primary sex characteristics and continued to decline with additional surgeries on secondary sex characteristics.[26]

Overall, most of the studies comparing pre- and postoperative data on quality of life, body image/satisfaction, and overall psychological functioning among individuals with gender dysphoria suggest that GAS leads to multiple, significant psychological benefits.

Comparing Data on Between-Group Differences

The authors' search yielded 17 studies comparing between-group differences on psychological functioning for individuals with and without gender-affirming surgical interventions (**see Table 2**). Twelve of the identified studies compared various aspects of psychological well-being between transgender individuals who did or did not undergo "gender/sex reassignment surgeries (GRS)," including breast augmentation, mastectomy, chest reconstruction, surgical voice feminization, craniofacial reconstructive surgery, vaginoplasty, and phalloplasty.[29–40] Three of the 17 studies specifically compared differences between transgender participants who did or did not undergo chest reconstruction surgeries (CRS).[41–43] One study specifically compared quality of life among participants with no past GAS, with facial feminization surgery (FFS) only, with genital surgery (GS) only, or with both FFS and GS.[44] One study compared psychological and social functioning among transgender men who did or did not receive genital surgery.[45] More than 25 different measurements of psychological functioning were used across studies. The most common measurement tools were the Abbreviated World Health Organization Quality of Life Assessment (WHOQOL-BREF), Short Form-36 Health Survey (SF-36), BIS, Beck Anxiety Inventory (BAI), and SCL-90.

The studies included in **Table 2** measured a broader range of psychological constructs compared with the studies with pre- and postoperative data included in **Table 1**. Several of these studies also showed differing psychological benefits by specific gender-affirming medical intervention. One study found that GRS had the most significant impact on reducing depressive symptoms and SI for transgender women and men. Participants with both gender-affirming hormones and surgery on the chest and genitals had the greatest impact on reducing SI compared with those without medical intervention, affirming hormones without GAS, or a history of affirming hormones with only chest or genital surgery.[39] Another study found that transgender men and women who had undergone GRS reported the lowest rate of social anxiety symptoms compared with those who had not undergone any GAS or who were still considering GAS.[29] Findings by Testa and colleagues[38] demonstrated how experiencing gender "nonaffirmation" increases body dissatisfaction, which was correlated with greater likelihood of eating disorder symptoms. Furthermore, chest surgery was specifically found to significantly reduce body dissatisfaction and lower levels of eating disorder symptoms. In a sample of 208 transgender men, gender-affirming hormones alleviated symptoms of depression, anxiety, and anger, whereas chest reconstruction surgery only had a significant benefit on body dissatisfaction.[41]

Multiple studies found that body image and satisfaction rates were higher among those who had received GAS compared with those who had not.[34,36–38,42] One study of both transgender men and women found that body dissatisfaction, gender dysphoria, and psychological functioning were significantly better among those who had received GRS compared with those without GAS. More specifically, Olson-Kennedy and colleagues[42] also found that chest dysphoria and the associated body distress was significantly lower among transgender men who had undergone chest reconstruction surgery compared with those who had not. Differences by surgical procedure were found in a study comparing the body image of transgender men. Participants who had undergone phalloplasty did not report more positive body image compared with those without phalloplasty. Hysterectomy was associated with significantly more positive body image compared with those without hysterectomy.[30] van de Grift and colleagues[40] also reported significant improvements in both gender dysphoria and body dissatisfaction among transgender men and women after GRS compared those with no medical intervention or gender-affirming hormones alone.

Despite the aforementioned significant psychological benefits, some studies included did not demonstrate significant improvements in psychological functioning. Motmans and colleagues[33] compared quality of life between transgender men and women with and without GRS. The differences between groups were nonsignificant and transgender men specifically reported lower quality of life compared with both the general population and transgender women. Another study found that quality of life was significantly lower among transgender women with or without GAS compared with the general population. Although the transgender women who had received GRS, facial feminization surgery (FFS), or both reported better quality of life compared with those without any GAS, the difference was not statistically significant.[44] One study found that depressive symptoms were worse in a group of transgender men postgenital surgery compared with those who had not received genital surgery.[45]

Although most of the studies demonstrated a trend of better mental health among individuals who undergo GAS compared with those without GAS, the statistical significance of these findings varied and many studies found psychological well-being to still be poor post-GAS compared with the general population.

DISCUSSION AND IMPLICATIONS FOR FUTURE RESEARCH

There is a paucity of research examining how psychological functioning is affected by GAS. The aim of this review was to examine the existing literature on the psychological impact of GAS to understand to what extent these interventions may improve the psychological well-being of individuals with gender dysphoria. Overall, most studies included in this review found that many GAS have a significant, positive impact on several constructs associated with psychological well-being. Findings from this review suggest that individuals with gender dysphoria who undergo facial feminization or masculinization, vocal feminization, breast augmentation, mastectomy, chest reconstruction, metoidioplasty, orchiectomy, salpingo-oophorectomy, vaginoplasty, or phalloplasty may experience significant improvements in quality of life, body image/satisfaction, and overall psychiatric functioning.

Findings from this review also indicate that there may be some variability in the impact of specific gender-affirming medical interventions on psychological well-being, and as more individuals access their preferred medical interventions, future research should focus on understanding how specific GAS affect mental health over time. Past research has demonstrated the increased prevalence of co-occurring mental health difficulties among individuals with gender dysphoria compared with those without gender dysphoria.[2,3] The improvements in psychological well-being after GAS illustrated in this review are particularly important to understand the need for improved access to gender-affirming care in order to reduce the psychiatric burden on this community. In order to maximize the psychological benefits of GAS, further research is necessary to identify mediating factors that can inform the development and improvement of additional interventions, such as psychotherapy and systemic policy changes.

Although this review indicates that psychological functioning improves after GAS, it cannot reach firm predictive conclusions about these improvements due to the methodological variability of studies included. The studies in **Table 1** with both pre- and postoperative data utilize more robust methodology, and, therefore, more sound conclusions can be made about the impact of GAS on psychological functioning. Most of the studies using pre- and postoperative measurement of psychological functioning found significant psychological benefits after GAS. However, the 2 studies that demonstrated the least significant improvements in psychological well-being

illustrate important factors to be considered in the assessment of psychological functioning pre- and post-GAS[13,14]: (1) very few studies available collect prospective data over multiple points of time postoperatively. It is possible that trends in long-term psychological benefits from GAS are underrepresented in the current research due to a very small number of studies collecting ongoing prospective data post-operatively. Because baseline psychiatric burden is greater among individuals with gender dysphoria compared with the general population,[2–5] it is possible that significant improvements demonstrated in the research early postoperatively can be explained by initial benefits from treatment compared with baseline. More longitudinal research is necessary to understand the psychological benefits of GAS in the long term. (2) The scarcity of research on the psychological benefits of GAS is further complicated by the variability of assessment procedures for psychological well-being. As noted previously, the studies compared in both **Tables 1** and **2** used inconsistent measurement tools to assess the various components of psychological well-being. The variety of measurement tools limits the extent to which generalizations can be made between studies. In order to better assess the psychological benefits of GAS across health care settings, professionals providing gender-affirming services must apply and develop standardized assessments of psychiatric functioning. More research is necessary to validate the use of existing standard assessments of psychological functioning with individuals with gender dysphoria. Furthermore, it may be important for the next version of the WPATH SOC to provide recommendations regarding the use of specific measurement tools for mental health providers.

Overall, this review indicates that GAS may lead to multiple psychological benefits for individuals with gender dysphoria. Future research must focus on standardizing the assessment of psychological functioning pre- and post-GAS to gather longitudinal data that will allow for more definitive conclusions to be made about factors that contribute to the psychological benefits of GAS.

SUPPLEMENTARY DATA

See Appendix 1 online at theclinics.com.

REFERENCES

1. American Psychiatric Association diagnostic and statistical manual of mental disorders (DSM-5). Washington, DC: American Psychiatric Publishing; 2013.

2. de Vries AL, Doreleijers TA, Steensma TD, et al. Psychiatric comorbidity in gender dysphoric adolescents. J Child Pscyhol Psychiatry 2011;52: 1195–202.

3. Carmel TC, Erickson-Schroth L. Mental health and the transgender population. J Psychosoc Nurs Ment Health Serv 2016;54(12):44–8.

4. Dhejne C, Van Vlerken R, Heylens G, et al. Mental health and gender dysphoria: a review of the literature. Int Rev Psychiatry 2016;28:44–57.

5. Millet N, Longworth J, Arcelus J. Prevalence of anxiety symptoms and disorders in the transgender population: a systematic review of the literature. Int J Transgend 2016;18:27–38.

6. Hendricks ML, Testa RJ. A conceptual framework for clinical work with transgender and gender nonconforming clients: an adaptation of the Minority Stress Model. Prof Psychol Res Pract 2012;43(5):460–7.

7. Olson KR, Durwood L, DeMeules M, et al. Mental health of transgender children who are supported in their identities. Pediatrics 2016;137:e20153223.

8. Flores AR, Herman JL, Gates GJ, et al. How many adults identify as transgender in the United States. Retrieved from the Williams Institute website. Available at: http://williamsinstitute.law.ucla.edu/wp-content/uploads/Gates-How-Many-People-LGBT-Apr-2016.pdf. Accessed January 17, 2019.

9. Lane M, Ives GC, Sluiter EC, et al. Trends in gender-affirming surgery in insured patients in the United States. Plast Reconstr Surg Glob Open 2018;6(4): e1738.

10. Hadj-Moussa M, Ohl DA, Kuzon WM Jr. Feminizing genital gender-confirmation surgery. Sex Med Rev 2018;6(3):457–68.e2.

11. Hadj-Moussa M, Agarwal S, Ohl DA, et al. Masculinizing genital gender confirmation surgery. Sex Med Rev 2018. https://doi.org/10.1016/j.sxmr.2018.06.004.

12. Coleman E, Bockting W, Botzer M, et al. Standards of care for the health of transsexual, transgender, and gender-nonconforming people, version 7. Int J Transgend 2012;13(4):165–232.

13. Agarwal CA, Scheefer MF, Wright LN, et al. Quality of life improvement after chest wall masculinization in female-to-male transgender patients: a prospective study using the BREAST-Q and Body Uneasiness Test. J Plast Reconstr Aesthet Surg 2018;71(5):651–7.

14. Cardoso da Silva D, Schwarz K, Fontanari AM, et al. WHOQOL-100 before and after sex reassignment surgery in Brazilian male-to-female transsexual individuals. J Sex Med 2016;13(6):988–93.

15. de Vries AL, McGuire JK, Steensma TD, et al. Young adult psychological outcome after puberty suppression and gender reassignment. Pediatrics 2014; 134(4):696–704.

16. Isung J, Mollermark C, Farnebo F, et al. Craniofacial reconstructive surgery improves appearance congruence in male-to-female transsexual patients. Arch Sex Behav 2017;46(6):1573–6.

17. Mora E, Cobeta I, Becerra A, et al. Comparison of cricothyroid approximation and glottoplasty for surgical voice feminization in male-to-female transsexuals. Laryngoscope 2018;128(9):2101–9.

18. Papadopulos NA, Zavlin D, Lelle JD, et al. Male-to-female sex reassignment surgery using the combined technique leads to increased quality of life in a prospective study. Plast Reconstr Surg 2017; 140(2):286–94.

19. Lindqvist EK, Sigurjonsson H, Mollermark C, et al. Quality of life improves early after gender reassignment surgery in transgender women (vol 40, pg 223, 2017). Eur J Plast Surg 2017;40(3):227.

20. van de Grift TC, Pigot GLS, Boudhan S, et al. A longitudinal study of motivations before and psychosexual outcomes after genital gender-confirming surgery in transmen. J Sex Med 2017; 14(12):1621–8.

21. Becker I, Auer M, Barkmann C, et al. A cross-sectional multicenter study of multidimensional body image in adolescents and adults with gender dysphoria before and after transition-related medical interventions. Arch Sex Behav 2018;47(8):2335–47.

22. Cohen-Kettenis PT, Van Goozen SHM. Sex reassignment of adolescent transsexuals: a follow-up study. J Am Acad Child Adolesc Psychiatry 1997;36(2): 263–71.

23. van de Grift TC, Kreukels BP, Elfering L, et al. Body image in transmen: multidimensional measurement and the effects of mastectomy. J Sex Med 2016; 13(11):1778–86.

24. Weigert R, Frison E, Sessiecq Q, et al. Patient satisfaction with breasts and psychosocial, sexual, and physical well-being after breast augmentation in male-to-female transsexuals. Plast Reconstr Surg 2013;132(6):1421–9.

25. Heylens G, Verroken C, De Cock S, et al. Effects of different steps in gender reassignment therapy on psychopathology: a prospective study of persons with a gender identity disorder. J Sex Med 2014; 11(1):119–26.

26. Mueller A, Quadros C, Schwarz K, et al. Rumination as a marker of psychological improvement in transsexual women postoperative. Transgend Health 2016;1(1):274–8.

27. Smith YL, Cohen L, Cohen-Kettenis PT. Postoperative psychological functioning of adolescent transsexuals: a Rorschach study. Arch Sex Behav 2002; 31(3):255–61.

28. Udeze B, Abdelmawla N, Khoosal D, et al. Psychological functions in male-to-female transsexual people before and after surgery. Sex Relation Ther 2008; 23(2):141–5.

29. Butler RM, Horenstein A, Gitlin M, et al. Social anxiety among transgender and gender nonconforming

individuals: The role of gender-affirming medical interventions. J Abnorm Psychol 2019;128(1):25–31.

30. Fleming MZ, MacGowan BR, Robinson L, et al. The body image of the postoperative female-to-male transsexual. J Consult Clin Psychol 1982;50(3): 461–2.

31. Jellestad L, Jaggi T, Corbisiero S, et al. Quality of life in transitioned trans persons: a retrospective cross-sectional cohort study. Biomed Res Int 2018;2018: 8684625.

32. Kraemer B, Delsignore A, Schnyder U, et al. Body image and transsexualism. Psychopathology 2008; 41(2):96–100.

33. Motmans J, Meier P, Ponnet K, et al. Female and male transgender quality of life: socioeconomic and medical differences. J Sex Med 2012;9(3): 743–50.

34. Owen-Smith AA, Gerth J, Sineath RC, et al. Association between gender confirmation treatments and perceived gender congruence, body image satisfaction, and mental health in a cohort of transgender individuals. J Sex Med 2018;15(4):591–600.

35. Ozata Yildizhan B, Yuksel S, Avayu M, et al. Effects of gender reassignment on quality of life and mental health in people with gender Dysphoria. Turk Psikiyatri Derg 2018;29(1):11–21.

36. Simbar M, Nazarpour S, Mirzababaie M, et al. Quality of life and body image of individuals with gender Dysphoria. J Sex Marital Ther 2018;44(6):1–10.

37. Smith YLS, Van Goozen SHM, Cohen-Kettenis PT. Adolescents with gender identity disorder who were accepted or rejected for sex reassignment surgery: a prospective follow-up study. J Am Acad Child Adolesc Psychiatry 2001;40(4): 472–81.

38. Testa RJ, Rider GN, Haug NA, et al. Gender confirming medical interventions and eating disorder symptoms among transgender individuals. Health Psychol 2017;36(10):927–36.

39. Tucker RP, Testa RJ, Simpson TL, et al. Hormone therapy, gender affirmation surgery, and their association with recent suicidal ideation and depression symptoms in transgender veterans. Psychol Med 2018;48(14):2329–36.

40. van de Grift TC, Elaut E, Cerwenka SC, et al. Effects of medical interventions on gender Dysphoria and body image: a follow-up study. Psychosom Med 2017;79(7):815–23.

41. Davis SA, Meier S. Effects of testosterone treatment and chest reconstruction surgery on mental health and sexuality in female-to-male transgender people. Int J Sex Health 2014;26(2):113–28.

42. Olson-Kennedy J, Warus J, Okonta V, et al. Chest reconstruction and chest dysphoria in transmasculine minors and young adults comparisons of nonsurgical and postsurgical cohorts. JAMA Pediatr 2018;172(5):431–6.

43. van de Grift TC, Elfering L, Greijdanus M, et al. Subcutaneous mastectomy improves satisfaction with body and psychosocial function in trans men: findings of a cross-sectional study using the BODY-Q chest module. Plast Reconstr Surg 2018;142(5): 1125–32.

44. Ainsworth TA, Spiegel JH. Quality of life of individuals with and without facial feminization surgery or gender reassignment surgery. Qual Life Res 2010; 19(7):1019–24.

45. Barrett J. Psychological and social function before and after phalloplasty. Int J Transgend 1998;2(1).

Fertility Preservation in Male to Female Transgender Patients

Check for updates

Wen Liu, MD, MPH[a], Michael L. Schulster, MD[a], Joseph P. Alukal, MD[b], Bobby B. Najari, MD, MSc[a,c],*

KEYWORDS

- Transgender health • Gender dysphoria • Fertility preservation • Gender-affirming therapy
- Sperm cryopreservation

KEY POINTS

- Hormonal (spironolactone, cyproterone acetate, GnRH agonists, estrogen) and surgical (penectomy, vaginoplasty, orchiectomy) treatments for gender affirmation in transgender patients may compromise fertility.
- Sperm cryopreservation via ejaculation, electroejaculation, or surgical testicular sperm extraction is a well-established method of FP.
- Sperm can be used for intrauterine insemination if sufficient or in vitro fertilization with intracytoplasmic sperm injection if lower quality/quantity (testicular sperm).
- Restoration of fertility after hormonal treatment may be bolstered by use of selective estrogen receptor modulators (clomiphene citrate) and human chorionic gonadotropin.

INTRODUCTION

Gender diversity reflects the wide spectrum of ways in which personal gender identification may differ from sex assigned at birth. This incongruity can lead to clinically significant emotional and physical distress manifesting in gender dysphoria,[1] which has replaced the prior diagnosis of gender identity disorder in the most recent *Diagnostic and Statistical Manual of Mental Disorders*, version 5.[2]

The care of transgender patients is complex and requires coordination not only across medical, mental health, and surgical specialties, but also with such domains as social, educational, and employment.[3] The multidimensionality of such care, in conjunction with increased public visibility of gender diversity and societal shifts in opinion, has resulted in the formation of several multidisciplinary gender clinics to better serve transgender patients, especially the more vulnerable youth and adolescent population.[4] It is increasingly critical for all providers to have an understanding of the treatment options for gender dysphoria in patients wishing to undergo gender-affirming interventions and the role of fertility preservation (FP) in the transgender population.

BACKGROUND

Currently, medical and mental health clinicians frequently reference guidelines from the World Professional Association of Transgender Health[5] and the Endocrine Society[6] for the care of transgender,

---

[a] Department of Urology, NYU Langone Medical Center, New York University School of Medicine, 222 East 41st Street, New York, NY 10017, USA; [b] Department of Urology, New York Presbyterian Hospital, Columbia University Medical Center, 161 Fort Washington Avenue, New York, NY 10032, USA; [c] Department of Population Health, NYU Langone Medical Center, New York University School of Medicine, 227 East 30th Street, New York, NY 10016, USA
* Corresponding author. 222 East 41st Street, 11th Floor, New York, NY 10017.
E-mail address: bobby.najari@nyulangone.org

Urol Clin N Am 46 (2019) 487–493
https://doi.org/10.1016/j.ucl.2019.07.003
0094-0143/19/© 2019 Elsevier Inc. All rights reserved.

transsexual, and gender-nonconforming individuals. In prepubertal gender-diverse patients, treatments for gender dysphoria include psychoeducation, changing external gender expression (social gender transition), and support against potential stigma or discrimination.[3,7] For those patients undergoing initial pubertal changes, gonadotropin-releasing hormone (GnRH) analogues may be used to reversibly suppress the production of sex hormones, thus halting puberty.[8] This serves several purposes including the reduction of feelings of gender dysphoria associated with the physical changes of puberty, increasing the time for patients to undergo comprehensive evaluations, and allows demonstration of the persistence of the patient's desire for further treatments that would be irreversible.

THE EFFECT OF HORMONAL THERAPY ON FERTILITY

Hormonal interventions for transgender individuals include cross-sex hormones to facilitate congruent secondary sex characteristic development and target the hypothalamic-pituitary-gonadal (HPG) axis (**Fig. 1**). Typically, downregulation of the HPG axis is achieved with antiandrogens (spironolactone, cyproterone acetate, or GnRH agonists) with feminization by estrogens.[9] Estrogen therapy in transgender women

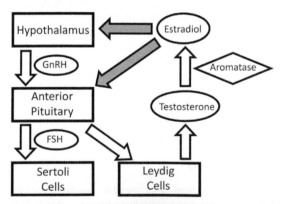

Fig. 1. HPG axis. The hypothalamus releases GnRH, which stimulates the anterior pituitary to secrete luteinizing hormone and follicle-stimulating hormone (FSH). In males, luteinizing hormone increases the production and release of testosterone from Leydig cells in the testes and FSH facilitates Sertoli cells to support and maintain spermatogenesis. Aromatase facilitates the conversion of testosterone into estradiol, which forms a negative feedback loop at the level of the hypothalamus to inhibit GnRH production and at the anterior pituitary, with downregulation of spermatogenesis and antiandrogenic effects. White arrows indicate activation, gray arrows indicate inhibition.

suppresses gonadotropin levels, which decreases testosterone levels and subsequently reduces sperm counts and motility.[9–11] After long-standing estrogen treatment, Leydig cells appear to become dedifferentiated and Sertoli cells resemble immature precursor cells.[12,13] Overall, spermatogenesis is suppressed during hormonal therapy; however, the long-term effects of this hormonal manipulation are not well understood. It is also unclear how long one must discontinue hormones to recover adequate gonadal function for fertility. Some reports have found that within weeks of discontinuing hormones before examining the testes, spermatogenesis has returned to normal along with normal Leydig cells.[14] Other studies of testes examined after orchiectomy during gender-confirmation surgery report smaller diameters and expanded interstitium of seminiferous tubules, hypoplastic germ cells, hypoplastic or absent Leydig cells, and hyperplastic epididymis.[15]

Gender-affirming surgical procedures, such as penectomy and orchiectomy for transgender women or hysterectomy and bilateral oophorectomy for transgender men, would lead to irreversible sterility. To that end, and based on expert consensus, one criteria before undergoing these irreversible interventions is that patients must live in a role congruent with their gender identity for at least 1 year. This allows time to experience the physical and social adjustments associated with living in their desired gender role.[5,6] However, because many patients may be young when they choose to pursue gender transitioning, the compromise of future fertility may not otherwise be at the forefront of their immediate concerns. Additionally, there are a multitude of barriers to accessing proper fertility consultation services, patient awareness notwithstanding. Thus, it is of the utmost importance for providers taking care of the transgender population to discuss the potential loss of fertility with many gender-affirming treatments. Furthermore, offering FP services before such interventions is key to improving the chances of preserving future fertility.

FERTILITY PRESERVATION
Rationale

FP aims to increase and optimize the opportunity for individuals to produce genetic offspring when fertility may be compromised. Historically, gender transition with hormonal or surgical therapies meant loss of reproductive potential, and despite significant advances in assisted-reproductive technologies (ART), this remains the case in many countries. Those who fall outside of the heteronormative idea of a family have been denied access to ART as a result of legal, ethical, or accessibility barriers.[16] For example, gay and lesbian couples have struggled with the stigma and lack of social acceptance of having children. Past arguments center around the welfare of children raised by gay or lesbian couples alongside fears that psychological and social problems may arise. However, these preconceived notions and purported harm have not been demonstrated in the literature.[17–20] Accordingly, the Ethics Committee of the American Society for Reproductive Medicine argues that there is no ethical basis on which gay or lesbian couples should be denied access to ART.[21]

More recently, as social acceptability of gender-nonconformance has increased, a similar ethical debate surrounding transgender reproductive rights and equality has ensued.[22] Achieving parenthood in and of itself is affirming to transgender patients.[23] Among transgender adults, surveys show that about half of men and women wish to have biologic children[24–26] and more than a third would have considered FP, if the technology had been available to them. Many gender-affirmed transwomen also expressed regret that they could not have their own biologic children.[26] A multicenter study in Germany[27] found that although transmen had higher desire for children pretreatment, 25% of transmen and transwomen wanted children currently, and this increased to almost 70% and 50% for future interest in having children. Equal proportions of participants had at least thought about gamete preservation (76%), although only 9.6% and 3.1% of transwomen and transmen had gone through with FP, respectively.

Although there are less data regarding children raised by transgender parents, several studies show that these children are not at increased risk of harm psychologically, developmentally, or sexually.[19,28,29] A study following 52 children born via direct sperm insemination in couples with a transgender man have found normal development without major psychological disorders or gender dysphoria.[30] In fact, the American Society for Reproductive Medicine Ethics Committee has also published statements supporting the right to access fertility services regardless of sexual orientation.[31] The Endocrine Society also recommends full counseling about FP for patients seeking gender-affirming treatment before initiating such interventions.[32] Despite statements by professional organizations and experts, in certain countries (eg, France and the Netherlands), only transgender men and their female partners can undergo donor insemination, because ART is not legalized for nonheterosexual couples.[33] In other countries, such as Poland and Finland, a mental disorder diagnosis or gender-reassignment surgery is required for legal gender recognition.[34] A US World Wide Web–based survey found that 76% of 986 respondents thought physicians should assist transgender people to have biologic children; however, a lower percentage (60%) thought they should help minors preserve gametes before transitioning or help transgender men carry pregnancies.[35]

Utilization

Overall, data about FP in transgender patients are limited; however, several studies have demonstrated low use of FP among transgender patients. The largest study to date of transgender adolescents[36] described the clinicodemographics and outcomes of FP consultation in 105 patients and found low rates of FP use overall. About 12% of the adolescents (seven transgender women, six transgender men) were seen by a fertility specialist, with 5% undergoing successful gamete cryopreservation (four completing sperm cryopreservation and one completing oocyte cryopreservation). Patient-specific barriers included cost and invasiveness of procedures, such as ovarian hyperstimulation and egg retrieval. In a similar cohort of 73 adolescents with gender dysphoria seeking hormone therapy, Nahata and colleagues[37] found higher rates of FP counseling (98.6%) before treatment, although with only two patients attempting FP (2.8%, both transgender females). Reasons for declining FP included desire to adopt (45.2%), no child wish (21.9%), cost (8.2%), discomfort of masturbation (1.4%), and potential hormonal treatment delay (1.4%). Both studies of transgender youth demonstrated rates lower than those in the adult transgender population. Several possible reasons may account for this difference, including high rates of depression and suicidality linked to a sense of a hopeless foreshortened future, family rejection, and societal pressures impacting ideas on what a family unit should encompass. In addition to these reasons high rates of body dysphoria can create an urgency for hormonal intervention in adolescent transgender patients who would be more open to exploring reproductive desires only after receiving medical gender-affirming treatments, despite the challenges this can pose.[37] Although patients are more often transitioning at younger ages, it is particularly difficult for this group to make reproductive choices before deciding on treatments that often permanently alter their reproductive potential.[38]

FERTILITY PRESERVATION METHODS
Methods

In transgender women (ie, male-to-female), FP options include sperm cryopreservation, a well-established and generally widely available method,[39] and more experimental techniques for prepubertal patients or those with azoospermia, such as cryopreservation of testicular tissue or spermatogonium stem cells.[40] In general, sperm should be collected before starting hormone therapy or after discontinuation when sperm counts recover. Sperm collected for cryopreservation may be obtained through ejaculation through self-stimulation, ejaculation through penile vibratory stimulation or transrectal electrostimulation, or surgical testicular extraction (testicular sperm extraction), the latter two being preferred for those who experience worsening gender dysphoria through the act of masturbation or for those with erectile and ejaculatory dysfunction.[41] Once collected, the sperm may then be used with female partners for intrauterine insemination if the ejaculated sperm is of sufficient quality and quantity, whereas in vitro fertilization with intracytoplasmic sperm injection should be used if sperm is of lower quality or limited, such as testicular sperm. With male partners, ART requires an oocyte donor and surrogate.[42] Of note, there may be less gender dysphoria with respect to ejaculation for harvesting sperm in transgender women compared with menstruation and ovulation for transgender men.[43]

In patients with immature sperm or no sperm, testicular tissue cryopreservation is a theoretic future option that may be performed at the time of gender-reassignment surgery, with subsequent autoimplantation of testicular grafts at a later time.[44,45] Alternatively, spermatogonium stem cells isolated from testicular tissue may be directly injected into the testes or matured in vitro with special three-dimensional or organ cultures.[46,47] Thus far, only successful development of hybrid embryos after fertilization of mouse oocytes has been demonstrated.[48] Overall, these techniques are considered investigational and are associated with lower success rates of sperm harvest.[40] Along these investigational lines, testicular tissue cryopreservation has been offered to cisgendered boys with childhood cancers requiring gonadotoxic chemotherapies under research protocols investigating maintenance of reproductive potential, although future fertility is not guaranteed.[49]

Fertility Preservation Before Hormonal Therapy Initiation

In light of the rising incidence of transgender sperm banking overall, studies have examined semen parameters in transgender patients alone and compared with healthy cisgender males. A case series found a high incidence of oligozoospermia (28%), asthenozoospermia (31%), and teratozoospermia (31%) in transgender women, for which the authors often recommended pursuing in vitro fertilization/intracytoplasmic sperm injection rather than intrauterine insemination.[50] Similar abnormal parameters were demonstrated in a retrospective study by Li and coworkers[51] wherein banked sperm from hormone naive transgender women had lower median sperm concentration (14.2×10^6/mL vs 19.2×10^6/mL), sperm count (55.7×10^6 vs 69.5×10^6), total motile sperm count (35.0×10^6 vs 42.0×10^6), and post-thaw semen parameters (sperm count, motility, and total motile sperm count) compared with healthy cisgender control subjects. Although there were no statistically significant differences in ejaculatory volume and percent motility, a higher rate of oligozoospermia was also observed in transwomen (53.8% vs 38.3%). Practitioners should counsel patients that multiple FP attempts may be necessary to optimize future fertility potential.

Fertility Preservation After Hormonal Therapy Initiation

Given that testosterone's impact on the HPG axis is mediated through estradiol, the World Health Organization's testosterone contraception trials provide the most robust data on the reproductive impact of suppressing the HPG axis with exogenous hormones. These studies demonstrated that exogenous testosterone resulted in azoospermia in 75% of men after 6 months of use.[52,53] In an integrated analysis of 1549 men from 30 male hormonal contraceptive studies, the median time to fertility recovery after discontinuation of androgen treatment, as measured by sperm concentration of greater than 20 million/mL, was 3.4 months,[54] with 100% of men recovered by 24 months.[54]

Not surprisingly, semen samples from transgender women collected after hormonal therapy initiation demonstrate abnormal semen parameters (lower motility, total motile count, and concentration).[55] In transgender women undergoing gender-affirming surgery (ie, orchiectomy), maturation arrest was seen in 80% of patients, with histologic changes including decreased diameter of seminiferous tubules (82% of patients), hypoplasia (32% of testes) or absence of Leydig cells (53%), and epididymal hyperplasia (20% of testes).[15] Those who had discontinued hormones before cryopreservation were similar to those who had never used hormone therapy.[55]

In cismen, human chorionic gonadotropin (hCG), which is structurally similar to luteinizing hormone, and clomiphene citrate (CC), a selective estrogen receptor modulator that inhibits negative feedback by estrogen thereby raising GnRH and testosterone levels, are effective at restoring spermatogenesis after exogenous testosterone therapy.[56,57] In fact, a case series of hypogonadal cismen undergoing testosterone-replacement therapy with concomitant low-dose hCG, demonstrated no changes in semen parameters or azoospermia.[58] Despite this, there are case reports of this hCG protocol still resulting in azoospermia, although exogenous hormone cessation and treatment with CC and hCG can restore spermatogenesis and fertility even in these men.[59] Another retrospective series of 66 cismen with testosterone-associated infertility found that the use of high-dose hCG and/or selective estrogen receptor modulator resulted in 69.7% of men achieving total motile count of greater than 5 million sperm within 12 months of stopping testosterone and initiating hCG/selective estrogen receptor modulator therapy.[60] Given the similar effects of exogenous estradiol on the HPG axis, it is possible that CC and/or hCG may hasten the recovery of spermatogenesis in transgender men who are interested in FP after initiating hormonal therapy.

SUMMARY

Overall, more research is needed in transgender health, with a conspicuous absence of data regarding fertility. A comprehensive review of the literature focused on transgender health found that out of about 2400 articles published before 2016, only 22 (0.9%) focused on transgender reproduction and fertility, of which most were bioethical articles, with few clinical studies.[61] As more transgender people pursue medical and surgical gender-affirming treatments at younger ages, it is imperative that the medical community understand the side effects and risks associated with providing care to a vulnerable patient population. Communication with a multidisciplinary team of providers for transgender patients on diagnosis, and before hormone treatment or sterilizing surgeries, is paramount to maintaining reproductive potential in patients who may have significant barriers to access of FP services. Although there are successful and established options for FP, the ultimate method used is an informed decision based on patient age, preference, partner, cost, availability, and current law. The therapeutic approach is thus multipronged and requires significant coordination and discussion with the patient to ensure the greatest chances of success.

REFERENCES

1. Gooren LJ. Clinical practice. Care of transsexual persons. N Engl J Med 2011;364(13):1251–7.
2. Diagnostic and statistical manual of mental disorders: DSM-5. Arlington (VA): American Psychiatric Association, DSM-5 Task Force; 2013.
3. Grant J, Mottet L, Tanis J. Injustice at every turn: a report of the national transgender discrimination survey. Washington, DC: National Center for Transgender Equality and National Gay and Lesbian Task Force; 2011.
4. Chen D, Hidalgo MA, Leibowitz S, et al. Multidisciplinary care for gender-diverse youth: a narrative review and unique model of gender-affirming care. Transgend Health 2016;1(1):117–23.
5. Coleman E, Bockting W, Botzer M, et al. Standards of care for the health of transsexual, transgender, and gender-nonconforming people, Version 7. Int J Transgend 2012;13(4):165–232.
6. Hembree WC, Cohen-Kettenis PT, Gooren L, et al. Endocrine treatment of gender-dysphoric/gender-incongruent persons: an Endocrine Society clinical practice guideline. J Clin Endocrinol Metab 2017; 102(11):3869–903.
7. Adelson SL. Practice parameter on gay, lesbian, or bisexual sexual orientation, gender nonconformity, and gender discordance in children and adolescents. J Am Acad Child Adolesc Psychiatry 2012; 51(9):957–74.
8. Light AD, Zimbrunes SE, Gomez-Lobo V. Reproductive and obstetrical care for transgender patients. Curr Obstet Gynecol Rep 2017;6(2):149–55.
9. Schneider F, Kliesch S, Schlatt S, et al. Andrology of male-to-female transsexuals: influence of cross-sex hormone therapy on testicular function. Andrology 2017;5(5):873–80.
10. Lubbert H, Leo-Rossberg I, Hammerstein J. Effects of ethinyl estradiol on semen quality and various hormonal parameters in a eugonadal male. Fertil Steril 1992;58(3):603–8.
11. Maxwell S, Noyes N, Keefe D, et al. Pregnancy outcomes after fertility preservation in transgender men. Obstet Gynecol 2017;129(6):1031–4.
12. Schulze C. Response of the human testis to long-term estrogen treatment: morphology of Sertoli cells, Leydig cells and spermatogonial stem cells. Cell Tissue Res 1988;251(1):31–43.
13. Payer AF, Meyer WJ 3rd, Walker PA. The ultrastructural response of human Leydig cells to exogenous estrogens. Andrologia 1979;11(6):423–36.
14. Schneider F, Neuhaus N, Wistuba J, et al. Testicular functions and clinical characterization of patients with gender dysphoria (GD) undergoing sex reassignment surgery (SRS). J Sex Med 2015;12(11):2190–200.
15. Matoso A, Khandakar B, Yuan S, et al. Spectrum of findings in orchiectomy specimens of persons

undergoing gender confirmation surgery. Hum Pathol 2018;76:91–9.

16. Condat A, Mendes N, Drouineaud V, et al. Biotechnologies that empower transgender persons to self-actualize as individuals, partners, spouses, and parents are defining new ways to conceive a child: psychological considerations and ethical issues. Philos Ethics Humanit Med 2018;13(1):1.

17. Paige RU. Proceedings of the American Psychological Association, Incorporated, for the legislative year 2004. Minutes of the meeting of the Council of Representatives July 28 & 30, 2004 Honolulu (HI). American Psychologist. 60(5), 2005.

18. Greenfeld DA. Gay male couples and assisted reproduction: should we assist? Fertil Steril 2007; 88(1):18–20.

19. Green R. Sexual identity of 37 children raised by homosexual or transsexual parents. Am J Psychiatry 1978;135(6):692–7.

20. Green R. Transsexuals' children. Int J Transgend 1998;2(4).

21. Ethics Committee of American Society for Reproductive Medicine. Access to fertility treatment by gays, lesbians, and unmarried persons: a committee opinion. Fertil Steril 2013;100(6):1524–7.

22. T'Sjoen G, Van Caenegem E, Wierckx K. Transgenderism and reproduction. Curr Opin Endocrinol Diabetes Obes 2013;20(6):575–9.

23. Murphy TF. Assisted gestation and transgender women. Bioethics 2015;29(6):389–97.

24. Tornello SL, Bos H. Parenting intentions among transgender individuals. LGBT Health 2017;4(2): 115–20.

25. Wierckx K, Van Caenegem E, Pennings G, et al. Reproductive wish in transsexual men. Hum Reprod 2012;27(2):483–7.

26. De Sutter P, Verschoor A, Hotimsky A, et al. The desire to have children and the preservation of fertility in transsexual women: a survey. Int J Transgend 2002;6(3).

27. Auer MK, Fuss J, Nieder TO, et al. Desire to have children among transgender people in Germany: a cross-sectional multi-center study. J Sex Med 2018;15(5):757–67.

28. White T, Ettner R. Adaptation and adjustment in children of transsexual parents. Eur Child Adolesc Psychiatry 2007;16(4):215–21.

29. De Wert G, Dondorp W, Shenfield F, et al. ESHRE task force on ethics and law 23: medically assisted reproduction in singles, lesbian and gay couples, and transsexual peopledagger. Hum Reprod 2014; 29(9):1859–65.

30. Chiland C, Clouet AM, Golse B, et al. New type of family: transmen as fathers thanks to donor sperm insemination. A 12-year follow-up exploratory study of their children. Neuropsychiatrie de l'enfance et de l. Adolescence 2013;61:365–70.

31. Ethics Committee of the American Society for Reproductive Medicine. Access to fertility services by transgender persons: an Ethics Committee opinion. Fertil Steril 2015;104(5):1111–5.

32. Panagiotakopoulos L. Transgender medicine: puberty suppression. Rev Endocr Metab Disord 2018;19(3):221–5.

33. Jouannet P. Issues surrounding the preservation and subsequent use of transsexual persons' gametes. Bull Acad Natl Med 2014;198(3):613–31.

34. Rowlands S, Amy JJ. Preserving the reproductive potential of transgender and intersex people. Eur J Contracep Reprod Health Care 2018;23(1):58–63.

35. Goldman RH, Kaser DJ, Missmer SA, et al. Fertility treatment for the transgender community: a public opinion study. J Assist Reprod Genet 2017;34(11): 1457–67.

36. Chen D, Simons L, Johnson EK, et al. Fertility preservation for transgender adolescents. J Adolesc Health 2017;61(1):120–3.

37. Nahata L, Tishelman AC, Caltabellotta NM, et al. Low fertility preservation utilization among transgender youth. J Adolesc Health 2017;61(1):40–4.

38. Johnson EK, Finlayson C, Rowell EE, et al. Fertility preservation for pediatric patients: current state and future possibilities. J Urol 2017;198(1):186–94.

39. Johnson MD, Cooper AR, Jungheim ES, et al. Sperm banking for fertility preservation: a 20-year experience. Eur J Obstet Gynecol Reprod Biol 2013; 170(1):177–82.

40. Martinez F. Update on fertility preservation from the Barcelona International Society for Fertility Preservation-ESHRE-ASRM 2015 expert meeting: indications, results and future perspectives. Hum Reprod 2017;32(9):1802–11.

41. Abram McBride J, Lipshultz LI. Male fertility preservation. Curr Urol Rep 2018;19(7):49.

42. De Roo C, Tilleman K, T'Sjoen G, et al. Fertility options in transgender people. Int Rev Psychiatry 2016;28(1):112–9.

43. Mitu K. Transgender reproductive choice and fertility preservation. AMA J Ethics 2016;18(11):1119–25.

44. Goossens E, Van Saen D, Tournaye H. Spermatogonial stem cell preservation and transplantation: from research to clinic. Hum Reprod 2013;28(4): 897–907.

45. Mattawanon N, Spencer JB, Schirmer DA 3rd, et al. Fertility preservation options in transgender people: a review. Rev Endocr Metab Disord 2018;19(3): 231–42.

46. Mulder CL, Zheng Y, Jan SZ, et al. Spermatogonial stem cell autotransplantation and germline genomic editing: a future cure for spermatogenic failure and prevention of transmission of genomic diseases. Hum Reprod Update 2016;22(5):561–73.

47. Sadri-Ardekani H, Atala A. Testicular tissue cryopreservation and spermatogonial stem cell

transplantation to restore fertility: from bench to bedside. Stem Cell Res Ther 2014;5(3):68.

48. Sun M, Yuan Q, Niu M, et al. Efficient generation of functional haploid spermatids from human germline stem cells by three-dimensional-induced system. Cell Death Differ 2018;25(4):747–64.

49. Ho WLC, Bourne H, Gook D, et al. A short report on current fertility preservation strategies for boys. Clin Endocrinol (Oxf) 2017;87(3):279–85.

50. Hamada A, Kingsberg S, Wierckx K, et al. Semen characteristics of transwomen referred for sperm banking before sex transition: a case series. Andrologia 2015;47(7):832–8.

51. Li K, Rodriguez D, Gabrielsen JS, et al. Sperm cryopreservation of transgender individuals: trends and findings in the past decade. Andrology 2018;6(6):860–4.

52. Contraceptive efficacy of testosterone-induced azoospermia in normal men. World Health Organization Task Force on methods for the regulation of male fertility. Lancet 1990;336(8721):955–9.

53. Contraceptive efficacy of testosterone-induced azoospermia and oligozoospermia in normal men. Fertil Steril 1996;65(4):821–9.

54. Liu PY, Swerdloff RS, Christenson PD, et al. Rate, extent, and modifiers of spermatogenic recovery after hormonal male contraception: an integrated analysis. Lancet 2006;367(9520):1412–20.

55. Adeleye AJ, Reid G, Kao C-N, et al. Semen parameters among transgender women with a history of hormonal treatment. Urology 2019;124:136–41.

56. Wenker EP, Dupree JM, Langille GM, et al. The use of HCG-based combination therapy for recovery of spermatogenesis after testosterone use. J Sex Med 2015;12(6):1334–7.

57. Rahnema CD, Lipshultz LI, Crosnoe LE, et al. Anabolic steroid-induced hypogonadism: diagnosis and treatment. Fertil Steril 2014;101(5):1271–9.

58. Hsieh TC, Pastuszak AW, Hwang K, et al. Concomitant intramuscular human chorionic gonadotropin preserves spermatogenesis in men undergoing testosterone replacement therapy. J Urol 2013;189(2):647–50.

59. Najari B. Azoospermia with testosterone therapy despite concomitant intramuscular human chorionic gonadotropin: NYU case of the month, July 2018. Rev Urol 2018;20(3):137–9.

60. Kohn TP, Louis MR, Pickett SM, et al. Age and duration of testosterone therapy predict time to return of sperm count after human chorionic gonadotropin therapy. Fertil Steril 2017;107(2):351–7.e1.

61. Wanta JW, Unger CA. Review of the transgender literature: where do we go from here? Transgend Health 2017;2(1):119–28.

A Discussion of Options, Outcomes, and Future Recommendations for Fertility Preservation for Transmasculine Individuals

Jennifer K. Blakemore, MD[a],*, Gwendolyn P. Quinn, PhD[b],
M. Elizabeth Fino, MD[a]

KEYWORDS

- Transmale • Fertility preservation • Oocyte cryopreservation • Embryo cryopreservation
- Ovarian tissue cryopreservation

KEY POINTS

- Counseling about reproductive health and fertility preservation before gender affirmation or puberty suppression is recommended.
- Fertility preservation options for transmen include oocyte cryopreservation, embryo cryopreservation, and ovarian tissue cryopreservation.
- Creating a strong network of providers and patient support will help provide better opportunities for the trans community.

INTRODUCTION

For many transgender people, the decision to undergo gender affirmation, or the transition from female to male, occurs during the reproductive lifespan. However, the rates of referral to fertility specialists, or reproductive endocrinologists, are currently low. These specialists offer important counseling on the fertility, family building, and reproductive health issues that may affect people assigned female at birth, as they affirm their gender.[1] This article provides background on the scope of fertility preservation and its specific application to those transitioning from female to male gender. It considers the barriers to referral and treatment for fertility counseling, as well as reviewing some of the authors' own outcomes with

respect to family building for this unique patient population. It concludes by providing insights on the future scope of the field and suggestions for how best to create a comprehensive team for transmasculine patients.

WHAT IS FERTILITY PRESERVATION?

Defined broadly, fertility preservation, refers to medical interventions used to cyropreserve, or freeze, gametes (oocytes or spermatocytes), embryos (an oocyte fertilized by a single spermatocyte), or gonadal tissue (ovarian and testicular) before the effects of time, disease, or medical treatment that may alter reproductive capacity. As time and technology have advanced, so too have the options and indications for fertility

Disclosures: All authors have no commercial or financial conflicts of interest or funding sources.
[a] New York University Langone Fertility Center, 660 First Avenue, Fifth Floor, New York, NY 10016, USA;
[b] Department of Obstetrics and Gynecology, New York University School of Medicine, 462 First Avenue, NBV 9N1-C, New York, NY 10016, USA
* Corresponding author.
E-mail address: Jennifer.Blakemore@nyulangone.org

Urol Clin N Am 46 (2019) 495–503
https://doi.org/10.1016/j.ucl.2019.07.014
0094-0143/19/© 2019 Elsevier Inc. All rights reserved.

preservation. Indications now include cancer and the gonadotoxic treatments of chemotherapy and radiation, autoimmune disease, hematopoietic stem cell transplant, medical conditions causing premature ovarian insufficiency (eg, Turner syndrome), fragile X premutation carriers, age-related decline or delayed childbearing, and most recently transgender persons before medical and/or surgical therapy.[2] Pregnancy outcomes among patients who return to use their cryopreserved tissues vary depending on indication, age, and type of preserved tissue, but live births have been reported among all forms of cryopreservation and across many medical indications.[2] In addition, the cumulative live-birth rate has been increasing in parallel with the technology; specifically with the introduction of the process of gamete vitrification. Vitrification reduces the fragility seen with slow freezing, reducing the large water content in the cells and ice crystal formation.[3]

For many patients undergoing fertility preservation, the discussion and counseling for preservation happen concurrently with the discussion and counseling for life-altering diagnoses and treatments. Particularly because patients often receive these diagnoses at a young age, treatment must be approached carefully and holistically. As quality of life in patients who may have reduced fertility from medical or surgical transition improves, there often comes an increased desire for family building.[4] There are fewer data evaluating reproductive regret in the transgender community among those who do not undergo fertility preservation; however, there is strong evidence of such regret in patients after cancer treatment who did not use fertility preservation.[5,6] Given the complexities of these situations, the American Society for Reproductive Medicine (ASRM) recommends counseling by a reproductive endocrinologist before any potentially fertility-altering treatment.[7]

For transmasculine individuals, fertility after medical treatment likely depends on type (puberty blockers and/or gender-affirming hormones; discussed later) and duration of use (prepubertal or postpubertal initiation). In addition to histologic data supporting that oocytes retain the ability to undergo meiosis after exposure to testosterone,[8] there have also been pregnancies (both spontaneous and with use of assisted reproduction) in transmen who had previously used gender-affirming hormones.[9] In addition, surgical affirmation may include a hysterectomy and bilateral salpingo-oophorectomy (removal of the uterus, tubes, and ovaries), resulting in permanent loss of fertility unless preservation is chosen a priori. These examples are just glimpses into the mobilizing evidence that transmen do not have to face a choice between gender affirmation and fertility, once considered a given. Discussion and counseling regarding fertility preservation and family building before affirmation procedures can offer transmen not only a chance but also a choice.

GUIDELINES TO TREATMENT OF TRANSMASCULINE INDIVIDUALS

In 2017, the Endocrine Society published an updated clinical practice guideline on treatment of individuals with gender dysphoria. These guidelines helped to establish an improved framework for treatment requiring a comprehensive health care team.[10] The update highlights the changes to the diagnostic classifications of gender dysphoria and outlines criteria and recommendations for the 2 mainstays of endocrine treatment: (1) puberty blockers, and (2) gender-affirming hormones. Puberty blockers, usually in the form of a gonadotropin-releasing hormone (GnRH) agonist, suppress transmen's hypothalamic-pituitary-gonadal axis to suppress the sex hormones, estrogens, that would be endogenously secreted. As a result, the processes of initiating the secondary sex characteristics in contrast with the patient's affirmed gender identity, such as breast development and menstruation, are inhibited. Gender-affirming hormones (for transmasculine individuals, the administration of testosterone or occasionally medroxyprogesterone to help with menstrual suppression) are also used to suppress endogenous estrogens and maintain testosterone levels to enhance male secondary sex characteristics, such as facial hair.

The Endocrine Society also provides recommendations for timing of treatment. Specifically, they recommend against puberty blockers and gender-affirming hormones in prepubertal children with gender dysphoria.[10] The guidelines from the Endocrine Society advocate waiting until a clinically appropriate time after the patient has the mental capacity to understand risks and benefits to any treatment, but before the advent of gender-affirming hormones. They recommend, ideally, that the person should be more than 16 years of age. The guidelines also advise that patients who desire surgical transition have satisfaction with hormonal transition for at least 1 year and be at least 18 years of age, especially when considering hysterectomy and/or gonadectomy.

Other organizations also provide guidance regarding the appropriate treatment and care for transgender individuals. The World Professional Association for Transgender Health (WPATH) is an international, multidisciplinary association that advocates for and works toward providing excellent health care for all gender-nonconforming individuals. In 2009, the WPATH published the seventh edition of the Standards of Care for the health of Transsexual, Transgender, and Gender Nonconforming People (SOC).[11] In this version of the SOC, 2 principles are further highlighted: (1) many transgender people want to have children, and (2) discussions by any health care professional initiating therapy about potential risks and options for preservation of fertility before treatment are imperative.

There are 3 critical aspects about fertility counseling in this patient population, specifically counseling that occurs before initiation of gender-affirming treatment. First, the impact of such treatment on fertility may vary largely depending on the age at which treatment begins. For example, a prepubertal individual who starts pubertal blockers or gender-affirming hormones may never develop reproductive function. In contrast, a postpubertal adult may have the ability to stop gender-affirming hormones and regain reproductive function, but this reappearance is not guaranteed.[12] Second, starting treatment does not preclude transgender persons from sexually transmitted infections or unintended pregnancy, and counseling of safe sexual health practices is equally important, especially in adolescent and young adult patients. Third, even with the most careful plan, transgender individuals are also susceptible to the same infertility issues that affect cisgender individuals. Therefore, planning and counseling for options must be expertly individualized.

The consensus from these professional organizations, the Endocrine Society, the WPATH, as well as ASRM, is that counseling regarding fertility and fertility preservation before puberty suppression in adolescents or hormonal or surgical therapy in adolescents and adults is not only recommended but essential.

FERTILITY PRESERVATION OPTIONS FOR TRANSMASCULINE INDIVIDUALS

There are 3 mainstays of fertility preservation accessible for transmasculine persons. Within that framework, the availability of each option depends on age and, potentially, region of the United States.[13] These options are discussed individually (**Table 1**).

Oocyte cryopreservation is an option that involves controlled ovarian hyperstimulation, similar to the process used for elective egg freezing and in vitro fertilization (IVF) following egg thaw at the time of desired pregnancy.[14] Transmasculine patients use daily injectable gonadotropin hormones for 10 to 12 days to stimulate the ovaries to mature multiple oocytes, compared with the maturation of a single oocyte that happens in a natural cycle. Response is monitored with transvaginal (or abdominal) ultrasonography (**Fig. 1**) and serum hormone levels approximately every 2 days. GnRH antagonists are another injectable medication used to prevent natural ovulation until follicles achieve appropriate size. When ready, injectable GnRH agonists or compounded human chorionic gonadotropins are used to trigger the oocyte maturation process and a transvaginal aspiration procedure under sedation is used to retrieve the oocytes (**Figs. 2** and **3**). Retrieved oocytes (**Fig. 4**) are evaluated under a microscope and those that have reached maturity, determined by visualization of extrusion of a polar body confirming completion of metaphase II of meiosis, undergo vitrification and are stored in a tank of liquid nitrogen until the patient is ready to return.[15] Oocytes that have not completed maturation (metaphase 1 or germinal vesicle stage) can also undergo cryopreservation, but their later use depends on the technology of in vitro maturation, which holds promise but does not currently have high success rates. Once the patient returns to use the oocytes, they are removed from the liquid nitrogen and undergo a warming process before fertilization to create embryos for transfer into the uterus of a patient, partner, or gestational carrier. Oocyte cryopreservation is the method of choice for adolescents.[7] However, it requires the patient to be postpubertal, which roughly correlates with a minimum of Tanner stage 4 in the case of adolescents. This requirement poses a conflict for adolescents considering initiation of pubertal blockers at Tanner stage 2. As current technology stands, the initiation of pubertal blockers before the maturation of the hypothalamic-pituitary- ovarian (HPO) axis, negates the opportunity for oocyte cryopreservation at that time. If pubertal blockers are initiated at this stage, the adolescent may again have the opportunity for oocyte cryopreservation after stopping pubertal blockers but will need to await maturation of the HPO axis along with pubertal progression and its undesired side effects of breast growth and menstruation. The timing of this maturation is unpredictable and is in conflict with the goals of pubertal blockers and subsequent gender-affirming hormones. Newer data show that the use of testosterone as treatment of gender dysphoria does not affect ovarian reserve[16,17] and transmen willing to discontinue testosterone therapy are candidates for oocyte cryopreservation. The optimal length of time to

Table 1
Fertility preservation options for transmen

FP Option	Tissue Type	Procedure	Age Restrictions	Considerations	How It Would Be Used in the Future
Oocyte cryopreservation	Oocyte	Controlled ovarian hyperstimulation with administration of gonadotropin hormone with transvaginal oocyte aspiration (egg retrieval)	Must be at least Tanner stage 4	Emerging evidence that this is an available option to patients who are willing to stop gender-affirming hormones for a short period of time	Warming of oocytes to then fertilize with donor or partner sperm to create embryos for transfer into patients' uterus, partner uterus, or gestational carrier
Embryo cryopreservation	Embryos	Same as oocyte cyropreservation with subsequent insemination of oocytes with spermatocytes before vitrification	Same as oocyte cyropreservation, generally reserved for older populations given readiness to create embryos	Same as oocyte cryopreservation, requires sperm from a partner, anonymous donor, or directed donor at time of procedure	Warming of embryos for transfer into patients' uterus, partner uterus, or gestational carrier
Ovarian tissue cryopreservation	Ovarian tissue	No hormonal preparation; removal of portion or whole ovary via laparoscopy or laparotomy	All ages, including prepubertal	Currently experimental; tissue harvesting can happen at time of oophorectomy for surgical affirming treatment	Goal: in vitro maturation of oocytes, fertilization by partner or donor sperm to create embryos for transfer into a uterus, or for tissue retransplant

Abbreviation: FP, fertility preservation.

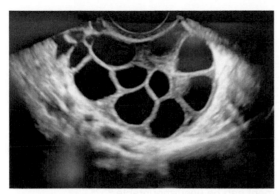

Fig. 1. Ultrasonography image of ovary with multiple stimulated follicles that contain oocytes.

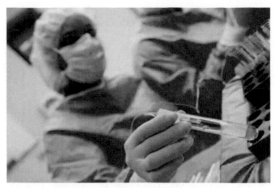

Fig. 3. An oocyte aspiration collection tube.

discontinue testosterone therapy before fertility preservation is unknown,[12,18] but transmen can restart testosterone therapy once menstruation occurs after oocyte aspiration. For adolescents treated with pubertal blockers followed by testosterone therapy, it is not known whether the HPO axis will respond to ovarian stimulation after cessation of testosterone, and, if so, what length of time would be required after cessation of testosterone to initiate ovarian stimulation. This point of counseling is important for all transgender people considering the option of pubertal blockers. In addition, note that the number of oocytes necessary to cryopreserve future fertility depends on many factors, including age, ovarian reserve, and desired family size,[15] and individualized optimal results may take more than 1 cycle.

Embryo cryopreservation starts with same process as oocyte cryopreservation but, once mature oocytes are retrieved, they are inseminated with sperm on the same day to create embryos, which are vitrified for future use. The sperm can come from a partner, an anonymous donor (sperm

bank), or a known donor. Embryos (**Fig. 5**) can be stored for as long as needed and high pregnancy and live-birth rates have been shown in both conventional IVF and in fertility preservation.[2,19] In all cases, the use of a partner's sperm or donor sperm to create embryos requires careful counseling. The partner must sign consents as an intended parent to (1) confirm the plan to create embryos, (2) confirm the plan for embryo transfer, and (3) confirm disposition for disposal if death or separation were to occur.

The third option, ovarian tissue cryopreservation, is currently experimental. Ovarian tissue cryopreservation involves resection of a portion of the ovary, or the entire ovary, which is subsequently cryopreserved.[15] The procedure does not require preparation with hormonal stimulation nor is it restricted by age, puberty, or partner status. It can be performed at the same time as gender-

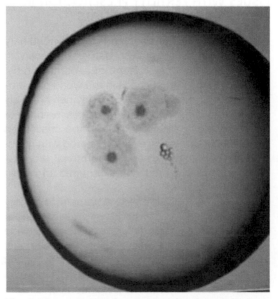

Fig. 4. Three retrieved oocytes under the microscope.

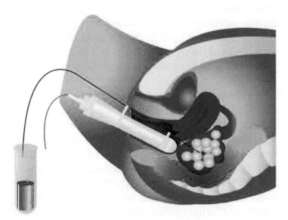

Fig. 2. The technique of oocyte aspiration.

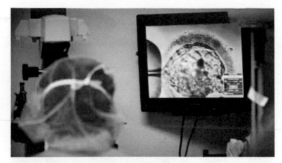

Fig. 5. An evaluation of an embryo in the laboratory before vitrification. (*Courtesy of* Juliana Thomas, New York, NY.)

affirming surgery.[20] There has been evidence of natural conception after retransplant of ovarian tissue, mostly in patients with cancer,[21] for those who chose natural conception. In vitro maturation of mature oocytes from immature or primordial follicles or germ cells to produce a live birth is still in the early stages of research[22] but has not yet been applied to the transgender fertility preservation population. Similarly, the concept of encapsulated in vitro follicle growth under investigation by Woodruff and colleagues[23,24] offers hope for the future in transgender fertility preservation. This innovative research may provide for the development of an artificial ovary that can be used to mature oocytes taken from prepubertal ovarian tissue without ever transplanting the ovary back into the body.[25] These options, although young and complex, remain exciting areas of research.[14]

ATTITUDES, PERCEPTIONS, AND ETHICAL ISSUES WITH FERTILITY PRESERVATION IN TRANSMASCULINE INDIVIDUALS

It is well-known that trans and gender-nonbinary individuals experience many barriers to receiving adequate health care, a fact that is perhaps most apparent in the unmet needs in the world of reproductive and sexual health.[26,27] Transmen are likely one of the most underserved in this arena. For transmen there are differences in the challenges for fertility preservation even compared with transwomen, particularly given the hormonal preparation and invasive procedures required to obtain gametes or tissue.

One of the most prominent barriers to fertility preservation is cost. Fertility preservation is expensive and most insurance plans provide either limited or, in many cases, no coverage. This barrier can be especially prohibitive for young people, who face a potentially longer time with storage fees; may have lower incomes; and, in the case of transgender persons, who may also

be facing expenses related to treatment of gender affirmation.[27,28] It has been shown that use of fertility preservation is especially low in the adolescent and young adult population,[1] despite many studies showing that the desire for fertility preservation and family building is high.[29] Furthermore, although fertility preservation in the transgender population is generally supported by public opinion,[30] social support depends on the individual's personal situation and environment. The availability of such support is immensely helpful; in its absence, the obstacles to successful treatment can be unsurmountable.[31,32]

Another unique barrier for transmen is that the process of oocyte and embryo cryopreservation is a highly feminizing experience. It requires administration of hormones to increase the endogenous levels and, consequently, feminizing effects of estrogens as well as multiple transvaginal (or abdominal) ultrasonography scans. Transmen desiring cryopreservation who are on testosterone are required to stop the affirming hormone treatment and resume menses before starting the process. In all cases, the process has potential to amplify the gender dysphoria that is diminished via gender affirmation.[33] There are options to help minimize some of the gender incongruence when in cycle. For one, the addition of an aromatase inhibitor, such as letrozole, which, when taken daily during a cycle, can reduce the amount of estrogen produced. There is documented success with fertility preservation cycles with letrozole in the breast cancer population[34] and so its use has been extrapolated to transmale patients using fertility preservation. In addition, transabdominal ultrasonography can sometimes be used in place of the transvaginal technique as long as the ovaries can be visualized. Although these temporizing measures are useful, it does not negate the overt feminizing tone of transmale fertility preservation, which is a unique part of the necessary counseling performed by reproductive endocrinologists. Although this feminizing aspect of fertility preservation can be difficult, patients can be comforted and reassured that the process is short term (2–3 weeks) and undesirable hormonal side effects are temporary.

Given this backdrop, health care providers in the trans community can experience challenges with regard to fertility preservation. A recent study of provider perceptions and attitudes showed that many providers considered themselves unqualified to discuss fertility preservation based on lack of knowledge or inability to refer.[35] There is wide variation in practice behavior regarding discussion of fertility preservation by health care providers with the trans community, which offers an important area of education and improvement to benefit this patient population.[36]

For many patients, adoption, donor gametes, and surrogacy may be viewed as preferable options for building a family, as well as a way to avoid some of the barriers referenced throughout this article. Even when these options are preferred or selected from the outset and remain attractive options, it is essential for patients to discuss family building and reproductive health with a specialist to avoid reproductive regret.[5,6] This requirement highlights the need for improved information access for referral to reproductive endocrinologists before any treatment.[33,37]

PREGNANCY OUTCOMES FROM TRANSMEN WHO HAVE UNDERGONE FERTILITY PRESERVATION

The use of fertility preservation by transmen is increasing[38] and there are increasing data on transmale pregnancies.[9] The unique pathway to pregnancy after fertility preservation and some of the associated issues represented by cases from our own institution are discussed here.

A case series published by Maxwell and colleagues[39] in 2017 describes 3 transmen, aged 17 years (case 1), 30 years (case 2), and 32 years (case 3), who presented for consultation for fertility preservation before initiating gender-affirming hormones and successfully underwent oocyte cryopreservation with 17, 45, and 13 mature oocytes cryopreserved respectively. Case 2 returned 8 years after initiating testosterone desiring embryo creation with plan to transfer to his cisgender female partner. During preconception genetic carrier screening, the patient was found to carry a fragile X premutation and he and his partner elected for embryo creation with preimplantation genetic testing for both aneuploidy and the fragile X. A single euploid unaffected embryo was subsequently warmed and transferred into the patients' partner, resulting in a live birth. Case 3 returned 5 years after cryopreservation desiring embryo creation and transfer to his cisgender female partner. His 13 mature oocytes plus 6 immature oocytes were thawed, fertilized, and resulted in 6 embryos or blastocysts. Of these 6 embryos, 1 embryo was transferred after 5 days of culture and the remaining 5 embryos were vitrified. The transferred embryo resulted in a biochemical pregnancy. Two months later, the couple returned and thawed 2 more of the previously vitrified 5 embryos, which resulted in a dichorionic-diamniotic twin pregnancy with subsequent live births. Case 1 has not yet returned to the clinic and his oocytes remain cryopreserved.

These cases show the variability in the pathway to pregnancy even after fertility preservation and again highlight the importance of individualized counseling by a reproductive endocrinologist.

RECOMMENDATIONS FOR THE FUTURE OF FERTILITY PRESERVATION IN TRANSMASCULINE INDIVIDUALS

Fertility preservation has come a long way since its inception, and the subgroup focused on cancer, oncofertility, is a microcosm for the field at large. In 2018, the American Society of Clinical Oncology (ASCO) published updated guidelines promoting the importance and necessity of fertility preservation discussion and referral in patients with cancer.[40] Moreover, there are principles and guidelines recommending that cancer centers ensure the provision of both adequate and excellent care, which includes (1) providing education on cancer-related infertility and fertility preservation; (2) providing printed resources; (3) notifying patients in writing about risks of cancer treatment and documenting that counseling; (4) referring patients to reproductive specialists; and (5) having a policy stating their commitment as an institution to the fertility needs of their patients.[41] The goal of these guidelines and center of excellence designations was to further standardize and improve the process of fertility preservation and counseling in this vulnerable population.

The authors argue that the same parallels can and should be drawn to the transgender community. All health care providers, psychologists, psychiatrists, endocrinologists, primary care providers, surgeons, and social workers engaged in providing care to transgender persons should receive training and education in fertility preservation options. In addition, providers should be prepared with a list of reproductive endocrinologists who they can refer to, or people they can contact to help with referral. The authors recognize that not all providers have direct access to a fertility program or a fertility specialist with experience in transgender fertility preservation at their institution or even in their city or state. We urge providers to create relationships both nearby and across the country to cultivate a network of support that will help patients receive superior care from a diverse and comprehensive health care team. As with most networks, patient experience travels quickly via word of mouth and, more modernly, through social media and other electronic media, and these channels can also be used to help cultivate a strong network and make outreach easy for provider to provider.

SUMMARY

Discussion of fertility preservation is an important step for all transmasculine individuals considering hormones as part of their transitions, and such discussions are recommended by most affiliated professional organizations. This article provides an assessment of the scope, barriers, outcomes, and future of fertility preservation for transmasculine patients. Whether the preservation services are used or not, referral is a vital component to the discussion of risks and benefits before any gender-affirming treatment.

REFERENCES

1. Nahata L, Tishelman AC, Caltabellotta NM, et al. Low fertility preservation utilization among transgender youth. J Adolesc Health 2017;61(1):40–4.
2. Martinez F. Update on fertility preservation from the Barcelona International Society for Fertility Preservation – ESHRE-ASRM 2015 expert meeting: indications, results and future perspective. Fertil Steril 2017;108(3):407–15.
3. Dolmans M, Manavella DD. Recent advances in fertility preservation. J Obstet Gynaecol Res 2019; 45(2):266–79.
4. Wierckx K, Van Caenegem C, Pennings G, et al. Reproductive wish in transsexual men. Hum Reprod 2012;27(2):483–7.
5. Letourneau JM, Ebbel EE, Katz PP, et al. Pretreatment fertility counseling and fertility preservation improve quality of life in reproductive age women with cancer. Cancer 2011;118(6):1710–7.
6. Benedict C, Thom B, Kelvin JF. Young adult female cancer survivors' decision regret about fertility preservation. J Adolesc Young Adult Oncol 2015;4(4): 213–8.
7. Ethics Committee of the American Society for Reproductive Medicine. Fertility Preservation and reproduction in patients facing gonadotoxic therapies: a committee opinion. Fertil Steril 2013;100(5): 1224–31.
8. Lierman S, Tilleman K, Braeckmans K, et al. Fertility preservation for trans men: frozen-thawed in vitro matured oocytes collected at the time of ovarian tissue processing exhibit normal meiotic spindles. J Assist Reprod Genet 2017;34(11):1449–56.
9. Light AD, Obedin-Maliver J, Sevelius JM, et al. Transgender men who experienced pregnancy after female-to-male gender transitioning. Obstet Gynecol 2014;124(6):1120–7.
10. Hembree WC, Cohen-Kettenis PT, Gooren L, et al. Endocrine Treatment of Gender-Dysphoric/Gender-Incongruent Persons: An Endocrine Society Clinical Practice Guideline. J Clin Endocrinol Metab 2017; 102(11):3869–903.
11. World Professional Association for Transgender health. Standards of Care Version 7. Available at: https://www.wpath.org/publications/soc. Accessed February 18, 2019.
12. Ethics Committee of the American Society for Reproductive Medicine. Access to fertility services by Transgender persons: an Ethics Committee opinion. Fertil Steril 2015;104(5):1111–5.
13. Johnson EK, Finlayson C. Preservation of fertility potential for gender and sex diverse individuals. Transgend Health 2016;1(1):41–4.
14. Wallace SA, Blough KL, Kondapalli LA. Fertility preservation in the transgender patient: expanding oncofertility care beyond cancer. Gynecol Endocrinol 2014;30(12):868–71.
15. Mattawanon N, Spencer JB, Schirmer DA, et al. Fertility preservation options in transgender people: a review. Rev Endocr Metab Disord 2018;19(3): 231–42.
16. De Roo C, Lierman S, Tilleman K, et al. Ovarian tissue cryopreservation in female-to-male transgender people: insight into ovarian histology and physiology after prolonged androgen treatment. Reprod Biomed Online 2017;34(6):557–66.
17. Rodriguez-Wallberg KA, Dhejne C, Stefenson M, et al. Preserving eggs for men's fertility. A pilot experience with fertility preservation for female-to-male transsexuals in Sweden. Fertil Steril 2014;102(3): e160–1.
18. Neblett MF, Hipp HS. Fertility considerations in transgender persons. Endocrinol Metab Clin North Am 2019. https://doi.org/10.1016/j.ecl.2019.02.003.
19. Bedoschi G, Oktay K. Current approach to fertility preservation by embryo cryopreservation. Fertil Steril 2014;99(6):1496–502.
20. Van Den Broecke R, Van Der Elst J, Liu J, et al. The female-to-male transsexual patient: a source of human ovarian cortical tissue for experimental use. Hum Reprod 2001;16:145–7.
21. Gellert SE, Pors SE, Kristensen SG, et al. Transplantation of frozen-thawed ovarian tissue: an update on worldwide activity published in peer-reviewed papers and on the Danish cohort. J Assist Reprod Genet 2018;35(4):561–70.
22. Kawamura K, Cheng Y, Suzuki N, et al. Hippo signaling disruption and Akt stimulation of ovarian follicles for infertility treatment. Proc Natl Acad Sci U S A 2013;110(43):17474–9.
23. Laronda MM, Jakus AE, Whelan KA, et al. Initiation of puberty in mice following decellularized ovary transplant. Biomaterials 2015;50:20–9.
24. Skory RM, Xu Y, Shea LD, et al. Engineering the ovarian cycle using in vitro follicle culture. Hum Reprod 2015;30(6):1386–95.
25. Xu M, Kreeger PK, Shea LD, et al. Tissue-engineered follicles produce live, fertile offspring. Tissue Eng 2006;12(10):2739–46.

26. Wingo E, Ingraham N, Roberts SCM. Reproductive health care priorities and barriers to effective care for LGBTQ people assigned female at birth: a qualitative study. Womens Health Issues 2018;28(4):350–7.

27. Mitu K. transgender reproductive choice and fertility preservation. AMA J Ethics 2016;18(11):1119–25.

28. Nixon L. The right to (trans) parent: a reproductive justice approach to reproductive rights, fertility and family-building issues facing transgender people. Wm & Mary J Women & L 2013;20(1):72–103.

29. Auer MK, Fuss J, Nieder TO, et al. Desire to have children among transgender people in germany: a cross-sectional multi-center study. J Sex Med 2018;15(5):757–67.

30. Goldman RH, Kaser DJ, Missmer SA, et al. Fertility treatment for the transgender community: a public opinion study. J Assist Reprod Genet 2017;34(11):1457–67.

31. Quinn GP, Sampson A, Campo-Englestein L. Familial discordance regarding fertility preservation for a transgender teen: an ethical case study. J Clin Ethics 2018;29(4):261–5.

32. Leonardi M, Frecker H, Scheim AI, et al. Reproductive Health Considerations in sexual and/or gender minority adolescents. J Pediatr Adolesc Gynecol 2019;32(1):15–20.

33. Armuand G, Dhejne C, Olofsson JI, et al. Transgender men's experiences of fertility preservation: a qualitative study. Hum Reprod 2017;32(2):383–90.

34. Azim AA, Constantini-Ferrando M, Oktay K. Safety of fertility preservation by ovarian stimulation with letrozole and gonadotropin in patients with breast cancer: a prospective controlled study. J Clin Oncol 2008;26(16):2630–5.

35. Tishelman AC, Sutter M, Chen D, et al. Health care provider perceptions of fertility preservation barriers and challenges with transgender patients and families: qualitative responses to an international survey. J Assist Reprod Genet 2019;36(3):579–88.

36. Chen D, Kolbuck VD, Sutter ME, et al. Knowledge, Practice behaviors, and perceived barriers to fertility care among providers of transgender healthcare. J Adolesc Health 2019;64(2):226–34.

37. Chen D, Matson M, Macapagal K, et al. Attitudes toward fertility and reproductive health among transgender and gender-nonconforming adolescents. J Adolesc Health 2018;63(1):62–8.

38. Chen D, Bernardi LA, Pavone M, et al. Oocyte cryopreservation among transmasculine youth: a case series. J Assist Reprod Genet 2018;35(11):2057–61.

39. Maxwell S, Noyes N, Keefe D, et al. Pregnancy outcomes after fertility preservation in transgender men. Obstet Gynecol 2017;129(6):1031–4.

40. Oktay K, Harvey BE, Partridge AH, et al. Fertility preservation in patients with cancer: ASCO Clinical Practice Guideline Update. J Clin Oncol 2018;36(19):1994–2001.

41. Reinecke JD, Kelvin JF, Arvey SR, et al. implementing a systematic approach to meeting patients' cancer and fertility needs: a review of the fertile hope centers of excellence program. J Oncol Pract 2012;8(5):303–8.

Orchiectomy as Bridge or Alternative to Vaginoplasty

Marah C. Hehemann, MD[a], Thomas J. Walsh, MD, MS[b],*

KEYWORDS

- Transgender • Gender dysphoria • Sex reassignment surgery • Orchiectomy • Gender identity

KEY POINTS

- Simple orchiectomy for gender affirmation is a low-risk, minimally invasive, generalizable procedure that eliminates circulating endogenous testosterone, allowing reduced hormonal supplementation.
- This procedure serves as a step in definitive phenotypic transition while maximally preserving healthy tissue for future genital reconstructive surgery.
- Orchiectomy should be offered routinely as a bridge or alternative to vaginoplasty, particularly in the setting of limited access to specialized centers for transgender surgery.

INTRODUCTION

Gender dysphoria denotes the experience of distress caused by incongruence between genotypically determined gender and experienced gender.[1] An estimated 1.4 million adults, or 0.6% of the United States population, identify as transgender, although these figures may be underestimated given marginalization and limited access to health care experienced by transgender individuals.[2–4] Although transgender identities exist on a broad spectrum, including nonbinary categories, the largest proportion of transgender individuals identify as male to female, or transfemale.[2,3]

In 2012, the World Professional Association for Transgender Health (WPATH) published the Standards of Care (SOC) for the Health of Transsexual, Transgender, and Gender Nonconforming People, which provides a framework around which health care providers can deliver safe and effective care to transgender individuals.[4] Care of transitioning transfemale patients requires a multidisciplinary approach, involving input from mental health,

psychiatry, endocrinology, preventive medicine, as well as possible involvement of surgical services, including plastic surgery, otolaryngology, gynecology, and urology.[4–7] Gender-confirming treatments include hormone therapy and surgical management of the chest and genitalia (so-called top and bottom gender-affirming surgeries [GASs], respectively), along with adjunctive treatments, including facial and laryngeal surgery, voice therapy, and hair removal.[3,8]

By definition, GASs are designed to reduce or alleviate the distress associated with gender dysphoria by bringing these patient's physical appearance further in accord with their gender identities. Certain surgeries are also performed with the goals of generating a physiologic change to optimize transition, or creating a functional modification for the patient, such as vaginoplasty to allow receptive intercourse. Gender-affirming orchiectomy has the distinct physiologic goal of reducing the need for antiandrogen treatments, such as spironolactone, which are required of many transwomen with intact testicles. In addition,

---

Disclosures/Conflicts of Interest: None.
[a] Division of Urology, NorthShore University HealthSystem, 2180 Pfingsten Road, #3000, Glenview, IL 60026, USA; [b] Department of Urology, University of Washington, 1959 Northeast Pacific Street, BB-1121, Box 356510, Seattle, WA 98195, USA
* Corresponding author.
E-mail address: Walsht@uw.edu

Urol Clin N Am 46 (2019) 505–510
https://doi.org/10.1016/j.ucl.2019.07.005
0094-0143/19/© 2019 Elsevier Inc. All rights reserved.

for many patients, orchiectomy represents a conservative step in the process of surgical feminization, helping to mitigate the distress of intact male gonads. It is essential that surgical care should be tailored to each individual patient, because not all patients desire, need, or qualify for each form of GAS.[8]

This article reviews the history of orchiectomy for gender affirmation, eligibility criteria for genital GAS, intentions of orchiectomy as a bridge or alternative to vaginoplasty, and recommendations for preoperative counseling. The surgical technique used by surgeons at our institution is described here along with postoperative considerations.

HISTORICAL PERSPECTIVES ON ORCHIECTOMY FOR GENDER AFFIRMATION

Although diagnostic terminology related to gender dysphoria has only been refined in the past several decades, the notion of fluid gender identity that exists along a continuum from male to female has existed for centuries. One of the earliest known examples of gender nonconformity in North America occurred well before the United States established independence. A servant living in Jamestown in the 1620s, known as both Thomas and Thomasine Hall, claimed to be both man and woman. After much speculation and examination, Hall was eventually ordered by the court to don specific articles of clothing, and was subject to lifelong ridicule and shaming.[9]

It was not until 300 years later that Magnus Hirschfield, a German physician and sexologist, authored *Transvestites*, thereby bringing the concept of gender fluidity into the medical literature.[9] He later founded the Hirschfield Institute for Sexual Science in Berlin, where he performed the first reported genital gender-confirmation surgery on Dorchen Richter, a German individual assigned male gender at birth, but who reportedly experienced the desire to be female since childhood. Richter underwent bilateral orchiectomy in 1922 and had further genital gender-affirming surgery, including penectomy, in 1931.[9]

Hirschfield's concepts and treatment strategies were carried on in the United States by Dr Harry Benjamin who wrote *The Transsexual Phenomenon* in 1966, raising awareness among clinicians about the potential benefits of gender-affirming surgery.[10] This publication marked an awakening among the United States medical community, after which the Johns Hopkins University became the first of many institutions to open a gender identity clinic.[11] Programs dedicated to diagnosing and treating transgender individuals, as well as conducting research related to transsexuality and gender dysphoria, were soon established nationwide, including at the University of Minnesota, Stanford University, and the University of Washington.[9,12] Outcomes studies on the psychological benefits of gender-affirmation surgery and improvement in subjective well-being confirmed the importance of offering surgical treatment to transgender patients.[11,13] It is estimated that, by the end of the 1970s, more than 1000 Americans had undergone GAS at a major university hospital.[12]

In 1978, Benjamin founded the Harry Benjamin International Gender Dysphoria Association (which would later become WPATH), and, shortly thereafter, published the first version of the *Standards of Care for Gender Dysphoric Persons*.[8,9] However, it was not until 2012 that the US Department of Health and Human Services highlighted policy protecting transgender individuals from discrimination based on gender identity at the hands of health insurance companies, and, in 2014, repealed the 1989 decision that banned genital reconstruction for so-called transsexualism.[14] The term gender dysphoria was only recently (2013) added to the *Diagnostic and Statistical Manual of Mental Disorders, Fifth Edition*, providing recognition of the distress experienced by individuals with gender dysphoria as a condition.[1] It is clear that while the arc of United States public policy on transgender health care slowly bends toward acceptance, patients continue to face significant barriers to care.

ELIGIBILITY CRITERIA FOR GENITAL GENDER-AFFIRMING SURGERY

Despite the advancement of research in transgender medicine and policy protections for transgender patients, there remains a deficiency in knowledge among practicing surgeons about SOC guidelines and factors that must be satisfied before offering genital GAS. These criteria have been refined over time since Harry Benjamin published the first SOC, but remain stringent with regard to insurance carrier requirements.[15]

According to current WPATH SOC recommendations, patients seeking genital reconstruction for the purpose of gender affirmation must (1) have persistent, well-documented gender dysphoria; (2) have capacity to provide fully informed consent for treatment; (3) be of adult age in a given country; (4) have well-controlled medical or mental health conditions; (5) have 2 referrals from qualified mental health providers; (6) have been treated for 12 continuous months with hormone therapy in accordance with the patient's medical transition goals (provided there are no contraindications); and (7) have lived continuously for at least 12 months in the gender role that is congruent with the gender identity.[4]

The WPATH SOC address the ethical quandaries surgeons may encounter regarding genital GAS by recommending physicians meet transgender patients with empathy and respect, remembering the potential for harm by denying access to appropriate treatments.[4] For many patients, surgical modification to establish greater congruence with gender identity is the only means by which they can experience amelioration of gender dysphoria–related distress. Urologists and other surgeons should be encouraged to work closely with the other members of the multidisciplinary team involved in each patient's care.

GOALS AND BENEFITS OF BILATERAL ORCHIECTOMY
Hormone Reduction

Medical hormone therapy serves to minimize secondary sexual characteristics of biological gender by suppressing endogenous sex hormones, and to maximize the secondary sex characteristics congruent with gender identity by supplementing cross-sex hormones.[16] The goal of antiandrogen medication is to reduce serum testosterone to biological female levels (<55 ng/dL).[16] When combined with estrogen supplementation, this regimen allows for initiation of biological phenotypic transition.

Spironolactone, the most commonly used antiandrogen by providers in the United States, has several commonly known side effects, including dehydration, hypotension, and electrolyte derangement (including life threatening hyperkalemia), and risks interaction with numerous foods.[17] Lesser known adverse reactions include gastric bleeding, hematologic dyscrasia, neurotoxicity, and cutaneous reactions, including Stevens-Johnson syndrome.[17] Its use is contraindicated in patients with renal failure and adrenal insufficiency caused by Addison disease, and it must be used with caution in patients with liver disease.[17]

Simple orchiectomy offers transwomen the least invasive means of eliminating the major source of circulating endogenous testosterone. For most, this allows the discontinuation of antiandrogen therapy and a possible reduction in estrogen requirement by up to 25% to 50%.[18] Orchiectomy affords the avoidance of potentially harmful adverse effects of antiandrogen therapy, and for elimination of endogenous androgens in transwomen with contraindications to medical therapy.

Accessible Feminizing Genital Gender-Affirming Surgery

Cited barriers to transgender genital GAS include limited geographic distribution of programs offering gender-confirmation surgery and surgeon inexperience with GAS.[14] However, the technique described later for simple orchiectomy is a straightforward outpatient procedure that does not require training beyond that of a general urologist. The operation is generalizable and can be performed even in rural settings without surgical subspecialists or the presence of a multidisciplinary team. Furthermore, in our experience, this technique has been successfully performed entirely under local anesthesia, and is feasible using monitored anesthesia care.

For transwomen who wish to proceed with genital GAS to reduce antiandrogen use, or to begin phenotypic transition, simple orchiectomy can be readily achieved with little preparation other than meeting the aforementioned WPATH criteria. Unlike vulvoplasty or vaginoplasty, simple orchiectomy can be performed without prior scrotal electrolysis, which is a barrier to surgical care for some transwomen. Orchiectomy offers an accessible form of GAS, which has been shown to improve body-congruence scores and quality of life, and reduce depression and anxiety compared with nontreated individuals with gender dysphoria.[19–21]

Minimize Surgical Risk and Maximize Future Feminizing Surgery

Karim and colleagues[22] described the primary goal of genital reconstruction in transwomen as creation of a feminine-appearing perineogenital complex, including a neovagina and a downwardly pointing, shortened neourethra. Although the highly specialized surgical techniques required to accomplish this goal have been refined for decades, full transfemale genital reconstruction remains fraught with risks and potential complications, such as graft contraction, suboptimal sensation, urethral stenosis, fistulization, vaginal or labial necrosis, and rectal injury.[23] In addition, transwomen contemplating vaginoplasty are confronted with the possibility of lifelong daily neovaginal dilation.[24] For individuals with concerns regarding or at high risk for surgical complications, for those who do not seek receptive vaginal intercourse, or for those who do not wish to adhere to daily neovaginal maintenance, bilateral orchiectomy offers an alternative to genital reconstruction.

It should be noted that, unlike patients who elect to undergo vulvoplasty, neovagina creation after bilateral orchiectomy is still feasible.[5] As described later, our technique offers maximal preservation of penoscrotal skin, which may later be pedicalized for use as a skin flap.[10,12] The avoidance of tissue destruction is critical to simple orchiectomy as a bridge to future GAS.

SURGICAL CONSIDERATIONS AND TECHNIQUE
Preoperative Considerations

Bilateral simple orchiectomy is considered to be of low operative complexity, and, with this in mind, standard preoperative evaluation should be conducted with regard to patient safety.[25] Most individuals undergoing genital GAS are concurrently receiving estrogen therapy, so special consideration should be given to intraoperative venous thromboembolism (VTE) prophylaxis. Estrogen therapy is associated with a 1% to 6.2% increased risk of VTE, particularly in patients who are smokers, immobilized, more than 40 years old, or have a thrombophilic disorder.[26] The authors therefore recommend routine use of sequential compression devices, despite the reported short duration of surgery (mean duration 29 minutes in a small series).[27] Although surgical duration is brief, it is imperative to maintain safety as a priority in this high-risk population.

Some clinicians advocate cessation of hormone therapy before surgery because of a theoretic bleeding risk.[26] However, this risk has not been substantiated in the literature and we therefore do not recommend cessation of hormone therapy, which can detract from the goals of reducing overall virilization.[28] Furthermore, the surgical bleeding risk during simple bilateral orchiectomy is exceedingly low, such that we would not consider full anticoagulation to be a contraindication to surgery.

Intraoperative Technique

The principles of our technique for simple orchiectomy are 2-fold: (1) eliminate bilateral testes and spermatic cords to maximally debulk the scrotum, and (2) optimize tissue preservation of scrotal skin and dartos for future reconstructive GAS.[29] The technique for gender-affirming orchiectomy differs significantly from radical orchiectomy for oncologic purposes.

Bilateral spermatic cord blocks are applied using 0.5% bupivacaine without epinephrine. The median raphe incision site is also anesthetized. One testis is elevated against the median raphe and a 3-cm to 4-cm longitudinal skin incision is made along the raphe. Sharp, direct dissection is carried down to the avascular plane of the tunica vaginalis, which allows complete mobilization of the spermatic cord. Care is taken to mobilize only the spermatic cord and tunica vaginalis, allowing preservation of scrotal fat and fascia for potential future use.

The spermatic cord is exposed in entirety using gentle retraction at the level of the superficial inguinal ring. The external spermatic fascia is opened circumferentially using surgical electrocautery, and cord contents are ligated in 2 parts using 2-0 silk stick tie and proximal free tie. Hemostasis is evaluated and cord blocks are readministered before release of cord stumps. The opening of the external fascia allows full retraction of spermatic cord into the retroperitoneum on ligation of cord contents and release of the cord stump. This technique prevents residual tissue in the inguinal and scrotal regions. The contralateral testis is approached similarly and delivered through the same midline incision. The procedure is repeated on the contralateral testis and cord.

Closure is accomplished in 2 layers. First, absorbable suture is used in a running, locking fashion to reapproximate the dartos layer, including scrotal septum. Skin is closed using Monocryl suture in a running mattress fashion. Using a midline scrotal approach allows the surgeon to recreate scrotal symmetry and to minimize aberrant scarring.

Although there are no studies evaluating the incidence of testicular cancer in transwomen, animal studies have shown a possible link between estrogen and testicular cancer.[30] In addition, there are 2 published case reports of transwomen diagnosed with testicular cancer, although both patients were observed to have palpable testicular masses on preoperative examination.[31,32] Given the low overall incidence of testicular cancer and absence of reported incidental, clinically imperceptible masses, the authors feel that routine use of transscrotal orchiectomy is safe and does not pose an oncologic risk.

POSTOPERATIVE EXPECTATIONS

Awareness of the physiologic and psychological outcomes after genital GAS is a critical portion of counseling patients contemplating reconstructive surgery. In a study of 697 patients, including 350 transwomen, 4 validated instruments (the Transgender Congruence Scale, Revised Physical Self-Perception Profile, Center for Epidemiologic Studies Depression Scale, and the Beck Anxiety Index) were used to compare body congruence, body image satisfaction depression, and anxiety among transgender individuals in various stages of transition.[19] The investigators found that body-gender congruence and body image satisfaction increased with the extent of gender-confirming treatment, whereas depression and anxiety significantly declined. Transwomen who had undergone partial bottom surgery (orchiectomy) scored similarly with regard to body congruence compared with their counterparts who had undergone definitive bottom surgery (vaginoplasty).[19] The investigators concluded that withholding gender-confirming treatments until depression and anxiety are treated is counterproductive because these treatments alleviate distress, depression, and anxiety related to gender dysphoria. Iranian and Turkish studies have also confirmed improvements in quality of life and body image, as well as reduction in gender-related discrimination and victimization after GAS.[33,34]

Importantly, regret after GAS is rare, occurring in 0% to 3.8% of patients.[35–37] In a study of 6793 transgender patients attending a single Dutch gender identity clinic, only 0.6% of transwomen expressed regret after undergoing gonadectomy.[35] Factors associated with regret include insufficient social or familial support, late-onset gender transition, coexistent mental health diagnoses, poor cosmetic outcome, poor sexual function, and noncompliance with WPATH SOC guidelines.[36–38] Adherence to SOC guidelines is paramount to treatment success.

There exists a paucity of studies directly addressing sexual function and desire after simple orchiectomy without feminizing reconstruction. However, Wierckx and colleagues[39] investigated sexual desire in a cohort of transgender individuals at various stages of transition. Most transwomen (83.4%) never or rarely experienced sexual desire, and 22.1% met criteria for hypoactive sexual desire disorder (HSDD). Transwomen who had completed genital GAS (including orchiectomy, penectomy, and vaginoplasty) had a higher prevalence of HSDD and more commonly described a decrease in sexual desire after gender-confirming surgery than transmen, who were found to have an increase in desire. Patients should be counseled about the potential for diminished sexual desire after orchiectomy, and HSDD should be addressed by the mental health providers on the patient's care team.

SUMMARY

Simple orchiectomy for gender affirmation is a low-risk, minimally invasive, generalizable procedure that eliminates circulating endogenous testosterone, allowing reduced hormonal supplementation. This procedure serves as a step in definitive phenotypic transition while maximally preserving healthy tissue for future genital reconstructive surgery. Orchiectomy should be offered routinely as a bridge or alternative to vaginoplasty, particularly in the setting of limited access to specialized centers for transgender surgery.

REFERENCES

1. American Psychiatric Association. Diagnostic and statistical manual of mental disorders. 5th edition. Arlington (VA): American Psychiatric Publishing; 2013.
2. Arcelus J, Bouman WP, Van Den Noortgate W, et al. Systematic review and meta-analysis of prevalence studies in transsexualism. Eur Psychiatry 2015; 30(6):807–15.
3. Reisner SL, Radix A, Deutsch MB. Integrated and gender-affirming transgender clinical care and research. J Acquir Immune Defic Syndr 2016; 72(Suppl 3):235.
4. Coleman E, Bockting W, Botzer M, et al. Standards of care for the health of transsexual, transgender, and gender-nonconforming people, version 7. Int J Transgend 2012;13(4):165–232.
5. Jiang D, Witten J, Berli J, et al. Does depth matter? factors affecting choice of vulvoplasty over vaginoplasty as gender-affirming genital surgery for transgender women. J Sex Med 2018;15(6):902–6.
6. Klein DA, Paradise SL, Goodwin ET. Caring for transgender and gender-diverse persons: What clinicians should know. Am Fam Physician 2018;98(11):645–53.
7. Wylie K, Knudson G, Khan SI, et al. Serving transgender people: clinical care considerations and service delivery models in transgender health. Lancet 2016;388(10042):401–11.
8. Berli JU, Knudson G, Fraser L, et al. What surgeons need to know about gender confirmation surgery when providing care for transgender individuals: a review. JAMA Surg 2017;152(4):394–400.
9. Beemyn G. Transgender history in the United States. In: Erickson-Schroth L, editor. Trans bodies, trans selves. Oxford: a resource for the transgender community. Oxford University Press; 2014.
10. Selvaggi G, Ceulemans P, De Cuypere G, et al. Gender identity disorder: general overview and surgical treatment for vaginoplasty in male-to-female transsexuals. Plast Reconstr Surg 2005;116(6):145e.
11. Edgerton MT. The role of surgery in the treatment of transsexualism. Ann Plast Surg 1984;13(6):473–81.
12. Frey JD, Poudrier G, Thomson JE, et al. A historical review of gender-affirming medicine: focus on genital reconstruction surgery. J Sex Med 2017;14(8): 991–1002.
13. Edgerton MT, Knorr NJ, Callison JR. The surgical treatment of transsexual patients. limitations and indications. Plast Reconstr Surg 1970;45(1):38–46.
14. Weissler JM, Chang BL, Carney MJ, et al. Gender-affirming surgery in persons with gender dysphoria. Plast Reconstr Surg 2018;141(3):396e.
15. Colebunders B, Brondeel S, D'Arpa S, et al. An update on the surgical treatment for transgender patients. Sex Med Rev 2017;5(1):103–9.
16. Hadj-Moussa M, Ohl DA, Kuzon WM Jr. Evaluation and treatment of gender dysphoria to prepare for

gender confirmation surgery. Sex Med Rev 2018; 6(4):607–17.

17. Pfizer Inc. Aldactone (spironolactone) [package insert] New York: 2018.

18. Kent MA, Winoker JS, Grotas AB. Effects of feminizing hormones on sperm production and malignant changes: microscopic examination of post orchiectomy specimens in transwomen. Urology 2018;121:93–6.

19. Owen-Smith AA, Gerth J, Sineath RC, et al. Association between gender confirmation treatments and perceived gender congruence, body image satisfaction, and mental health in a cohort of transgender individuals. J Sex Med 2018;15(4):591–600.

20. van de Grift TC, Elaut E, Cerwenka SC, et al. Effects of medical interventions on gender dysphoria and body image: a follow-up study. Psychosom Med 2017;79(7):815–23.

21. Papadopulos NA, Lelle JD, Zavlin D, et al. Quality of life and patient satisfaction following male-to-female sex reassignment surgery. J Sex Med 2017;14(5): 721–30.

22. Karim RB, Hage JJ, Mulder JW. Neovaginoplasty in male transsexuals: review of surgical techniques and recommendations regarding eligibility. Ann Plast Surg 1996;37(6):669–75.

23. van der Sluis WB, Bouman MB, Buncamper ME, et al. Clinical characteristics and management of neovaginal fistulas after vaginoplasty in transgender women. Obstet Gynecol 2016;127(6):1118–26.

24. Buncamper ME, van der Sluis WB, van der Pas RS, et al. Surgical outcome after penile inversion vaginoplasty: a retrospective study of 475 transgender women. Plast Reconstr Surg 2016;138(5):999–1007.

25. Aust JB, Henderson W, Khuri S, et al. The impact of operative complexity on patient risk factors. Ann Surg 2005;241(6):8.

26. Schneider F, Kliesch S, Schlatt S, et al. Andrology of male-to-female transsexuals: influence of cross-sex hormone therapy on testicular function. Andrology 2017;5(5):873–80.

27. Bapat S, Mahajan PM, Bhave AA, et al. Prospective randomised controlled trial comparing sub-epididymal orchiectomy versus conventional orchiectomy in metastatic carcinoma of prostate. Indian J Surg 2011;73(3):175–7.

28. Schneider F, Neuhaus N, Wistuba J, et al. Testicular functions and clinical characterization of patients with gender dysphoria (GD) undergoing sex reassignment surgery (SRS). J Sex Med 2015;12(11): 2190–200.

29. Dy GW, Brisbane WG, Walsh TJ. Surgical technique: simple orchiectomy for transgender patients 2017.

30. Andervont HB, Dunn TB, Canter HY. Susceptibility of agent-free inbred mice and their F 1 hybrids to estrogen-induced mammary tumors. J Natl Cancer Inst 1958;21(4):783–811.

31. Wolf-Gould CS, Wolf-Gould CH. A transgender woman with testicular cancer: a new twist on an old problem. LGBT Health 2016;3(1):90–5.

32. Kobori Y, Suzuki K, Iwahata T, et al. Mature testicular teratoma with positive estrogen receptor beta expression in a transgendered individual on cross-sex hormonal therapy: a case report. LGBT Health 2015;2(1):81–3.

33. Simbar M, Nazarpour S, Mirzababaie M, et al. Quality of life and body image of individuals with gender dysphoria. J Sex Marital Ther 2018;44(6):523–32.

34. Ozata Yildizhan B, Yuksel S, Avayu M, et al. Effects of gender reassignment on quality of life and mental health in people with gender dysphoria. Turk Psikiyatri Derg 2018;29(1):11–21.

35. Wiepjes CM, Nota NM, de Blok CJM, et al. The amsterdam cohort of gender dysphoria study (1972-2015): trends in prevalence, treatment, and regrets. J Sex Med 2018;15(4):582–90.

36. Lawrence AA. Factors associated with satisfaction or regret following male-to-female sex reassignment surgery. Arch Sex Behav 2003;32(4):299–315.

37. Landen M, Walinder J, Hambert G, et al. Factors predictive of regret in sex reassignment. Acta Psychiatr Scand 1998;97(4):284–9.

38. Djordjevic ML, Bizic MR, Duisin D, et al. Reversal surgery in regretful male-to-female transsexuals after sex reassignment surgery. J Sex Med 2016; 13(6):1000–7.

39. Wierckx K, Elaut E, Declercq E, et al. Prevalence of cardiovascular disease and cancer during cross-sex hormone therapy in a large cohort of trans persons: a case-control study. Eur J Endocrinol 2013; 169(4):471–8.

Penile Inversion Vaginoplasty Technique

Poone Shoureshi, MD[a], Daniel Dugi III, MD[b],*

KEYWORDS

- Gender-affirming surgery • Penile inversion • Vaginoplasty • Neoclitoris • Skin graft

KEY POINTS

- Patient preparation surgery includes mental health, social, and medical evaluations. Patients must be nicotine-free and be counseled for appropriate expectations of surgical results.
- Genital skin is used as flaps or grafts in constructing the vulva and neovaginal canal. A small amount of scrotal skin is used to construct the labia major; the rest may be used as a skin graft for neovaginal construction.
- The neoclitoris is constructed from the glans penis on the dorsal neurovascular pedicle. The lower nerve density of the glans penis versus the glans clitoris means that the neoclitoris will be larger than a native clitoris.
- The urethra is extensively reconstructed for appropriate location of the neomeatus and resection of redundant spongiosum.

INTRODUCTION

Gender-affirming vaginoplasty is a surgery to create the female vulva and vaginal canal for those people assigned male sex at birth with gender dysphoria. Creation of the vulva, or external female genitalia, includes removing the testicles and portions of the penis and creation of a neoclitoris, labia minora, labia majora, perineal urethral position, and a neovaginal canal. Although vulvar and vaginal canal construction may be considered separately, this articles discusses the construction of both the vulva and vaginal canal from genital skin, or penile inversion vaginoplasty. With this technique, the penile skin is separated from the deep structures of the penis, and the penile skin flap is inverted into a cavity created between the prostate and rectum. The technique was first described by Gillies and Millard in 1957,[1] but it was the Moroccan gynecologist Dr Georges Burou who independently developed the technique and popularized it through his high surgical volume.[2]

Many surgeons have made improvements and modifications over the years; this article describes the authors' technique with their own modifications, built on the wisdom and experience of many others.

PATIENT SELECTION AND ELIGIBILITY

Patients seeking gender-affirming vaginoplasty must have well-documented gender dysphoria and be mentally, physically, and socially ready for surgery. The authors follow guidelines put forth by the World Professional Association for Transgender Health (WPATH). The WPATH *Standards of Care*[3] outlines requirements that must be met prior to performing surgical treatment of gender dysphoria, written with the intention of maintaining flexibility in application. The authors currently use *Standards of Care*, version 7 (https://www.wpath.org/publications/soc).[3] These selection criteria are discussed further in Ian T. Nolan and colleagues' article, "Considerations in

No disclosures.
[a] Department of Urology, Oregon Health & Science University, 3303 Southwest Bond Avenue, CH-10-U, Portland, OR 97210, USA; [b] Department of Urology, Transgender Health Program, Oregon Health & Science University, 3303 Southwest Bond Avenue, CH-10-U, Portland, OR 97210, USA
* Corresponding author.
E-mail address: dugi@ohsu.edu

Urol Clin N Am 46 (2019) 511–525
https://doi.org/10.1016/j.ucl.2019.07.006
0094-0143/19/© 2019 Elsevier Inc. All rights reserved.

Gender Affirming Surgery: Demographic Trends," in this issue.

Medical Fitness

The usual concerns of medical fitness for any major surgery apply. Vaginoplasty, however, is a major reconstructive surgery, with tissue transfers that require optimal healing potential and blood supply, more so than for a solely extirpative procedure. Due to the increased risk of tissue necrosis and graft failure in active nicotine users,[4] the authors require all patients to cease all nicotine use at least 6 weeks before and after surgery, and preoperative laboratory test are used to check for nicotine and metabolites. Additionally, chronic anticoagulation may increase the risk of bleeding postoperatively, which can increase the risk of skin graft failure if a hematoma forms beneath a graft.

Surgical site infections and poor healing generally are associated with poor diabetic control.[5,6] The authors use a hemoglobin A_{1C} level of 6.5 as an upper limit and strictly adhere to this, because the worst wound complications observed have been in diabetics. As with any selection criteria, some patients may never be able to reach a target goal that makes them eligible for surgery.[7] The relative risk of surgical complications must be balanced with the risk of not providing important, sometimes life-saving, surgical therapy.

Obese patients are at increased risk of perioperative surgical morbidity from anesthesia, potential positioning injury, and postoperative surgical complications, such as wound infection and breakdown.[8] One recent study found higher complication rates with body mass index (BMI) over 35.[9] Anecdotally, many surgeons around the world have described BMI limits of 28 to 35. Not surprisingly, vaginoplasty is technically harder in obese patients, especially the dissection of the neovaginal canal. The authors do not use a formal BMI cutoff because individual body fat distribution is highly variable, and even some patients with very high BMI may have favorable body fat distribution for perineal surgery. The authors recommend that patients target a BMI of 35 or less and that some patients above this may not be ready for surgery. The authors try to say "yes" whenever possible, recognizing the difficulty patients have in achieving and maintaining weight loss[10] to access surgery.

A patient's prior medical history may affect if a neovaginal canal may safely be dissected. Patients who have a history of radical prostatectomy or pelvic radiation[11] are at increased risk of injury to the rectum with subsequent rectoneovaginal fistula formation due to scarring in the rectoprostatic space. Additionally, they may be at increased of urinary incontinence[12] from further disruption of the urinary continence mechanisms from the dissection. After vaginoplasty, when the proximal corpus spongiosum is no longer available to place an artificial urinary sphincter, the best surgical options for stress urinary incontinence are no longer possible. For these reasons, the authors do not offer vaginal canal construction post-prostatectomy or after radiation therapy for prostate or rectal cancer but instead offer gender-affirming vulvoplasty,[13] surgery without the construction of the neovaginal canal.

Additionally, patients must be willing and able to perform regular dilation of the neovagina after surgery, most intensely in the first year after surgery (discussed later). Patients must have access to a private area for self-dilation, the physical dexterity to perform dilation, and the dedication to this time-consuming and tedious maintenance regimen. The authors do not consider patients who are unable or unwilling to perform self-dilation eligible for vaginal canal construction, although they may be eligible for vulvoplasty.

PATIENT READINESS AND PREPARATION
Patient Expectations

Setting appropriate patient expectations for surgical outcomes is important for any operation, and this is especially true in gender-affirming surgery. High expectations of a natural appearance, coupled with the general population's low knowledge level of female vulvar anatomy,[14] can contribute to unmet expectations after surgery. In an attempt to help educate patients about the wide range of normal vulvar anatomy, at patient consultations and preoperative visits, the authors give patients 2 books to peruse while they wait: The Great Wall of Vagina by Jamie McCartney[15] and Womanhood: The Bare Reality by Laura Dodsworth.[16] Both have pictures demonstrating vulvas from people with a wide range of ages and body types, including transwomen, to illustrate that every person's vulva is unique.

Mental Health and Social Support

Vaginoplasty is a major surgery with significant recovery time, and patients must be medically, socially, and emotionally prepared for success. Patients sometimes express frustration at perceived gate-keeping in requiring mental health evaluation prior to surgery, something that most cis-gender patients undergoing surgery are not required to undergo. The authors emphasize the psychological stress of surgery and that this resource is something they wish cis-gender patients had for major surgery as well. Patients should have previously established access to mental health support in case it is needed postoperatively.

Patients must also have the housing stability and sufficient social support in their activities of daily living for recovery from a major surgery. Recovery requires typically 6 weeks to 8 weeks off from work, and this can be a significant financial stressor. The authors recommend patients have a support person to help reduce the need for extensive walking activities, such as grocery shopping, refilling prescriptions, etc.

Hair Removal

Scrotal and perineal skin is hair bearing, and full-thickness grafts or flaps that transfer this skin into the neovaginal canal transfer that skin's hair growth potential as well. Hair growth within in the neovagina can be bothersome for patients and is a common complaint.[17] Prior studies have shown that patients are dissatisfied when vaginal hair is present postoperatively.[18] Efforts to remove hair from the skin that lines the neovaginal space is thus needed. These may include electrolysis or laser hair removal,[19] both of which may take several months.

Pelvic Floor Physical Therapy

Creation of the neovaginal canal requires dissection of a path through the pelvic floor muscles and into the pelvis. Patients then have to interact with their altered pelvic floor anatomy to perform neovaginal dilation postoperatively. This is something many patients express anxiety about, and most people have little awareness of the pelvic floor or its function.[20] The authors have found an approximately 40% rate of preexisting pelvic floor dysfunction, which can be improved significantly with pelvic floor physical therapy before surgery.[21] The authors strongly believe that pelvic floor education is important for helping patients prepare for and accomplish neovaginal dilation after surgery, and at their institution all patients planned for vaginoplasty are referred to pelvic floor physical therapy both before and after vaginoplasty.

SURGICAL TECHNIQUE
Overview

The phrase "penile inversion vaginoplasty" generally refers to the technique where at least part of the vaginal canal is made by advancing penile skin into the neovaginal space. The authors' technique uses excess scrotal and perineal skin as a graft to help line the neovaginal space. Management of genital skin use is a critical part of this surgery. Although vaginoplasty in total may seem complicated and foreign, it is really a collection of smaller procedures familiar to urologists: simple orchiectomy, penile disassembly, perineal exposure of the prostate, and perineal urethrostomy. Combining these with vaginal canal construction, clitoroplasty, and a natural-appearing aesthetic closure is the challenge of vaginoplasty.

Recommendations for operative preparation are found in **Box 1**. Surgical steps are found in **Box 2**.

Planning Skin Management: Early Versus Late Skin Excision

One of the first decisions involves skin incision pattern. Using excess scrotal and perineal skin as graft for the neovaginal lining, surgeons must decide what and how much skin is not needed for vulvar construction. In a majority of cases, the authors utilize **early skin excision**, with excision of skin to be used as a graft as the first step. This skin must be defatted and sewn into shape, which takes significant time. The benefit of early excision of this skin is that more time is available to prepare it for use as a skin graft (Dr Toby Meltzer, Scottsdale, Arizona; personal communication 2015). The downside is that surgeons must be confident in how much skin they are excising from the beginning, which takes experience.

An alternative technique begins with a midline incision from the tip of the perineal skin flap, across the scrotum, and up onto the penile shaft.[22] In this technique of **late skin excision**, the neovaginal space, the clitoris, and urethra are dissected and constructed prior to deciding how much of the scrotal and perineal skin to excision. The skin flaps

---

Box 1
Operative preparation

- Stop estrogen 2 weeks before surgery; may continue spironolactone/progesterone
- Magnesium citrate bowel preparation
- Intravenous cefazolin preincision
- Low-molecular-weight heparin and sequential compression devices preincision for thromboembolic prevention
- Low lithotomy position with attention to sacral padding and peroneal nerve protection
- Anus prepped into field to allow rectal examination

Box 2
Surgical steps of vaginoplasty at Oregon Health & Science University

- Skin incision and early excision of scrotal-perineal skin for graft preparation
- Bilateral simple orchiectomy
- Exposure of corpus spongiosum
- Dissection of neovaginal canal
- Distal skin incision and degloving of penis
- Incision of penile corpora and excision of spongiosum of penis
- Construction and fixation of clitoris
- Resection and reconstruction of urethra
- Preplacement of skin tube–anchoring sutures and incision for inset of clitorourethral complex
- Attachment of skin graft to penile skin flap and insertion of composite skin tube into neovaginal canal
- Final wound closure

are pulled into place and 2 large dog-ears of excess skin are excised and processed for use. The benefit of this approach is that it allows precise assessment of how much skin can be excised with acceptable wound tension. The downside is that the surgical team has to prepare this skin for use as a graft later in the operation, and there is more sewing with the 2 pieces of skin versus the single piece excised with early excision.

The authors routinely prefer the early excision technique, although in cases of very little genital skin, the authors occasionally use late skin excision for greatest flexibility. In some extreme cases, the authors have excised no genital skin at all, with all the vaginal canal made from extragenital skin graft.

Skin Incision Planning

The authors begin by palpating the perineal body and marking this level (**Fig. 1**). A small inverted U–shaped perineal skin flap based at the level of the perineal body is used to insert into the spatulated skin tube that later lines the vaginal canal (**Fig. 2**). For early skin excision, lateral incisions are marked just medial to the groin crease to help hide the incision along this natural skin fold as well as make sure that the penoscrotal skin flap has a very wide base to better preserve its vascular and lymphatic supply. The superior mark in the midline is at a level where the skin can be pulled down with acceptable tension to the perineal body mark, usually approximately 2 cm below the base of the penis. The skin inside these marks is excised for use as a graft. The midline ventral surface of the penile shaft skin is later incised as it is inserted into the neovaginal canal to reduce tension and avoid a kangaroo pouch effect.

For late skin incision, the authors make a midline incision from the tip of the perineal flap superiorly across the scrotum and onto the midshaft of the penis. Excess skin for graft use is excised after formation of the clitorourethral complex (discussed later).

VAGINAL CONSTRUCTION
Vaginal Canal Dissection

To create the neovaginal space, a plane must be developed between the lower urinary tract and rectum. The vaginal canal creation follows Hugh Hamptom Young's approach to perineal prostatectomy.[23] Dissection proceeds cautiously with bipolar scissors through the perineal body and onto the body of the prostate. A Lowsley prostatic retractor is helpful to identify the course of the urethra and the location of the body of the prostate (**Fig. 3**). Keep in mind, however, that the anorectal

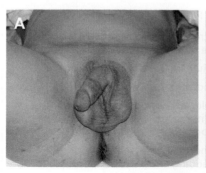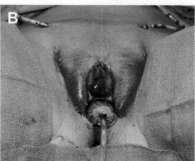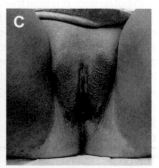

Fig. 1. Example patient before and after gender-affirming vaginoplasty. (*A*) Patient prior to surgery. The level of the perineal body is marked first. (*B*) Vulvar appearance at conclusion of surgery. (*C*) Vulvar appearance 6 months after surgery.

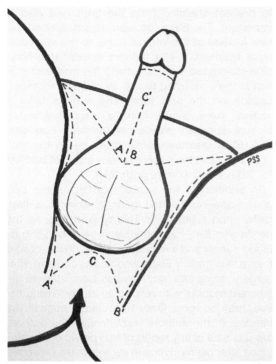

Fig. 2. Pattern of skin incisions. Hashed lines indicate areas of incisions. The scrotal and perineal skin within these lines will be excised and used as a graft. Tips of flaps (A, B, C) will insert into the corresponding positions (A′, B′, C′) during final closure.

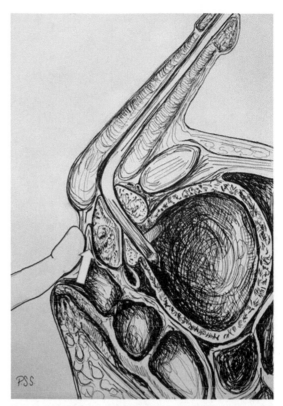

Fig. 3. Sagittal view of vaginal canal dissection with Lowsley retractor in place. Arrow indicates anorectal junction pulled up over prostate by Lowsley retraction.

junction is closely associated with the apex of the prostate and is at risk of injury, especially when the Lowsley retractor pulls this and the prostate more up into the wound.[24] Frequent palpation of the Lowsley retractor to identify the prostate and the area of the urinary sphincter as well as digital rectal examinations is helpful to guide safe dissection.

The authors partially divide the levator muscles (puborectalis and puboanalis) to widen the vaginal canal. Once the plane between the ventral rectal fascia (sometimes referred to as posterior Denonvilliers fascia) and prostate is developed, the authors use a custom skin graft mold/dilator (**Fig. 4**) to bluntly dissect up to the peritoneal reflection. The depth of the neovaginal space is measured from the apex to the entrance, below the base of the corpus spongiosum. This measurement is used to plan how much skin is needed to construct the skin tube used to make the neovagina later in the operation.

Lining the Neovaginal Space

The traditional description of penile inversion vaginoplasty uses the penile skin alone as a flap to line the vaginal canal. The penile skin flap has several advantages: it is sensate, thin, largely hairless,

well-vascularized, and elastic. The greatest limitation is its limited availability due to the range of penile lengths and/or prior circumcision. A full-thickness skin graft can make up the difference between what the penile skin can provide and what is needed. No difference has been found in vaginal depth or patient satisfaction after healing when using only penile skin versus including a graft in addition.[25] In contrast to this study from Amsterdam where a graft was only used in 32% of cases, the authors have used a graft nearly all cases to date. In the authors' center, more than 80% of patients are circumcised, which significantly reduces the amount of penile skin available. Obesity also increases the distance from the skin surface to the neovaginal space, increasing how much skin is needed.

Because the penile skin is based significantly cephalad from the neovaginal opening, some surgeons mobilize the penile skin flap attached to the prepubic and lower abdominal skin from its attachment to the lower body wall to advance it inferiorly into the vaginal canal.[26,27] In the authors' hands, this is variably effective, and the skin tends to retract back toward its original position over the course of healing, changing the aesthetic result

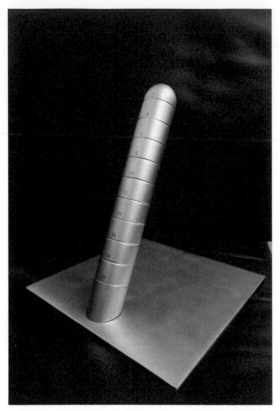

Fig. 4. Oregon Health & Science University vaginoplasty mold. The post is detachable from the base, 3.5 cm in diameter/11 cm in circumference, and marked every 2 cm. The post is used for blunt dissection of the vaginal canal and later reattached to the base for sewing the skin graft into the correct shape.

and potentially putting more tension on the skin flap. The authors no longer use this technique, instead trying to minimize tension on the penile skin flap. This means, however, that less penile skin flap reaches into the neovaginal canal, and more of the vaginal canal must come from skin graft.

Once the clitoral and urethral position have been finalized (discussed later), the authors measure how much penile skin reaches into the neovaginal canal and then subtract this from the depth of the vaginal canal to determine how much graft is needed. Occasionally, there is not enough genital skin to fully cover the canal as either graft or flap. In those cases, an additional full-thickness skin graft[28] is harvested from the area near the iliac crest, bilaterally if necessary. This skin usually is hairless, and the resulting scar is easily hidden beneath underwear or a swimsuit.

Skin grafts require meticulous preparation of the graft and graft bed,[29] with particular attention to hemostasis to avoid hematoma formation, which can cause graft failure. Immobilization of the graft

to prevent shearing from the graft bed also is important. The Belgrade team has described suture fixation of the vaginal canal to the sacrospinous ligament.[30] The authors instead use fibrin glue (discussed later) to adhere the graft and skin flap to the underlying tissue, as well as minimizing tension on the skin tube. The authors tailor a vaginal pack made from a vacuum-assisted closure sponge[31] inside polyurethane condoms (**Fig. 5**) to maintain gentle pressure on the skin graft and have the patient remain on strict bedrest for 5 days to maximize graft take.

In addition to the penile skin flap, some surgeons use scrotal and perineal skin as a flap, rather than a graft.[27,32] This type of flap, as the penile skin flap, has the advantage of bringing its blood supply and innervation, although it is bulkier than a skin graft.[33] Flaps also do not contract after surgery as grafts do. Genital skin, due to its inherent mobility with respect to its underlying tissue, may be more likely to prolapse outside the introitus in the authors' experience. The authors are unaware of any report of true pelvic organ prolapse after penile inversion vaginoplasty, however.

Recently, Jacoby and colleagues[34] have described their technique of a robotic approach to vaginal canal dissection and construction with the use of a peritoneal flap as the apex of the vaginal canal. This innovative approach has great potential both for primary and revision vaginoplasty. The use of a peritoneal flap may potentially decrease the need for skin grafts in creation of the vaginal canal.

Although not the focus of this article, the use of intestinal flaps for neovaginal canal construction also can be considered, commonly sigmoid colon or ileum.[35,36] It is worth keeping in mind that vulvar and vaginal canal construction can be considered separately, and the techniques (described later) for vulvar construction may be applicable

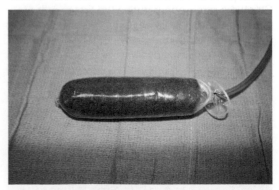

Fig. 5. Vaginal pack made from medium sized vacuum-assisted closure sponge and polyurethane condoms.

regardless of the tissue used for vaginal canal construction.

VULVAR CONSTRUCTION

Construction of the vulva involves removing the testicles and unneeded penile and urethral tissue, constructing the clitoris and urethral meatus, and wound closure. After excising the scrotal skin to be used for the skin graft, the testicles are mobilized to the external ring and suture ligate them en bloc. The corpus spongiosum is exposed to the base of the bulb and dissection of the vaginal canal begun. Once that is completed, the bulbospongiosus muscle is excised because it can cause an animation defect—bothersome perineal skin movement when patients contract their pelvic floor muscles—even without its previous attachment to the corpus spongiosum.

Penile Skin Use and Dissection

A priority of the authors' approach is to have the penile skin flap reach beneath the new urethral meatus to help form the introitus. In the authors' experience, there is a higher risk of introital stenosis when the penile skin flap does not reach the introitus and skin graft used for the vaginal canal forms the introitus. The irregular contour and fatty tissue of the perineum in this area are not always a good skin graft bed, which can lead to poor graft take and greater wound contraction. Whenever possible, the authors avoid skin graft extending outside the vaginal canal. This is not always possible, but this priority guides the choice of clitoroplasty technique, which in turn affects where the distal penile incision is made (discussed later).

A circumcising incision allows degloving of the penis. The distal incision location depends on clitoroplasty technique—one method of creating the clitoral hood and labia minora uses inner preputial skin or the skin distal to a prior circumcision's scar (discussed later). Otherwise, the incision is just proximal to the corona in circumcised patients. In uncircumcised patients, the incision is made at the reflection of inner and outer preputial skin. The authors do not believe the inner preputial skin can be used safely as part of the penile skin flap.

Preparation of Dorsal Neurovascular Bundle

One major goal of vaginoplasty to remove the erectile capabilities of the penis and construct a sensate clitoris from the glans penis based on a pedicle of the dorsal neurovascular bundle. The neurovascular bundle may be dissected from the underlying tunica albuginea, allowing the corpora to be excised. This approach is similar to elevation of the neurovascular bundle for Peyronie plaque incision and grafting,[37] although it must be done the full length of the penis.

The authors have found this approach slow, with risk of injury to the neurovascular bundle, and instead use a different approach. The neurovascular bundle is left intact on the tunica albuginea and after corporotomies, the inside spongiosum is removed.[38] An incision is made into the corporal space just lateral to the corpus spongiosum bilaterally from beneath the glans to the level of the corporal bifurcation. The dorsal nerves branch and course more ventrally than may be expected,[39] and the authors make the corporotomy just lateral to the urethra to maximally preserve that innervation. The spongiosum inside then is completely excised, along with the unneeded penile corpus spongiosum. The authors have been surprised to find the spongiosum often sweeps away from the underlying tunica easily (**Fig. 6**). Small perforating vessels are coagulated with bipolar diathermy. The bilateral unopened crura proximally are dilated, the proximal corporal arteries coagulated with bipolar diathermy, and the spaces are packed at this level with absorbable hemostatic agent. The space is closed with a modified purse-string suture closing both crura. Avoid any suture through the dorsal surface to prevent neurovascular injury.

In addition to a faster, less traumatic handling of the neurovascular bundle, the additional bulk of the folded tunica albuginea with this technique has an aesthetic benefit because it provides more volume in the area of the mons pubis,[38]

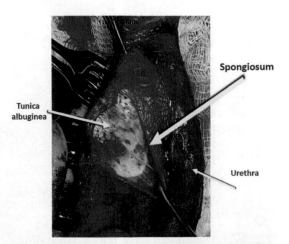

Fig. 6. Dissection of spongiosum from inside surface of tunica albuginea. Large arrow indicates spongiosum dissected off the inside surface of the tunica albuginea. Small arrow indicates the urethra within the corpus spongiosum.

which can otherwise have a hollow appearance after removal of the penile structures. More attention must be paid to hemostasis, however, because leaving the dorsal neurovascular bundle on the tunica means the corporal space cannot be completely closed.

Construction of the Neoclitoris, Clitoral Hood, and Labia Minora

Techniques of constructing a neoclitoris have evolved greatly. Despite the central importance of the clitoris to female genital anatomy and sexual function, some prominent surgeons in decades past did not form a neoclitoris.[40] Although a technique, similar to what the authors use currently, was described in 1976,[41] a variety of techniques, including deliberately transecting the dorsal nerve and creating the clitoris from a graft, were used in the past.[42] Creation of a neoclitoris on a dorsal neurovascular bundle pedicle was debated and only came into wider use in the 1990s.[43]

Many surgeons use a small portion of the dorsal glans to make the clitoris.[33] Recognizing that the nerve density of the glans penis may be only one-third or less than that of the glans clitoris,[44] the authors believe that more tissue is needed to keep adequate erogenous potential. They use the majority of the corona and excise the central portion of the glans, with the rationale that keeping the corona where nerves insert from the dorsal bundle is likely to permit the greatest erogenous sensation.

How surgeons fashion the clitoris may be influenced by how they plan to create a clitoral hood and labia minora. When a patient is uncircumcised or has adequate penile skin to reach beneath the new urethral meatus to the neovaginal introitus, the authors use inner preputial shaft skin left attached to the glans to make a clitoral hood and inner labia.[41,45] This inner preputial shaft skin can survive with perfusion from the dorsal neurovascular bundle.[46] This skin is the anatomic analog to the clitoral hood and in the authors' opinion the best tissue for clitoral hood formation.

When using inner preputial skin to construct a clitoral hood, the authors use most of the corona in forming the neoclitoris (**Fig. 7**). A small portion, 2-cm to 3-cm in length, is used to create the visible clitoris; folded together with the midline at the apex, this portion is 1 cm to 1.5 cm long. The rest of the corona is directed inferolaterally and anchored to the proximal crura just lateral to the urethra. With this tissue, the authors aim to recreate the clitoral frenulum, keeping more of this sensitive tissue in an attempt to mimic natural anatomic features. The attached preputial skin is later advanced downward on each side and secured to the urethral flap edges (discussed later).

When there is not adequate penile skin to use this technique, the authors use an extended urethral flap to construct the clitoral hood and inner labia[9] (**Fig. 8**). This allows the surgeon to use all the penile skin to try to reach the vaginal canal. In this case, the authors use the corona to make

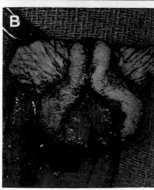
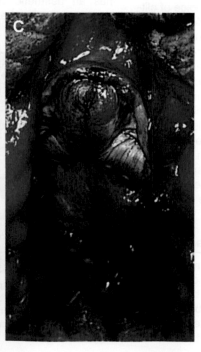
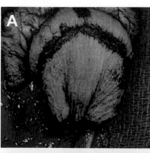

Fig. 7. Construction of neoclitoris from glans penis corona and cuff of preputial skin. (*A*) Area of glans inside marking is discarded. (*B*) Reshaping corona to make area of visible neoclitoris and clitoral frenulum with attached preputial skin for clitoral hood and inner labia. (*C*) Final appearance after anchoring of neoclitoris and urethroplasty.

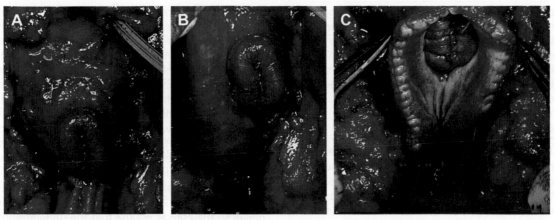

Fig. 8. Construction of neoclitoris with urethral flap as clitoral hood and inner labia. (*A*) Neoclitoris fixed in place after formation from corona of glans penis. (*B*) Bulbar urethral positioned next to the neoclitoris prior to dorsal urethrotomy for neoclitoral inset. (*C*) Final clitorourethral complex after neoclitoral inset, ventral urethrotomy, and urethroplasty.

a narrow, oval-shaped neoclitoris that is brought through the dorsal surface of an extended urethral flap. This technique can be reproduced consistently with little regard to penile skin length and provides a good aesthetic result, in the authors' opinion.

Positioning of the Neoclitoris

The correct anatomic position for the glans clitoris is atop the joining of the corporal crura, and a clitoral throne (Dr Stan Monstrey, Ghent, Belgium; personal communication 2015) is described as an anchoring point for the neoclitoris.[45,47] This may aesthetically be too inferior a position in some patients, however, due to the sexual dimorphism of the pelvis.[48] The pubic symphysis of the android pelvis is thicker than the gynecoid pelvis, and the distance from the joining of the crura to the top of the symphysis is greater than in the gynecoid pelvis. Therefore, in the gynecoid pelvis, the clitoris may be visibly closer to the top of the symphysis than if the neoclitoris is placed at the joining of the corpora cavernosa in the android pelvis. The authors usually anchor the clitoris slightly higher, with the adductor longus tendon as another anatomic landmark for placement of the top of the glans clitoris.

Once the clitoris has been constructed, the authors fold the previously opened tunica albuginea with intact neurovascular bundle and anchor the tunica beneath the neoclitoris to the edge of the proximal tunica bilaterally, just above where the corporal bodies join (**Fig. 9**). The authors include a piece of absorbable hemostatic material (Surgicel Fibrillar, Ethicon, Somerville, New Jersey) both to help with hemostatis and to soften the curvature at the apex of the folded neurovascular

bundle, with the intention that this is less traumatic to the nerves and blood vessels. Be aware that if a patient has computed tomographic/magnetic resonance imaging in the postoperative time

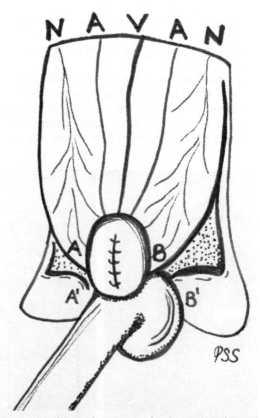

Fig. 9. Neoclitoris showing anchoring points (A to A′ and B to B′) to tunica albuginea of crura, superior to corpus spongiosum. N-A-V-A-N indicate relative positions of dorsal nerves (N), dorsal penile arteries (A), and dorsal penile vein (V).

period that this area may appear to radiologists as an abscess. The authors also anchor the apices of the folded tunica to the tissue around the symphysis to keep it in position, taking care not to put the tunica on stretch with these anchoring sutures because patients may complain of a feeling of the penis being stretched or tucked.

Drain Placement

The authors place the drains at this time, 2 15F round, channel drains 1 on each side of the folded bundle exiting in the suprapubic area just within the pubic hair line. The distal tips are positioned at the inferior-most portion of the outer labia closure during final wound closure.

Urethroplasty

Little is published on urethral reconstruction in vaginoplasty. Many patients report bother by urinary issues after vaginoplasty,[12] including 33% with a misdirected urine stream.[18] Urethral stenosis is one of the most common complications, approximately 15%.[49] Three factors guide the authors' handling of the urethra: positioning of the neomeatus, resection of redundant spongiosum beneath the neomeatus, and how much of the corpus spongiosum and urethral distal to the meatus is retained.

The positioning of the urethral meatus is an important consideration. The authors have heard multiple patients who have undergone vaginoplasty complain of their urine stream being directed too far forward and hitting the toilet seat while voiding. This, in combination with the authors' experience with perineal urethrostomy in cis-gender men with urethral stricture disease, has led to making the urethral meatus as low as possible, in direct line with the exit from the urinary sphincter (**Fig. 10**A). The authors believe this allows as straight a path as possible for the urine to exit. Although this may mean that the distance between the urethral meatus and clitoris is greater than in the native vulva, this is one of the choices to be made and compromises necessary in gender-affirming vulvar construction in the android pelvis. Leaving the urethra tubularized for a longer segment to bring it out closer to the clitoris means that the urine stream may be directed more anteriorly and there may be more corpus spongiosum left between the meatus and the vaginal introitus (discussed in the following paragraph).

Next, excessive spongiosum is resected from the base of the bulb beneath the new meatus (**Fig. 10**B, C). This is necessary because the corpus spongiosum is an erectile organ and engorges with sexual arousal, narrowing the vaginal introitus.[18,50] Removing the wide base of the bulbospongiosum shortens the visual distance between the meatus and the vaginal canal and creates a more natural-appearing introitus, in the authors' opinion. The authors split the spongiosum beneath the urethra at the level of the sphincter to the base of the spongiosum and then suture the tunica of the spongiosum to the urethral mucosa to create the new meatus. Next, the authors resect the redundant spongiosum laterally and then sew

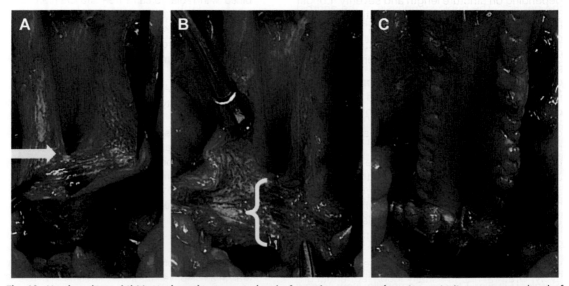

Fig. 10. Urethroplasty. (*A*) Ventral urethrotomy to level of membranous urethra. Arrow indicates area on level of membranous urethra. (*B*) Bracket indicates redundant spongiosum beneath level of future urethral meatus. (*C*) Urethral appearance after resection of redundant spongiosum and closure of urethra.

the cut edge of the tunica to the mucosal edge in running-locking fashion for hemostasis.

The authors use the urethral mucosa and corpus spongiosum to line the space between the neo-meatus and the neoclitoris[41,45] or as a longer flap to create the clitoral hood,[9] as discussed previously. In the first clitoroplasty method, the authors measure how much urethra and spongiosum is needed to fill the space beneath the clitoris and then excise the excess, close the edges, and attach the urethral flap to the base of the clitoris to form the clitorourethral complex. In the second clitorplasty method, the urethral flap envelops the clitoris to also form a clitoral hood and be the inner labia. The urethral flap provides a pink, mucosal surface to this area, which has a more natural appearance than when penile skin separates the urethral meatus and the neoclitoris.[51]

Composite Skin Tube Insertion and Wound Closure

Once the clitorourethral complex is formed, the authors prepare to place the neovaginal skin tube into position and pull the inverted penile skin tube downwards to measure how much can reach beneath the new urethral meatus, trying to minimize this downward tension. Two sutures are preplaced to anchor the skin tube to the tunica albuginea of the crura at the introitus using 2-0 long-lasting monofilament resorbable suture. In addition to reducing tension on the vaginal skin tube, these sutures help give definition between the inner vulva and the outer labia. A midline incision is made in the dorsal penile shaft skin to expose the clitorourethral complex. The authors then measure how much penile skin is present below the urethral meatus; this measurement is then subtracted from the depth of the neovaginal space to determine how much skin graft is necessary.

The skin graft, prepared on the surgical back table previously, is then trimmed to measure. The skin on top of the mold is inserted through the penile skin flap and sewn in place (**Fig. 11**) with interrupted absorbable sutures to avoid causing ischemia of the end of the skin tube with running sutures.

The neovaginal canal is then meticulously inspected for hemostasis. This is extremely important because anywhere that a blood clot forms between the graft and the surrounding tissue leads to graft failure in that location. Flaps also do not adhere to the surrounding tissue if a hematoma is present. The skin tube is sprayed with Artiss fibrin glue (Baxter International)—this product has lower thrombin concentration than typical

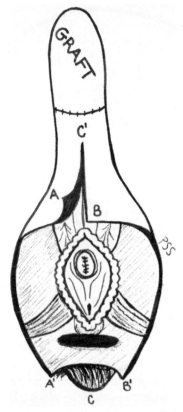

Fig. 11. Configuration of composite skin tube of penile skin and graft after construction of clitorourethral complex. (*A, B, C*) indicate tips of skin flaps that inset into their corresponding positions (*A', B', C'*).

fibrin sealant (ie, Tisseel, Baxter International), allowing greater time to position the skin prior to the fibrin clot forming.[52] The skin tube is inserted quickly into the canal (**Fig. 12**) and the vacuum previously applied to the vaginal pack is released. The preplaced sutures are tied down. The inferior surface of the skin tube is spatulated to the level of the perineal body to minimize tension on the tube, and the tip of the perineal skin flap is anchored to the perineal body and the apex of the spatulation of the skin tube. This anchoring provides another point of fixation of the skin tube and prevents the perineal flap and skin tube from retracting outward and partially covering the posterior introitus after healing. Wound closure begins with advancing the outer labia flap tips into their position. The rest of the wound closure proceeds after final positioning of the surgical drains.

Dressings and Hospital Stay

The authors place a Foley catheter and a tie-over dressing of nonadherent gauze with antibiotic ointment surrounding the vaginal pack, followed by a compressive dressing. Patients are kept

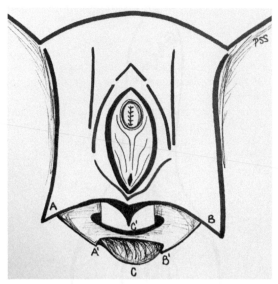

Fig. 12. Composite skin tube inverted and placed into neovaginal canal. (*A*, *B*, *C*) indicate tips of skin flaps that inset into their corresponding positions (*A'*, *B'*, *C'*).

on strict bedrest until postoperative day 5 with low-molecular-weight heparin and antibiotics while the vaginal pack is in place. The outer, compressive dressing is removed postoperative day 3. The remaining items all are removed postoperative day 5.

To remove the vaginal pack, its tubing is connected to wall suction to compress the dressing, the patient is coached on pelvic floor relaxation, and the pack gently withdrawn. Approximately 15% of patients experience urinary retention and need catheter replacement.[22] Most patients leave the hospital postoperative day 5.

POSTOPERATIVE CARE

The surgical team sees the patient at 2 weeks, 4 weeks, 6 weeks, 3 months, 6 months, and 1 year after surgery. Additional visits may be necessary to check on wound care or difficulty with neovaginal dilation.

Dilation of the Neovagina

The process of wound healing and secondary contraction of skin grafts can lead to stenosis of the neovaginal space in some patients. Many surgeons instruct patients to perform dilation of the neovaginal to prevent narrowing or stenosis; despite these efforts, vaginal stenosis has been reported in approximately 10%.[49]

Patients return to clinic for the first postoperative visit approximately 1 week after discharge. At this

time, patients are instructed how to perform dilation of the neovagina and provided with a set of dilators (Soul Source, www.soulsource.com; sizes P2, 1, 2, and 3). A smaller or larger dilator is available on request. Many surgeons begin dilation immediately after vaginal pack removal. Based on experience with external skin grafting and research showing secondary contraction of full-thickness skin grafts reaches a maximum after 1 month,[49] the authors instituted dilation approximately 2 weeks after surgery, believing this gives more time for postoperative pain and swelling to diminish and for further skin graft stabilization prior to dilation. Patients are instructed and then observed performing dilation on their own and asked to dilate for 30 minutes 3 times per day. They then have a follow-up appointment with pelvic floor physical therapy 1 week after they begin dilating and then again with the surgical team 1 week later.

As the neovagina passes through a new opening through the pelvic floor muscles, patients must learn to relax their pelvic floor in order to successfully perform dilation or have receptive vaginal intercourse. As discussed previously, the authors believe pelvic floor physical therapy is helpful and refer all patients before and after surgery.[21]

Although it would be convenient to provide a written schedule for how to progress to larger dilators, the authors have observed great variability in how patients progress. Patients are instructed to progress to the next larger dilator when their current dilator is no longer providing a stretch feeling.[21] Progression is characterized by overlaps in dilator size—patients may begin the session with a small dilator to help relax their pelvic floor and lubricate the neovagina before moving up to the larger dilator. If the larger dilator cannot be inserted to the maximal depth of the previously used dilator, patients are encouraged to continue to use the smaller dilator for a portion of the session to assure that the depth is maintained while still working on gaining width.

Many patients find it difficult to maintain dilation 3 times per day as they return to work, school, etc and frequently change to twice per day for several months. Once patients reach their goal size dilator and it no longer is difficult, they may begin to see if they can decrease the frequency of dilation. The authors encourage decreasing frequency of dilation gradually, with the ultimate goal of dilation only 1 time to 2 times per week or less to make sure depth and width are maintained. Anecdotally, patients have reported loss of vaginal width and depth if they stop dilating or having vaginal sexual activity, even many years after surgery.

Wound Healing

Minor wound separation is common,[53] especially in the area of the posterior introitus where wound tension tends to be highest. Most of these wounds respond to simple frequent dressing changes with dry fluffed cotton gauze and later silver nitrate treatment of granulation tissue. The authors instruct patients to expect tissue swelling to resolve gradually by 8 weeks to 12 weeks after surgery and do not offer aesthetic revisions until 6 months to 12 months after surgery because the appearance continues to mature and usually improves during this time.

COMPLICATIONS

Overall complication rates have been reported in meta-analysis as 32.5%,[49] although most are minor wound complications. Urethral stenosis was the most common complication requiring reoperation, at 15%. Serious complications, such as rectal injury and rectovaginal fistula, are fortunately uncommon but can be devastating for patients. Complications and management are discussed further in J.N. Schardein and colleagues's article, "Management of Vaginoplasty and Phalloplasty Complications," in this issue.

SEXUAL FUNCTION

The authors encourage patients to use a vibrator for self-stimulation of the clitoris, the area above the clitoris (where the neurovascular bundle is folded), or the vaginal canal as soon as they please once they begin dilation. The authors recommend they wait to manually stimulate the clitoris until enough time has passed to regain adequate tissue strength, 8 weeks to 12 weeks. The authors routinely recommend waiting 3 months after surgery to begin vaginal sexual activity and encourage patients to be mindful of how their dilation is progressing to predict how comfortable/safe vaginal sexual activity may be.

Patients do not have natural vaginal lubrication that is created by transudation of fluid into the vaginal lumen after pelvic vascular engorgement.[18] The authors counsel patients that they will need exogenous lubrication for sexual activity afterward. Many transwomen are bothered by this and think it is somehow unnatural; patients are further counseled that in the United States alone, the market for sexual lubrication is more than $500 million/year,[54] and that many people use extra lubrication. Anecdotally, some patients have reported self-lubrication; the authors presume that this may be fluid produced by the bulbourethral glands.

In the reported literature, there have been high rates of patient-reported orgasm, up to 85% in contemporary series.[55] Erogenous sensation comes from a combination of clitoral stimulation, the distal vaginal canal skin and introitus, and stimulation of the prostate.[55] Lawrence[56] provided a nuanced discussion of sexuality both before and after surgery. Although 82% of patients reported that orgasm was possible after surgery, only 48% were able to reach orgasm on at least half of their attempts. More than 50% reported that orgasms were substantially different from prior to their surgery. Hess and colleagues[57] reported a majority of patients felt their orgasms were more intense after vaginoplasty, and satisfaction with sexual activity was more associated with neoclitoral function than neovaginal depth. More research into sexuality and patient-reported outcome measures after gender-affirming surgery is needed, and there is much more to sexuality than genital anatomy alone.[58]

SUMMARY

Penile inversion vaginoplasty requires careful planning and use of genital skin to construct the vulva and neovaginal canal. The neoclitoris is constructed from the glans penis on a pedicle of the dorsal neurovascular bundle. Urethral reconstruction requires consideration of urethral positioning and how much urethral and spongiosal tissue to remove. Postoperatively, patients must spend significant time and effort in neovaginal dilation to prevent stenosis.

REFERENCES

1. Gillies H, Millard D. Genitalia. In: The principles and art of plastic surgery, vol. II. Boston: Little, Brown & Co; 1957. p. 368–88.
2. Hage JJ, Karim RB, Laub DR. On the origin of pedicled skin inversion vaginoplasty: life and work of Dr Georges Burou of Casablanca. Ann Plast Surg 2007;59(6):723.
3. Coleman E, Bockting W, Botzer M, et al. Standards of care for the health of transsexual, transgender, and gender-nonconforming people, version 7. Int J Transgend 2012;13(4):165–232.
4. Rinker B. The evils of nicotine: an evidence-based guide to smoking and plastic surgery. Ann Plast Surg 2013;70(5):599.
5. Rollins KE, Varadhan KK, Dhatariya K, et al. Systematic review of the impact of HbA1c on outcomes following surgery in patients with diabetes mellitus. Clin Nutr 2016;35(2):308–16.

6. Baltzis D, Eleftheriadou I, Veves A. Pathogenesis and treatment of impaired wound healing in diabetes mellitus: new insights. Adv Ther 2014;31(8):817–36.

7. Giori NJ, Ellerbe LS, Bowe T, et al. Many diabetic total joint arthroplasty candidates are unable to achieve a preoperative hemoglobin A1c Goal of 7% or less. J Bone Joint Surg Am 2014;96(6):500.

8. Wilson JA, Clark JJ. Obesity: impediment to postsurgical wound healing. Adv Skin Wound Care 2004; 17(8):426.

9. Massie JP, Morrison SD, Maasdam J, et al. Predictors of patient satisfaction and postoperative complications in penile inversion vaginoplasty. Plast Reconstr Surg 2018;141(6):911e.

10. Group T. Eight-year weight losses with an intensive lifestyle intervention: the look AHEAD study. Obesity 2014;22(1):5–13.

11. Gotto GT, Yunis L, Vora K, et al. Impact of prior prostate radiation on complications after radical prostatectomy. J Urol 2010;184(1):136–42.

12. Kuhn A, Hiltebrand R, Birkhäuser M. Do transsexuals have micturition disorders? Eur J Obstet Gynecol Reprod Biol 2007;131(2):226–30.

13. Jiang D, Witten J, Berli J, et al. Does depth matter? factors affecting choice of vulvoplasty over vaginoplasty as gender-affirming genital surgery for transgender women. J Sex Med 2018;15(6):902–6.

14. Sharp G, Tiggemann M. Educating women about normal female genital appearance variation. Body Image 2016;16:70–8.

15. McCartney, Jamie. The Great Wall of Vagina. Brighton, United Kingdon: Jamie McCartney, 2011.

16. Dodson, Laura. Womanhood. The Bare Reality. London: Pinter & Martin; 2019.

17. Suchak T, Hussey J, Takhar M, et al. Postoperative trans women in sexual health clinics: managing common problems after vaginoplasty. J Fam Plann Reprod Health Care 2015;41(4). https://doi.org/10.1136/jfprhc-2014-101091.

18. Lawrence AA. Patient-reported complications and functional outcomes of male-to-female sex reassignment surgery. Arch Sex Behav 2006;35(6):717–27.

19. Faurschou A, Haedersdal M. Laser and IPL technology in dermatology and aesthetic medicine. Berlin: Springer; 2010. p. 125–46. https://doi.org/10.1007/978-3-642-03438-1_9.

20. Berzuk K, Shay B. Effect of increasing awareness of pelvic floor muscle function on pelvic floor dysfunction: a randomized controlled trial. Int Urogynecol J 2015;26(6):837–44.

21. Jiang D, Gallagher S, Burchill L, et al. Implementation of a pelvic floor physical therapy program for transgender women undergoing gender-affirming vaginoplasty. Obstet Gynecol 2019;133:1003–11.

22. Buncamper ME, van der Sluis WB, van der Pas RS, et al. Surgical outcome after penile inversion vaginoplasty: a retrospective study of 475 transgender women. Plast Reconstr Surg 2016;138(5):999.

23. Young HH. Conservative perineal prostatectomy: presentation of new instruments and technic. J Am Med Assoc 1903;41:999–1009.

24. Melman A, Boczko J, Figueroa J, et al. Critical surgical techniques for radical perineal prostatectomy. J Urol 2004;171(2):786–90.

25. Buncamper ME, van der Sluis WB, de Vries M, et al. Penile inversion vaginoplasty with or without additional full-thickness skin graft: to graft or not to graft? Plast Reconstr Surg 2017;139(3):649e.

26. Wesser DR. A single stage operative technique for castration, vaginal construction and perineoplasty in transsexuals. Arch Sex Behav 1978;7(4):309–23.

27. Salim A, Poh M. Gender-affirming penile inversion vaginoplasty. Clin Plast Surg 2018;45(3):343–50.

28. Hage JJ, Karim RB. Abdominoplastic secondary full-thickness skin graft vaginoplasty for male-to-female transsexuals. Plast Reconstr Surg 1998; 101(6):1512–5.

29. Thakar HJ, Dugi DD. Practical plastic surgery: techniques for the reconstructive urologist. In: Brandes S, Morey A, editors. Advanced male urethral and genital reconstructive surgery. New York: Humana Press; 2013. p. 69–82.

30. Stanojevic DS, Djordjevic ML, Milosevic A, et al. Sacrospinous ligament fixation for neovaginal prolapse prevention in male-to-female surgery. Urology 2007;70(4):767–71.

31. Adamson CD, Naik BJ, Lynch DJ. The vacuum expandable condom mold: a simple vaginal stent for McIndoe-style vaginoplasty. Plast Reconstr Surg 2004;113(2):664.

32. Trombetta C. Management of gender dysphoria, a multidisciplinary approach. Milan: Springer; 2015. p. 93–104. https://doi.org/10.1007/978-88-470-5696-1_11.

33. Selvaggi G, Ceulemans P, Cuypere G, et al. Gender identity disorder: general overview and surgical treatment for vaginoplasty in male-to-female transsexuals. Plast Reconstr Surg 2005;116(6):135e.

34. Jacoby A, Maliha S, Granieri MA, et al. Robotic davydov peritoneal flap vaginoplasty for augmentation of vaginal depth in feminizing vaginoplasty. J Urol 2019. https://doi.org/10.1097/ju.0000000000000107.

35. Bizic M, Kojovic V, Duisin D, et al. An overview of neovaginal reconstruction options in male to female transsexuals. ScientificWorldJournal 2014;2014:1–8.

36. Bouman M, Zeijl M, Buncamper ME, et al. Intestinal vaginoplasty revisited: a review of surgical techniques, complications, and sexual function. J Sex Med 2014;11(7):1835–47.

37. Perovic SV, Djordjevic MLJ. The penile disassembly technique in the surgical treatment of Peyronie's disease. BJU Int 2001;88(7):731–8.

38. Soli M, Brunocilla E, Bertaccini A, et al. Original Research–Surgery: male to female gender reassignment: modified surgical technique for creating the neoclitoris and mons veneris. J Sex Med 2008;5(1):210–6.

39. Kozacioglu Z, Kiray A, Ergur I, et al. Anatomy of the dorsal nerve of the penis, clinical implications. Urology 2014;83(1):121–5.

40. Bouman F. Sex reassignment surgery in male to female transsexuals. Ann Plast Surg 1988;21(6):526–31.

41. Brown J. Creation of a functional clitoris and aesthetically pleasing introitus in sex conversion. Transactions of the Sixth International Congress of Plastic and Reconstructive Surgery. Paris, 1976. p. 654–5.

42. Hage JJ, Karim RB, Bloem JJ, et al. Sculpturing the neoclitoris in vaginoplasty for male-to-female transsexuals. Plast Reconstr Surg 1994;93(2):558.

43. Hage JJ, Karim RB. Sensate pedicled neoclitoroplasty for male transsexuals. Ann Plast Surg 1996;36(6):621–4.

44. Shih C, Cold CJ, Yang CC. Cutaneous corpuscular receptors of the human glans clitoris: descriptive characteristics and comparison with the glans penis. J Sex Med 2013;10(7):1783–9.

45. Opsomer D, Gast KM, Ramaut L, et al. Creation of clitoral hood and labia minora in penile inversion vaginoplasty in circumcised and uncircumcised transwomen. Plast Reconstr Surg 2018;142(5):729e.

46. Tuffaha SH, cks J, Shores JT, et al. Using the dorsal, cavernosal, and external pudendal arteries for penile transplantation: technical considerations and perfusion territories. Plast Reconstr Surg 2014;134(1):111e.

47. Schechter LS. Surgical management of the transgender patient. Philidelphia: Elsevier; 2016. p. 93–104. https://doi.org/10.1016/b978-0-323-48089-5.00005-3.

48. Fischer B, Mitteroecker P. Allometry and sexual dimorphism in the human pelvis. Anat Rec (Hoboken) 2017;300(4):698–705.

49. Dreher P, Edwards D, Hager S, et al. Complications of the neovagina in male-to-female transgender surgery: a systematic review and meta-analysis with discussion of management. Clin Anat 2018;31(2):191–9.

50. Karim R, Hage J, Bouman F, et al. The importance of near total resection of the corpus spongiosum and total resection of the corpora cavernosa in the surgery of male to female transsexuals. Ann Plast Surg 1991;26(6):554–7.

51. Wangjiraniran B, Selvaggi G, Chokrungvaranont P, et al. Male-to-female vaginoplasty: Preecha's surgical technique. J Plast Surg Hand Surg 2014;49(3):153–9.

52. Foster K, Greenhalgh D, Gamelli RL, et al. Efficacy and safety of a fibrin sealant for adherence of autologous skin grafts to burn wounds: results of a phase 3 clinical study. J Burn Care Res 2008;29(2):293.

53. Neto RR, Hintz F, Krege S, et al. Gender reassignment surgery - a 13 year review of surgical outcomes. Int Braz J Urol 2012;38(1):97–107.

54. Sexual lubricant market: global outlook and forecast 2017-2022. Arizton Advisory and Intelligence; 2017. Available at: www.arizton.com. Accessed March 10, 2019.

55. Selvaggi G, Monstrey S, Ceulemans P, et al. Genital sensitivity after sex reassignment surgery in transsexual patients. Ann Plast Surg 2007;58(4):427.

56. Lawrence AA. Sexuality before and after male-to-female sex reassignment surgery. Arch Sex Behav 2005;34(2):147–66.

57. Hess J, Henkel A, Bohr J, et al. Sexuality after male-to-female gender affirmation surgery. Biomed Res Int 2018;2018:1–7.

58. Basson R. Handbook of clinical neurology. Sect 2 Neural Substrate 2015;130:11–8.

Laparoscopic Intestinal Vaginoplasty in Transgender Women
An Update on Surgical Indications, Operative Technique, Perioperative Care, and Short- and Long-Term Postoperative Issues

Wouter B. van der Sluis, MD, PhD[a,b],*, Jurriaan B. Tuynman, MD, PhD[b,c],
Wilhelmus J.H.J. Meijerink, MD, PhD[b,c,d], Mark-Bram Bouman, MD, PhD[a,b]

KEYWORDS

- Vaginoplasty • Gender dysphoria • Transgender • Laparoscopy • Surgery
- Reconstructive surgical procedures • Sex reassignment procedures

KEY POINTS

- Intestinal vaginoplasty can be performed in transgender women in primary cases because of absence of sufficient penoscrotal skin, due to penoscrotal hypoplasia, circumcision, penile trauma with loss of penile skin quantity and/or quality, or when primary vaginoplasty has failed.
- It provides sufficient neovaginal depth without postoperative tissue shrinkage with self-lubricating qualities.
- Disadvantages of this procedure are the need for intraabdominal bowel surgery with intestinal anastomosis and concomitant risks. Long-term disadvantages are the risk on diversion neovaginitis, the risk on neovaginal inflammatory bowel disease, and the risk on neovaginal malignances.
- Major complications after intestinal vaginoplasty are rare but may occur.
- This type of surgery may be performed by an experienced surgical team with the right medical infrastructure and laparoscopic equipment.

INTRODUCTION

Surgical (re)construction of a vagina (vaginoplasty) is performed in biological women with congenital or postablative vaginal absence and in transgender women. In patients, who express the wish for vaginoplasty, vaginoplasty has a positive influence on sexual function, self-image, and general quality of life.[1–3] Different surgical techniques exist for this purpose. They can be divided according to the graft

Disclosure Statement: There are no commercial or financial conflicts of interest to report. No funding was received for the work.
[a] Department of Plastic, Reconstructive and Hand Surgery, Center of Expertise on Gender Dysphoria, Amsterdam University Medical Center, Location VUMC, Amsterdam, the Netherlands; [b] Center of Expertise on Gender Dysphoria, Amsterdam University Medical Center, Location VUMC, Amsterdam, the Netherlands; [c] Department of Surgery, Amsterdam University Medical Center, Location VUMC, Amsterdam, the Netherlands; [d] Department of Operation Rooms, Radboud University Medical Centre, Nijmegen, the Netherlands
* Corresponding author.
E-mail address: w.vandersluis@vumc.nl

Urol Clin N Am 46 (2019) 527–539
https://doi.org/10.1016/j.ucl.2019.07.007
0094-0143/19/© 2019 Elsevier Inc. All rights reserved.

used to line the (neo)vagina during the procedure. For transgender women, penile inversion vaginoplasty is the most commonly used procedure for vaginal construction.[4] Although different subtechniques for penile inversion vaginoplasty have been described, the common denominator is that the penile (and sometimes scrotal) skin is used to line the neovaginal cavity, which is created between bladder and rectum.[5–9]

In absence of sufficient penoscrotal skin, penile inversion vaginoplasty may not provide the postoperative neovaginal depth to enable neovaginal penetrative intercourse. In these patients, other surgical techniques are indicated. Techniques described for this purpose are full- or partial-thickness skin graft vaginoplasty, groin flap vaginoplasty, nongrafted vaginal depth augmentation, peritoneal vaginoplasty, and intestinal vaginoplasty.[10,11]

In intestinal vaginoplasty, an intestinal segment is isolated and transferred to the neovaginal cavity to form the neovaginal lining. Predominantly, sigmoid or ileal segments are used for this procedure.[11] A laparotomic, laparoscopy-assisted, total laparoscopic or robotic approach may be used for this procedure. An advantage of intestinal vaginoplasty is that it provides sufficient neovaginal depth without postoperative tissue shrinkage with self-lubricating qualities. Disadvantages of this procedure include the need for intraabdominal bowel surgery with intestinal anastomosis and concomitant risks. Long-term disadvantages are the risk on diversion neovaginitis, the risk on neovaginal inflammatory bowel disease, and the risk on neovaginal malignancies.

In this article, an update is provided on surgical (contra-)indications, operative technique, perioperative care, and short- and long-term postoperative issues.

INDICATIONS AND CONTRAINDICATIONS

For penile inversion vaginoplasty in transgender women, a sufficient amount of penoscrotal skin is needed. If not, the postoperative neovaginal depth is insufficient to enable neovaginal penetrative intercourse.

This is the case.

1. In penoscrotal hypoplasia because of biological variation and/or hormonal puberty inhibition,
2. In some patients with a history of circumcision,
3. In patients with a history of penile trauma with loss of penile skin quantity and/or quality, or
4. When vaginoplasty is performed as revision procedure when primary vaginoplasty has failed.

Different surgical strategies exist to overcome this problem. Penoscrotal vaginoplasty can be performed with additional neovaginal full- or partial-thickness skin grafting. Also, pedicled local flaps (lotus petal flaps, scrotal flaps) can be used to (additionally) line the neovaginal cavity. Peritoneal vaginoplasty is mentioned as surgical alternative.

Intestinal vaginoplasty is also an option in these patients. However, not all patients are candidates for this procedure. There are certain (relative) contraindications for performing this surgery: a history of extensive abdominal surgery, inflammatory bowel disease, colorectal carcinoma, or Lynch syndrome or the inability to safely undergo general anesthesia, smoking, and/or obesity (body mass index >30 kg/m^2).

PREOPERATIVE CARE

An experienced surgical team of a plastic and a colorectal surgeon, with the right medical infrastructure and laparoscopic equipment, is necessary to perform total laparoscopic intestinal vaginoplasty. In the Netherlands, this service has been centralized and has structured training pathway in place including theory, hands-on surgical cadaver training, and proctoring, to optimize outcomes. The authors advise adherence to and familiarity with the standards of care for the health of transgender and gender-nonconforming people.[12] In the preoperative phase, patients are counseled by a specialized psychologist with experience in the transgender care field to assess psychological eligibility. Sexual history, sexual expectations, and desires are explored. Intestinal vaginoplasty is indicated in patients who wish to engage in neovaginal penetrative sexual intercourse in the future. Preoperative evaluation of surgical eligibility is assessed by a gender surgeon and a gastrointestinal surgeon. Patients are informed about the possibility on postoperative complications, as mentioned later, and surgical alternatives. Informed consent is obtained. Preoperatively, all patients and surgical indications are discussed in a multidisciplinary patient consultation. Preoperative consultation of a pelvic floor physiotherapist is advised to facilitate an easier postoperative dilatation regime.[13] Coloscopy is performed preoperatively in all patients older than 40 years to check for unexpected findings.

SURGICAL TECHNIQUE

A laparotomic, laparoscopy-assisted, total laparoscopic or robotic approach may be used for this procedure.[14,15] In the authors' institution, the Amsterdam University Medical Center, location VU University, they have experience with total laparoscopic intestinal vaginoplasty. Minimal invasive surgery has shown to result in less postoperative pain, less wound-related complications, and a faster return to normal activities. The day before surgery, the patient receives full bowel preparation to clean the large bowel. Usually, 500 mg of metronidazole and 750 mg of cefuroxime are administered intravenously as perioperative antibiotic prophylaxis. Under general anesthesia, a bladder catheter is inserted. The patient is placed in lithotomy position with sufficient padding to prevent pressure injury. In the authors' center, the intraabdominal part of the procedure is performed by a gastrointestinal surgeon with advanced experience in laparoscopic surgery. The genital surgeon operates simultaneously with the gastrointestinal surgeon.

Primary Cases

Perineal surgery
Intersurgeon differences exist with regard to the genital surgical technique. Here, the authors describe their technique. First, a triangular full-thickness perineoscrotal flap is created. The bulbospongiosus muscle is dissected off the urethra. This muscle is left attached dorsally, for possible use later in the procedure. An incision is made in the midline raphe. Access to the plane of Denonvillier's fascia is obtained, after which blunt dissection is performed to the peritoneal fold. Meticulous effort is made not to lacerate the urethra (the urinary catheter may be of guidance in this process) and the rectum (a straight clamp with a gauze is placed in the rectum and rectal wall continuity is frequently checked by digital palpation). If the rectum is lacerated, the defect is oversewn immediately. Intraoperative rectal perforation is a predictor for rectoneovaginal fistula occurrence. Even when oversewn, approximately 20% of patients still develop a rectoneovaginal fistula.[16] In cases of rectal perforation, the bulbospongiosus muscle may be used as extra coverage on top of the defect, which may prevent rectoneovaginal fistula formation. A hemostatic gauze is placed in the neovaginal cavity to guide intraabdominal opening of the peritoneal fold and subsequent dissection of top of the neovaginal tunnel. From this point on, several surgical steps are taken identical to the penile inversion vaginoplasty method: shortening of the urethra and ventral spatulation; bilateral orchiectomy and removal of spermatic cord at the level of the superficial inguinal ring (all testicular resection specimens are sent for histopathologic examination); circumcision; and formation of the clitoris from the dorsal penile neurovascular bundle, clitoral hood, and labia minora. Corporal bodies

are resected. In the meantime, the gastrointestinal surgeon has generally finished isolating the pedicled intestinal segment and has brought the segment toward the perineal site. Then, the penile skin flap is inverted to the neovaginal meatus and is sewn to the intestinal segment in an exaggerated interdigitated fashion. This is done to prevent introital stenosis. A too superficial mucoepithelial junction creates an unaesthetic effect. At the end, labia majora are created by trimming scrotal skin.

Intraabdominal surgery
A total of 3 trocars are generally used in this procedure. Pneumoperitoneum is applied after open introduction of a 12-mm subumbilical trocar. After insufflation, the laparoscope is introduced and the abdomen is inspected for adhesions and particularities. Under direct vision, 2 extra trocars are introduced: one 5-mm right lateral trocar at umbilical height in the midclavicular line and one 12-mm in the right lower quadrant, lateral to the epigastric artery and vein. Trocar placement can vary due to individual patient factors, such as a history of intraabdominal surgery. The sigmoid segment is released from its lateral adhesions, and the mesosigmoid is mobilized completely. Careful inspection of the mesosigmoid is performed to identify the inferior mesenteric artery and its descending arteries, the left colic artery, the sigmoidal branches, and the superior rectal artery. The distal sigmoid is transected just proximal of the rectum and the mesosigmoid is transected to the sigmoid arterial base, allowing the sigmoid segment to be transferred toward the neovaginal cavity. The peritoneal fold is opened between bladder and rectum on guidance of the gauze in the neovaginal tunnel. The neovaginal gauze also prevents the pneumoperitoneum to be released. The distal end of the sigmoid segment is handed to the genital surgeon through the neovaginal tunnel. Care is taken that the vascular pedicle is free of tension and that the segment has no torsion.

Sigmoid arteries and the left colic artery provide blood to the sigmoid segment and are vital for tissue viability. However, some branches may have to be sacrificed in individual cases to allow for segment translocation. Sigmoid segment perfusion may be checked by inspection of arterial mesenterial and transverse pulsations. When there is doubt regarding segment viability, intraoperative use of indocyanine green fluorescence angiography may aid to determine if adequate perfusion exists in the sigmoid segment.[17]

Subsequent transection of the proximal sigmoid segment is performed at the appropriate level with

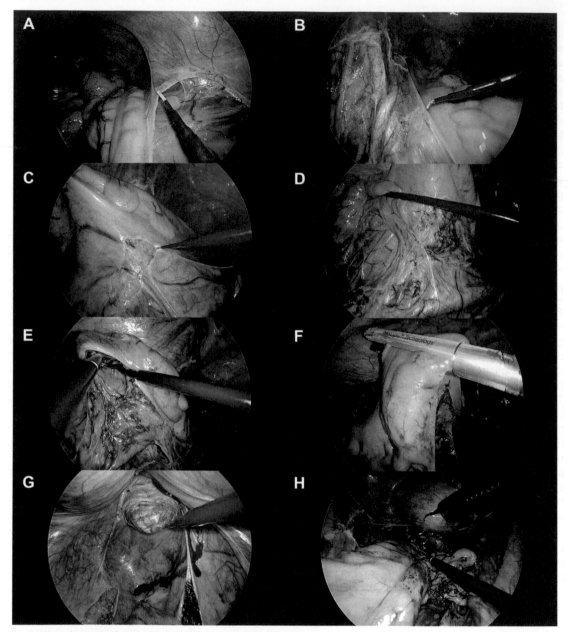

Fig. 1. Intraabdominal view of sigmoid vaginoplasty. (*A*) The sigmoid segment is released from its lateral adhesions. (*B*) Care is taken not to injure other structures, such as the ureter. (*C*) Transection of the mesosigmoid. (*D*) Inspection of the vascular anatomy, including the sigmoid artery. (*E*) Transection at the proper level. (*F*) Stapling of the distal part of the sigmoid segment. (*G*) Opening of the peritoneal fold. (*H*) The distal segment of the sigmoid is handed to the genital surgeon through the neovaginal tunnel. (*I*) Neovaginal depth is checked with the help of an illuminating dildo. (*J*) Vascularisation of the neovaginal segment is checked. (*K*) When there is doubt with regard to vascularisation, this may be checked by intraoperative indocyanine green real-time angiography. (*L*) Stapling of the proximal part of the sigmoid segment. (*M*) The neovaginal segment is fixed to the promontory. (*N*) Intraabdominal side-to-side stapled anastomosis. (*O*) The anastomosis is hand oversewn. (*P*) End result.

a stapler with respect to the marginal Drummond arcade. Generally a length of approximately 15 cm is regarded as an adequate segment length, and this can be checked intraoperatively by insertion of an illuminating dildo. To prevent postoperative neovaginal prolapse, the segment is fixated (neovaginopexy) to the promontory with nonresorbable sutures. Intestinal continuity is restored, commonly by stapled intraabdominal side-to-side anastomosis. For a visual representation of the intraabdominal part of the procedure, see **Fig. 1.**

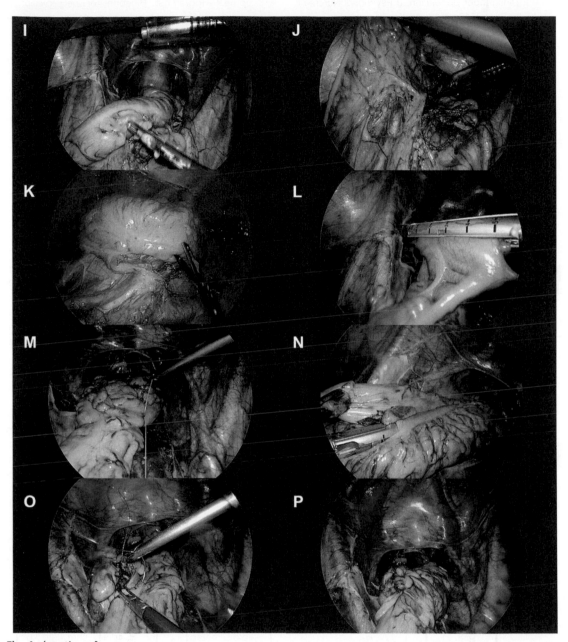

Fig. 1. (*continued*)

Revision Procedures

For revision vaginoplasty cases, traditionally, either full-thickness skin graft vaginoplasty or (laparoscopic) intestinal vaginoplasty were performed in our center. Now, however, because of a higher complication rate in the latter group, total laparoscopic intestinal vaginoplasty is the method of choice in these cases.[18] The use of laparoscopy provides adequate overview of the surgical area. Nonetheless, intestinal revision vaginoplasty is a demanding procedure for both the intraabdominal and the genital surgeons. The neovaginal cavity

has to be redissected, which can be performed simultaneously from the abdomen and the perineal site. When a previous full-thickness (penile) skin vaginoplasty has failed, contracted neovaginal remnants, sometimes even with inclusion cyst formation, are situated in the dissection plane of the neovaginal cavity and form stiff adherent tissue in which anatomic structures are hard to distinguish. Dissection in these cases can be demanding, and the risk on intraoperative rectal or urethral injury is higher.[18] When intestinal vaginoplasty is performed as revision after skin graft

Table 1
Overview of literature on surgical outcomes of intestinal vaginoplasty in transgender women published after 2000

Author, Year	n	Patients	Segment	Surgery	Neovaginal Depth (cm)	Complications
Krege et al,[35] 2001	3 transgender	Revision vaginoplasty	Ileum	NR	NR	NR
Kwun Kim et al,[36] 2003	28 transgender, 5 vaginal atresia, and 3 cervical cancer	For transgender patients, 14 revision and 14 primary	Sigmoid	Open	12	N = 2 Introital stenosis, for which Z-plasty and local flap N = 2 Meatal stenosis, for which surgical correction N = 1 Rectoneovaginal fistula, for which colostomy and fistula repair N = 3 Partial neovaginal prolapse, for which distal mucosal resection
Wedler et al,[37] 2004	9 transgender	Revision vaginoplasty	Sigmoid	Open (n = 2) and laparoscopic (n = 7) with intraabdominal anastomosis	NR	N = 1 Abdominal wall infection, for which antibiotics and drainage N = 2 Mucoepithelial junction stenosis, for which dilation under general anesthesia
Liguori et al,[38] 2005	5 transgender	Revision vaginoplasty	Ileum	Laparoscopic	13 cm (range 12.5–14)	N = 1 Urinary tract infection
Djordjevic et al,[39] 2011	Vaginal agenesis (N = 54), transgender (N = 27), and genital trauma (N = 5)	For transgender patients, all revision vaginoplasty	Sigmoid	Open	12	N = 7 Neovaginal prolapse, corrected by minor surgery N = 9 Introital stenosis, corrected by minor surgery
Morrisson et al,[24] 2015	83 transgender	Primary (N = 73) and revision (N = 13) vaginoplasty	Sigmoid	Open	NR	In the first postoperative year: protrusion (N = 5, 6%), urinary obstruction (N = 2, 2%), neovaginal stricture/stenosis (N = 16, 20%), rectoneovaginal fistula (N = 2, 2%),

					urethroneovaginal fistula (N = 1, 1%), bowel obstruction (N = 1, 1%) Long-term complications (>1 y): infection (N = 2, 2%), protrusion (N = 13, 16%), prolapse (N = 2, 2%), urinary obstruction (N = 1, 1%), neovaginal stricture/stenosis (N = 18, 22%), colitis (n = 2, 2%), urethral fistula (N = 1, 1%), bowel obstruction (N = 3, 4%)
van der Sluis et al,[25] 2016	Revision vaginoplasty	Sigmoid	14.5 (range 12–20)	Laparotomy (N = 20), laparoscopy assisted with extraabdominal anastomosis (N = 2) and laparoscopy with intraabdominal anastomosis (N = 2)	N = 1 Neovaginal segment necrosis, for which neovaginectomy N = 1 Neovaginal stenosis; during surgical correction a compromised vascular perfusion was observed, for which neovaginectomy N = 13 Introital stenosis, for which surgical correction N = 3 Meatal stenosis, for which meatoplasty N = 2 Partial (mucosal) prolapse, for which small excision N = 1 Total prolapse
Van der Sluis et al,[18] 2016	Revision vaginoplasty	Sigmoid	15.9 ± 1.4	Laparoscopically, intraabdominal anastomosis	N = 1 Intraoperative bladder neck trauma N = 2 Rectal perforations; in one patient oversewn without postoperative consequences, in one patient fecal peritonitis necessitated relaparoscopy, suturing of the perforation, and omentumplasty N = 1 Anastomotic stenosis, for which relaparotomy N = 1 Torsion of the small intestine, for which relaparoscopy

(continued on next page)

Table 1
(continued)

Author, Year	n	Patients	Segment	Surgery	Neovaginal Depth (cm)	Complications
Bouman et al,[40] 2016	42 transgender	Primary vaginoplasty	Sigmoid	Laparoscopically, intraabdominal anastomosis	16.3 ± 1.5	N = 1 Intraoperative rectal perforation, oversewn without long-term consequences N = 6 Introital stenosis, for which surgical correction N = 1 Minimal mucosal prolapse, for which excision under local anesthesia N = 1 anastomotic leakage, for which relaparoscopy N = 2 Postoperative bleeding, for which relaparoscopy N = 1 Death due to ESBL-positive necrotizing fasciitis leading to septic shock, with multiorgan failure
Manrique et al,[19] 2018	15 transgender	NR	Transverse colon	Laparoscopically	NR	N = 1 Introital stenosis N = 1 Excessive amount of secretions in the first month, which subsided later
van der sluis et al,[41] 2018	27 transgender and 5 nontransgender	Primary (n = 3) and revision (n = 29) vaginoplasty	Ileum	Laparoscopically (n = 7) or open (25)	13.2 ± 3.1	N = 1 Iatrogenic bladder damage N = 1 Intraoperative blood loss necessitating transfusion N = 4 Introital stenosis N = 1 Rectoneovaginal fistula, for which temporary ileostomy

Özkan et al,[42] 2018	34 Müllerian agenesis, 9 transgender	Revision vaginoplasty	Sigmoid	Open	11.7 ± 1.2	N = 1 Necrosis of the distal part of the rectosigmoid, for which debridement of the necrotic area and reconstruction with bilaterally raised local skin flaps
Salgado et al,[43] 2018	12 transgender	Primary vaginoplasty	Sigmoid	Laparoscopic with extraabdominal anastomosis	13.9 ± 2.0	N = 2 Ileus N = 1 Surgical site infection N = 1 Intraoperative bladder laceration N = 1 Deep venous thrombosis N = 1 Suspected pulmonary embolism No incidences of bowel injury, anastomotic leak, sigmoid necrosis, prolapse, diversion neovaginitis

Abbreviations: ESBL extended-spectrum beta-lactamase; NR not reported.

or penile inversion vaginoplasty, the neovagina is shortened to 2 to 4 cm from the introitus. The intestinal segment can be sutured to the remnants after cleaving levator muscles and scar tissue. When too much neovaginal tissue is left in place, dilation of the mucocutaneous junction becomes difficult with subsequent risk on stenosis. Harvesting of the intestinal segment is no different from primary cases. During the intraabdominal part of the surgery, secondary genital corrections can be performed if necessary.

Intestinal Segment Selection

Different intestinal segments may be used for vaginal reconstructive surgery. In transgender women, the commonest used segments are either sigmoid or ileum. Which segment provides the optimal result with regard to surgical complications, quality of life, sexual function, lubrication, discharge, and odor is unknown. The choice for a specific segment for intestinal vaginoplasty depends heavily on the surgeon's background and experience.[11] Different investigators prefer other segments, each with its advantages and disadvantages.[11,19,20] Generally, urologists tend to use the ileum, perhaps because they have experience with these grafts for bladder reconstructive surgery (Bricker procedure), whereas gastrointestinal surgeons tend to use sigmoid grafts. In the authors' institution, the sigmoid is preferred. However, if adequate mobilization of the sigmoid segment is not possible, there are no reservations to intraoperatively convert to ileal vaginoplasty. Advantages of the sigmoid comprise anatomic proximity and sufficient intestinal width. Disadvantages comprise the risk on neovaginal inflammatory bowel disease, such as ulcerative colitis, malignancies, and diversion neovaginitis.

Postoperative Instructions

In uncomplicated cases, patients are generally admitted to the hospital for 5 days. In literature, the average hospital stay is approximately 9 days.[11] At day 5, the urinary catheter is removed and patients are discharged when spontaneous voiding is possible.

At the first outpatient clinic visit, 3 weeks after surgery, introital dilation is practiced with the patient and continued hereafter for 30 minutes a day during 6 postoperative months. Patients are scheduled for postoperative outpatient visits at 3 weeks, 3 months, 6 months, and 1 year after surgery.

Postoperative Complications

In literature, more than thousand patients are described who underwent this procedure, most of them through laparotomic approach. All describe retrospective case series, most single-center. Major complications after intestinal vaginoplasty are rare but may occur. Postoperative necrotizing cellulitis and intestinal graft necrosis have been described in singular case reports.[21,22] In revision procedures, there is a higher chance of intra- and postoperative complications because of reasons described earlier. Intraoperative rectal perforation, which leads to a higher chance of rectoneovaginal fistula formation, occurs in less than 1% of primary cases and approximately 5% in revision procedures. Bowel anastomosis to restore intestinal continuity has a risk on anastomotic leakage or anastomotic stenosis, which is comparable to the general population after elective colorectal surgery. An overview of literature on surgical outcomes of intestinal vaginoplasty in transgender women is presented in **Table 1**.

PATIENT-REPORTED OUTCOMES

To date, there is a lack of validated questionnaires, focusing on patient-reported outcomes after gender-affirming surgery. This has led to the use of various self-created questionnaires or questionnaires aimed at different study populations in the gender surgery literature. This hinders comparison and appraisal of abovementioned outcomes. An international collaboration (Canada, Denmark, the Netherlands, and the USA) has been formed to address this specific problem. In the near future, the GENDER-Q will be available for this purpose.[23]

Generally, a lack of quality-of-life measures and patient-reported outcomes is observed in current literature on intestinal vaginoplasty in transgender women. An overview of short-term results is presented in **Table 2**. Data on long-term follow-up regarding patient-reported outcomes are scarce. Only 2 studies focused on long-term follow-up after intestinal vaginoplasty in this patient group. Both focused on patients who underwent GAS between 1980 and 2000.[24,25] Morrison and colleagues[24] described 83 patients who underwent primary (N = 70) or revision (N = 13) rectosigmoid vaginoplasty between 1978 and 2000. A total of 48 (58%) had complications, which consisted mainly of introital stenosis or excessive protrusion of the corpus spongiosum (see **Table 1**). A total of 21 patients filled in a self-made questionnaire, inquiring long-term satisfaction with the surgical procedure. On a five-point Likert scale, they scored satisfaction a mean score of 4.67, appearance 4.67, and sexual function 4.24. Van der Sluis and colleagues[25] identified 24 transgender women, who underwent intestinal vaginoplasty as revision procedure between 1980 and 2000. Nine patients

Table 2
Short-term patient-reported outcomes after sigmoid vaginoplasty in transgender women

Author, Year	n	Patients	Segment	PROM
Djordjevic et al,[39] 2011	Vaginal agenesis (N = 54), transgender (N = 27), and genital trauma (N = 5)	For transgender patients, all revision vaginoplasty	Sigmoid	FSFI ranged from 11.5 to 35.7 (mean 28.9) in the whole patient population. Sexual function was satisfactory in 21 (77.7%) and unsatisfactory in 6 (22.3%) transgender women. Of transgender women, mild depression, as defined by the Beck Depression Inventory, was observed in 4, moderate in 3, and severe in 1.
Bouman et al,[40] 2016	31 transgender	Primary vaginoplasty	Sigmoid	Life satisfaction scored a median of 8.0 (range = 4.0–10.0) on Cantril Ladder of Life Scale. Patients scored a mean total score of 27.7 ± 5.8 on the Satisfaction With Life Scale, which indicated high satisfaction with life, and a mean total score of 5.6 ± 1.4 on the Subjective Happiness Scale. Functionality was graded a median score of 8.0 of 10 (range = 1.0–10.0) and Esthetics was graded a score of 8.0 out of 10 (range = 3.0–10.0). The mean FSFI total score of sexually active transgender women was 26.0 ± 6.8.
Özkan et al,[42] 2018	34 Müllerian agenesis, 9 transgender	Revision vaginoplasty	Sigmoid	The mean score in 15 patients undergoing FSFI assessment was 29.5 (range 18–34.2).

Abbreviations: FSFI, female sexual function index; PROM, patient-reported outcome measure.

were traced after a median postoperative time of 29 years. They reported to be satisfied with life and scored 5.9 of 7 on a Subjective Happiness Scale. Neovaginal functionality was rated as 7.3 out of 10 and appearance as 7.4 of 10. Meanwhile, the surgical technique, somatic and psychological care, has changed considerably, so it remains to be seen if these results are extrapolatable to the transgender patient undergoing GAS currently.

LONG-TERM POSTOPERATIVE ISSUES
Diversion Neovaginitis of the Sigmoid Neovagina

Diversion colitis of the sigmoid neovagina ("diversion neovaginitis") has been described in varying levels of intensity after sigmoid vaginoplasty. Sigmoidal colonocytes obtain nutrients for their energy needs predominantly from the fecal stream and not from their blood supply. After surgical diversion from the fecal stream, nutrients are likely to be depleted over time. After sigmoid vaginoplasty, macro- and microscopic inflammatory

changes of the sigmoid neovagina are common and occur in most of the patients.[26,27] Most patients do not experience symptoms and only have minor inflammatory changes. However, some patients may experience a more severe manifestation with mucous discharge and malodor, which can be treated with topical short-chain fatty acids, coconut oil, and/or 5-aminosalicylic acid, but in the most severe form may even necessitate neovaginectomy.[28,29,30,31]

Neovaginal Cancer and Postoperative Surveillance

Cancer of the intestinal neovagina has been reported in singular case reports.[32–34] The overall incidence and prevalence are unknown. Patients may present with neovaginal discharge and/or a palpable neovaginal mass. In cases of intestinal neovaginal cancer, endoscopic examination of the native intestinal tract as oncological work-up is mandatory (and vice versa). A multidisciplinary approach (oncologists, oncological gastroenterologists, oncological surgeons, and reconstructive surgeons) is recommended when treating intestinal neovaginal cancer. To date, there is no clear guideline on postoperative cancer surveillance after intestinal vaginoplasty. Theoretically, a prolonged period of (mild) inflammation of the sigmoid neovagina, such as seems the case in long-term (mild) diversion neovaginitis, may lead to a higher risk on (inflammation-induced) sigmoid neovaginal malignancies. In these patients, and in patients with a genetically high cancer risk and/or with a history of (colorectal) malignancy, postoperative neovaginal cancer surveillance seems just.

SUMMARY

In this article, the authors provide an update on surgical indications, operative technique, pitfalls, perioperative care, and short- and long-term postoperative issues. Intestinal vaginoplasty is frequently performed as genital affirmation surgery in transgender women. In earlier years, it was predominantly used for revision cases. More recently, it is used for primary cases as well, for example, in cases with penoscrotal hypoplasia due to hormonal puberty blocking. This type of surgery may be performed by an experienced surgical team with the right medical infrastructure and laparoscopic equipment.

REFERENCES

1. Leclère FM, Casoli V, Weigert R. Outcome of vaginoplasty in male-to-female transgenders: a systematic review of surgical techniques. J Sex Med 2015;12: 1655–6.
2. Bizic MR, Stojanovic B, Djordjevic ML. Genital reconstruction for the transgendered individual. J Pediatr Urol 2017;13:446–52.
3. Colebunders B, Brondeel S, D'Arpa S, et al. An update on the surgical treatment for transgender patients. Sex Med Rev 2017;5:103–9.
4. Horbach SE, Bouman MB, Smit JM, et al. Outcome of vaginoplasty in male-to-female transgenders: a systematic review of surgical techniques. J Sex Med 2015;12:1499–512.
5. Perovic SV, Stanojevic DS, Djordjevic ML. Vaginoplasty in male transsexuals using penile skin and a urethral flap. BJU Int 2000;86:843–50.
6. Wangjiraniran B, Selvaggi G, Chokrungvaranont P, et al. Male-to-female vaginoplasty: Preecha's surgical technique. J Plast Surg Hand Surg 2015;49: 153–9.
7. Leclère FM, Casoli V, Baudet J, et al. Description of the baudet surgical technique and introduction of a systematic method for training surgeons to perform male-to-female sex reassignment surgery. Aesthet Plast Surg 2015;39:927–34.
8. Buncamper ME, van der Sluis WB, van der Pas RS, et al. Surgical outcome after penile inversion vaginoplasty: a retrospective study of 475 transgender women. Plast Reconstr Surg 2016;138:999–1007.
9. Gaither TW, Awad MA, Osterberg EC, et al. Postoperative complications following primary penile inversion vaginoplasty among 330 male-to-female transgender patients. J Urol 2018;199:760–5.
10. Reed HM, Yanes RE, Delto JC, et al. Non-grafted vaginal depth augmentation for transgender atresia, our experience and survey of related procedures. Aesthet Plast Surg 2015;39:733–44.
11. Bouman MB, van Zeijl MC, Buncamper ME, et al. Intestinal vaginoplasty revisited: a review of surgical techniques, complications, and sexual function. J Sex Med 2014;11:1835–47.
12. Coleman E, Bockting W, Botzer M, et al. Standards of care for the health of transsexual, transgender, and gender nonconforming people, 7th version. Int J Transgend 2011;13:165–232.
13. Manrique OJ, Adabi K, Huang TC, et al. Assessment of pelvic floor anatomy for male-to-female vaginoplasty and the role of physical therapy on functional and patient-reported outcomes. Ann Plast Surg 2018. https://doi.org/10.1097/SAP.0000000000001680.
14. Bouman MB, Buncamper ME, van der Sluis WB, et al. Total laparoscopic sigmoid vaginoplasty. Fertil Steril 2016;106:e22–3.
15. Kim C, Campbell B, Ferrer F. Robotic sigmoid vaginoplasty: a novel technique. Urology 2008;72: 847–9.
16. van der Sluis WB, Bouman MB, Buncamper ME, et al. Clinical characteristics and management of neovaginal fistulas after vaginoplasty in transgender women. Obstet Gynecol 2016;127:1118–26.
17. Claes KEY, Pattyn P, D'Arpa S, et al. Male-to-female gender confirmation surgery: intestinal vaginoplasty. Clin Plast Surg 2018;45:351–60.
18. Van der Sluis WB, Bouman MB, Buncamper ME, et al. Revision vaginoplasty: a comparison of surgical outcomes of laparoscopic intestinal versus perineal full-thickness skin graft vaginoplasty. Plast Reconstr Surg 2016;138:793–800.
19. Manrique OJ, Sabbagh MD, Ciudad P, et al. Gender-confirmation surgery using the pedicle transverse colon flap for vaginal reconstruction: a clinical outcome and sexual function evaluation study. Plast Reconstr Surg 2018;141:767–71.
20. van Hövell Tot Westerflier CVA, Meijerink WJHJ, Tuynman JB, et al. Gender-confirmation surgery using the pedicle transverse colon flap for vaginal reconstruction: a clinical outcome and sexual function evaluation study. Plast Reconstr Surg 2018; 142:605e–6e.
21. Negenborn VL, van der Sluis WB, Meijerink WJHJ, et al. Lethal necrotizing cellulitis caused by ESBL-producing E. Coli after laparoscopic intestinal

vaginoplasty. J Pediatr Adolesc Gynecol 2017;30: e19–21.

22. Thewjitcharoen Y, Srikummoon T, Srivajana N, et al. Hemorrhagic necrosis of small bowel following small bowel obstruction as a late complication of sex reassignment surgery-a gap in transgender care. J Surg Case Rep 2018;2018:rjy314.

23. Klassen AF, Kaur M, Johnson N, et al. International phase I study protocol to develop a patient-reported outcome measure for adolescents and adults receiving gender-affirming treatments (the GENDER-Q). BMJ Open 2018;8:e025435.

24. Morrison SD, Satterwhite T, Grant DW, et al. Long-term outcomes of rectosigmoid neocolporrhaphy in male-to-female gender reassignment surgery. Plast Reconstr Surg 2015;136:386–94.

25. van der Sluis WB, Bouman MB, de Boer NK, et al. Longterm follow-up of transgender women after secondary intestinal vaginoplasty. J Sex Med 2016;13: 702–10.

26. van der Sluis WB, Bouman MB, Meijerink WJHJ, et al. Diversion neovaginitis after sigmoid vaginoplasty: endoscopic and clinical characteristics. Fertil Steril 2016;105:834–9.e1.

27. van der Sluis WB, Neefjes-Borst EA, Bouman MB, et al. Morphological spectrum of neovaginitis in autologous sigmoid transplant patients. Histopathology 2016;68:1004–12.

28. van der Sluis WB, Bouman M, Meijerink W, et al. Refractory diversion neovaginitis in a sigmoid-colon-derived neovagina: clinical and histopathological considerations. Frontline Gastroenterol 2016;7: 227–30.

29. Zundler S, Dietz L, Matzel KE, et al. Successful long-term treatment of diversion colitis with topical coconut oil application. Am J Gastroenterol 2018;113: 1908–10.

30. Toolenaar TA, Freundt I, Huikeshoven FJ, et al. The occurrence of diversion colitis in patients with a sigmoid neovagina. Hum Pathol 1993;24:846–9.

31. Abbasakoor F, Mahon C, Boulos PB. Diversion colitis in sigmoid neovagina. Colorectal Dis 2004;6:290–1.

32. Schober JM. Cancer of the neovagina. J Pediatr Urol 2007;3:167–70.

33. Kita Y, Mori S, Baba K, et al. Mucinous adenocarcinoma emerging in sigmoid colon neovagina 40 years after its creation: a case report. World J Surg Oncol 2015;13:213.

34. Yamada K, Shida D, Kato T, et al. Adenocarcinoma arising in sigmoid colon neovagina 53 years after construction. World J Surg Oncol 2018;16:88.

35. Krege S, Bex A, Lümmen G, et al. Male-to-female transsexualism: a technique, results and long-term follow-up in 66 patients. BJU Int 2001;88:396–402.

36. Kwun Kim S, Hoon Park J, Cheol Lee K, et al. Long-term results in patients after rectosigmoid vaginoplasty. Plast Reconstr Surg 2003;112:143–51.

37. Wedler V, Meuli-Simmen C, Guggenheim M, et al. Laparoscopic technique for secondary vaginoplasty in male to female transsexuals using a modified vascularized pedicled sigmoid. Gynecol Obstet Invest 2004;57:181–5.

38. Liguori G, Trombetta C, Bucci S, et al. Laparoscopic mobilization of neovagina to assist secondary ileal vaginoplasty in male-to-female transsexuals. Urology 2005;66:293–8 [discussion: 298].

39. Djordjevic ML, Stanojevic DS, Bizic MR. Rectosigmoid vaginoplasty: clinical experience and outcomes in 86 cases. J Sex Med 2011;8:3487–94.

40. Bouman MB, van der Sluis WB, Buncamper ME, et al. Primary Total Laparoscopic Sigmoid Vaginoplasty in Transgender Women with Penoscrotal Hypoplasia: A Prospective Cohort Study of Surgical Outcomes and Follow-Up of 42 Patients. Plast Reconstr Surg 2016;138:614e–23e.

41. van der Sluis WB, Pavan N, Liguori G, et al. Ileal vaginoplasty as vaginal reconstruction in transgender women and patients with disorders of sex development: an international, multicentre, retrospective study on surgical characteristics and outcomes. BJU Int 2018;121:952–8.

42. Özkan Ö, Özkan Ö, Çinpolat A, et al. Vaginal reconstruction with the modified rectosigmoid colon: surgical technique, long-term results and sexual outcomes. J Plast Surg Hand Surg 2018;52:210–6.

43. Salgado CJ, Nugent A, Kuhn J, et al. Primary sigmoid vaginoplasty in transwomen: technique and outcomes. Biomed Res Int 2018;2018:4907208.

Vaginoplasty Modifications to Improve Vulvar Aesthetics

Suporn Watanyusakul, MD

KEYWORDS

- Vaginoplasty • Gender confirmation surgery • Male-to-female • Labia minora reconstruction
- Penile inversion • Preputial flap • Clitoroplasty • Gender dysphoria

KEY POINTS

- The author introduces a nonpenile inversion modification technique for vulvar aesthetic improvement using prepuce, and penile or scrotal skin to reconstruct the double surfaces of labia minora.
- The sensate clitoris, clitoral hood, and clitoral frenulum are constructed using the dorsal neurovascular whole glans penis preputial island flap.
- The simple full-thickness genital skin-mucosal graft vaginoplasty is used for the neovaginal wall lining.

INTRODUCTION

Male-to-female (MTF) gender confirmation surgery (GCS) is complex genital surgery, the outcome of which has an enormous psychological effect on the transwoman individual. Several vaginoplasty techniques including genital or nongenital skin grafts vaginoplasty, penile-scrotal skin flap inversion vaginoplasty, or pedicle intestinal vaginoplasty have been introduced since 1931 to reconstruct a functional vaginal canal.[1–6] The sensate clitoris reconstruction using the dorsal neurovascular glans penis flap was developed to introduce sexual sensation.[7,8] To date, penile skin inversion vaginoplasty (PIV) with the dorsal neurovascular glans penis clitoroplasty is the de facto choice in MTF GCS, which successfully provides sexual sensation and neovaginal depth.

Improvements to vulvar aesthetics, particularly the clitoral complex and labia minora reconstruction, are still difficult and remain the challenge of genital reconstructive surgeons. Several techniques exist to improve the clitoral complex and labia minora reconstruction; most are modified PIV and yield varied aesthetic results.[9–11]

BACKGROUND LEADING TO DEVELOPMENT OF THE AUTHOR'S TECHNIQUE

Between 1992 and 2000 the author had personal experience of MTF GCS in some 450 transwomen using the traditional PIV, modified with scrotal skin graft in cases of inadequate penile skin, and the dorsal neurovascular glans penis clitoroplasty. Generally these gave satisfactory neovaginal depth and sexual sensation results, but good vulvar aesthetic results were mostly not achieved because most penile tissue is consumed within the vaginal cavity in PIV. This leaves little to no surplus material to create a realistic vulvar appearance.

In preoperative surveys during 2014 to 2017, 580 patients prioritized their postoperative preferences to be

1. Sexual sensation 58.1% (n = 337)
2. Natural vulvar aesthetics 37.4% (n = 217)
3. Vaginal depth 4.5% (n = 26)

Sexual sensation and vulvar aesthetics are seen by most as being most important, whereas vaginal depth is generally the least important outcome to

Disclosure Statement: None.
Suporn Clinic, 938 Sukhumvit Road Bangplasoi, Muang District, Chonburi 20000, Thailand
E-mail address: drsuporn@yahoo.com

Urol Clin N Am 46 (2019) 541–554
https://doi.org/10.1016/j.ucl.2019.07.008
0094-0143/19/© 2019 Elsevier Inc. All rights reserved.

most patients, even though this had traditionally been the priority of the PIV technique. To improve vulvar aesthetics, the PIV technique was reviewed and revised by the author to prioritize material usage toward aesthetic appearance of the labia minora and construction of the clitoral complex in preference to achievement of vaginal depth.

GOALS OF VULVAR AESTHETIC APPEARANCE

The ideal aesthetic outcome of the reconstructed structures of female genitalia includes the following:

1. Clitoris should have a round/oval projection shape, located approximately 3 to 4 cm above the urethral orifice, covered with the clitoral hood dorsally, which splits into a clitoral frenulum connecting with the upper one-third part of labia minora on either side.
2. Labia minora must have a lip-like shape with the length running each side posteriorly from the clitoral region toward the bottom of the vagina. Labia minora need double surfaces; the inner surface of labia minora is hairless with a thin, pink color, whereas the outer surface is normal skin color and texture.
3. Urethral orifice is located near the vaginal entrance with minimum erectile tissue.
4. The constructed clitoris, clitoral hood, clitoral frenulum, labia minora, labia majora, urethral orifice, and vaginal introitus are all realistically placed in the correct three-dimensional planes.
5. Vaginal wall lining should be hairless, thin, and pink in color.

CHOICE OF DONOR TISSUE

For the best vulvar aesthetic reconstruction, each feature of the constructed female genitalia must be created from the most appropriate donor tissue of male genitalia to match typical color and tissue consistency.

1. The glans penis in a male is biologically homologous to the clitoris in female. The glans penis has about 10 times more volume than a typical clitoris, whereas there are fewer sexual sensory nerve endings than in a typical clitoris. Glans penis is considered as the most appropriate donor tissue for sensate clitoris reconstruction but reduction of glans penis to that of a typical clitoris size would also reduce postoperative sexual sensation. The author tries to keep the entire glans penis to preserve as much postoperative sexual sensation as possible.
2. The prepuce of penis is an extremely thin skin fold consisting of two layers of different color. The prepuce is hairless and contains no subcutaneous fat. The inner layer of the prepuce has similar texture, color, and quality as the inner surface of labia minora in a genetic female. Prepuce is also rich with innervated erogenous sensory receptors. The prepuce of penis is considered to be the most appropriate donor tissue for the inner surface of labia minora reconstruction, not only for the satisfactory aesthetic result but also for enhancement of sexual sensation.
3. The penile shaft skin has similar color and texture to the outer surface of natural labia minora and is considered as the most appropriate donor tissue to construct the outer surface of labia minora.
4. The scrotal skin in male genitalia has been used successfully as donor tissue for the reconstructed labia majora. With PIV, scrotal skin is always excess and excised. The excess scrotal skin is used as full-thickness graft addition with PIV by some surgeons for vaginal lining to attain adequate neovaginal depth.[9,12]

PRINCIPLE OF THE AUTHOR'S MALE-TO-FEMALE GENDER CONFIRMATION SURGICAL TECHNIQUE

In September 2000, the author originated the Suporn technique for MTF GCS using a dorsal neurovascular whole glans penis preputial island flap for sensate clitoris, clitoral hood, clitoral frenulum, and inner surface of labia minora reconstruction. To preserve sexual sensation as much as possible, the remaining glans penis tissue from the clitoris reconstruction is retained and named "the secondary sensate organ." The penile shaft skin flap is for the outer surface of labia minora reconstruction. The described labia minora reconstruction technique is known as "type A labia minora reconstruction" where adequate penile donor tissue is present. The technique was presented at the 27th Annual Scientific Meeting of The Royal College of Surgeons of Thailand on 26th July 2002, Na Chom Thian, Sattahip, Chonburi, Thailand.[13] Since its introduction, the technique has been used by the author on some 2700 transwomen.

Overcircumcision or penile-scrotal hypotrophy from hormone therapy, may lead to there being insufficient penile skin to construct the double surface of labia minora. In such cases an alternative "type B labia minora reconstruction" is applied, in which the inner surfaces of labia minora are constructed from existing penile skin and the outer surface from the medial part of scrotal skin flaps.

Because all or almost all penile skin is used for labia minora reconstruction, the remaining penile skin is inadequate in quality and quantity for neo-vaginal wall lining. Full-thickness genital skin-mucosal grafts harvested from excess scrotal skin, combined with the excess penile skin and urethral mucosa, are used for neovaginal wall lining in every case. This enables adequate neovaginal depth in all cases even with limited penile skin.[14]

The author's technique uses the following:

- *Dorsal neurovascular whole glans penis preputial island flap*: For sensate clitoris, clitoral hood, clitoral frenulum, secondary sensate organ, and internal surface of labia minora reconstruction.
- *Penile skin flap or scrotal skin flap*: For external surface of labia minora reconstruction.
- *Full-thickness scrotal skin, penile skin, urethral mucosa, with or without groin skin grafts*: For neovaginal wall lining.

Procedural steps are performed sequentially as follows:

1. Neovaginal cavity dissection
2. Orchidectomy
3. Penile skin flap dissection
4. Dorsal neurovascular whole glans penis preputial island flap dissection
5. Sensate clitoris, clitoral hood, clitoral frenulum, and secondary sensate organ reconstruction
6. Inset posterior perineal skin flap
7. Inner and outer surface of labia minora reconstruction
8. Labia majora reconstruction
9. Urethral reconstruction
10. Vaginal introitus reconstruction
11. Lining of vaginal cavity

The neovaginal cavity is carefully dissected between urethra-bladder and rectum guided by a silicone urinary catheter anteriorly and a guiding sponge stick in the rectum posteriorly. A vaginal cavity depth of at least 6 inches (15 cm) should be attained. Orchidectomy is performed, then bulbospongiosus muscle is excised.

The penis is pulled down to evaluate the adequacy of the donor penile tissue for the type of labia minora reconstruction choices. Circumferential incision is made at 3 to 4 cm from the corona of glans. The proximal penile skin is dissected off the penis superficial to buck fascia. Dorsal neurovascular whole glans penis preputial island flap is dissected from the tunica albuginea (**Fig. 1**).

A small strip (1 cm × 3 cm) of tunica albuginea that attaches to the dorsal neurovascular pedicle and the corona of glans is preserved for suspending the constructed clitoris at the best aesthetic

position. After the glans penis preputial flap is completely dissected off corpus cavernosa, the resected corpus cavernosum stump is resected and secured by 1–0 absorbable suture. The strip of tunica albuginea flap is fixed to periosteum of pubic tubercle on either side of the dorsal neurovascular pedicle with 4–0 absorbable suture to suspend the constructed clitoris in the right position 3 to 4 cm superior to the urethral orifice.

The glans penis is divided into three parts of which the middle part is used for sensate clitoris reconstruction. The lateral parts are sutured together and fixed to the corpus cavernosum stump, to become the secondary sensate organ. The preputial flap is divided on the dorsal side at midline just proximal to the corona of glans. The upper third part of each preputial flap is used to create the clitoral hood and clitoral frenulum. The lower two-thirds of preputial flap are used for the inner surface of labia minora reconstruction (**Figs. 2** and **3**).

The posteriorly narrow base perineal flap is inset to form the posterior aspect of the vaginal introitus. Urethral reconstruction is performed by everting the urethral mucosa to join the secondary sensate organ superiorly, the middle third part of the constructed inner surface of labia minora laterally, and the skin graft inferiorly.

In the type A procedure (adequate penile tissue), the inner surface of labia minora is reconstructed by suturing the volar rim of preputial flap to the constructed urethra and covering the lateral aspect of vaginal introitus (see **Fig. 3**F). The proximal penile skin flap is pulled down and divided in the midline (**Fig. 4**A). Each side of the divided skin flap is used for the outer surface of the labia minora reconstruction. The interlabial sulcus on either side are created to differentiate the labia minora from the labia majora. A 4–0 absorbing suture needle is used to pierce between the junction of penile skin flap and scrotal skin flap, with quilting fixed to the deep structures, such as corpora stump, crus of penis, and lateral aspect of neovagina introitus to create the deep interlabial sulcus on both sides (**Fig. 4**B). Both constructed inner and outer surface of labia minora are sutured together to form the double surfaces of labia minora (**Fig. 4**C).

In the type B procedure (limited donor penile tissue), all or almost existing penile skin is used for construction of clitoral hood, clitoral frenulum, and inner surface of labia minora. The scrotal skin flaps are pulled down, then a vertical 3- to 4-cm-long cut is made through all layers of the medial part of scrotal skin flap around 1 cm offset from the medial rim. This is to separate the scrotal

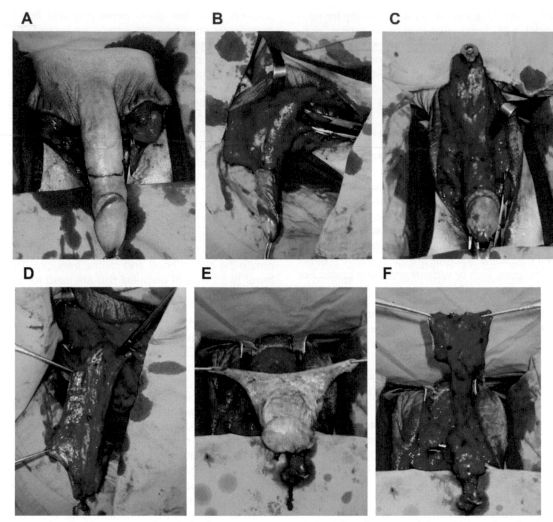

Fig. 1. The dorsal neurovascular whole glans penis preputial island flap dissection. (*A*) Marking and evaluation of penile skin. (*B*) Circumferential incision is made at 3 to 4 cm from the corona of glans. (*C*) The proximal penile skin is dissected off the penis superficial to buck fascia. (*D*) Dorsal neurovascular whole glans penis preputial island flap is dissected from the tunica albuginea. (*E*) The glans penis preputial flap is completely dissected. (*F*) A small strip of tunica albuginea that attaches to the dorsal neurovascular pedicle and the corona of glans is preserved.

skin flap into two flaps: the medial and the lateral scrotal skin flap. The medial scrotal skin flap is used for reconstruction of the outer surface of labia minora. A 4–0 absorbing suture needle is used to pierce between the medial and lateral scrotal skin flap and quilting fixed to the deep structures to create the deep interlabial sulcus on either side (**Fig. 5**). Labia majora are reconstructed from the lateral scrotal skin flap.

The vaginal introitus in Suporn technique is constructed with multiple skin flaps. A skin graft is never used to create the vaginal introitus to avoid scar contracture and unsightly scar. The inferior aspect (horizontal plane) of the vaginal introitus is lined by the posterior perineal skin flap. The superior aspect is everted urethral flap. Lateral aspects (vertical plane) of vaginal introitus on both sides are created by a penile skin flap, preputial flap, or scrotal skin flap.

The full-thickness genital skin-mucosal graft harvested from the excess scrotal skin, penile skin, or addition with urethral mucosa is used for neovaginal wall lining, which enables adequate neovaginal depth in all cases. The subcutaneous tissue and any hair follicles resident in all donor skins are excised completely to ensure a permanently hair-free vaginal cavity and sutured together to form a tubular skin on a plastic tube. The tubular skin is sutured to the neovaginal introitus, which is reconstructed from the urethral flap, penile skin flap, scrotal skin flap, and posterior perineal flap then inverted into the vaginal cavity with the dermis outside for full-thickness genital skin-mucosal graft vaginoplasty.

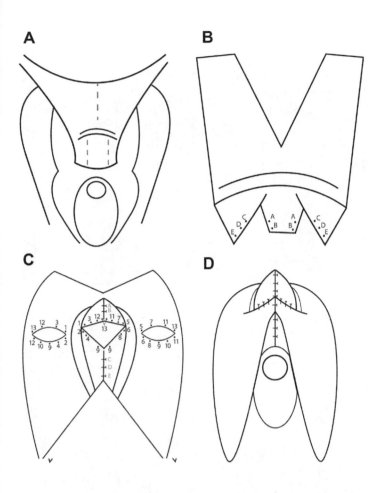

A

B

C

D

Fig. 2. Method for reconstruction of clitoral complex and inner surface of labia minora. (*A*) Mark and divide the glans penis into three flaps and prepuce into two flaps. (*B*) Clitoris and secondary sensate organ reconstruction is achieved by suturing the five pairs of the alphabetically marked points, starting by suturing point A with A then point B with B and repeating consecutively through points E. (*C*) The clitoral hood and clitoral frenulum reconstruction is achieved by suturing the numerically marked pairs of points sequentially from 1 through 13. (*D*) Outcome of the constructed clitoris, clitoral hood, clitoral frenulum, secondary sensate organ, and inner surface of labia minora.

The constructed neovagina is firmly packed with a roll of gauze soaked with povidone inside double condoms to hold in place and press the skin graft to the entire raw surface of the neovaginal cavity.

Patients are confined to bed for 4 to 5 days. The vaginal packing and urethral catheter are removed on Day 7. Patients are instructed how to care for the neovagina and instructed in the technique of vaginal dilation. The patient is scheduled to dilate the neovagina for 0.5 hour, two to three times daily, every day for 3 to 6 months then once a day until 1 year postoperative.

To maintain the integrity of a functionally deep neovaginal cavity, full preoperative understanding by the patient of the necessity for adequate dilation is essential. This is supplemented by encouragement and support by our team in the early postoperative period, and ongoing cooperation is given.

RESULTS

During 2014 to 2017, 580 cases of MTF GCS were performed on patients from 46 countries using the Suporn technique. Average age of the patients was 33 years (range, 18–65 years). Patients with prior circumcision numbered 249 (42.9%) and 19 (3.3%) had prior bilateral orchidectomy. Type A labia minora reconstruction was used in 424 patients (73.1%) and type B in 156 cases (26.9%).

VULVAR AESTHETICS OUTCOME

Goals of the ideal vulvar aesthetics outcome are successfully achieved by the author's technique.

1. The round projection shape of the clitoris with the clitoral hood superiorly and clitoral frenulum inferior-laterally is constructed (**Fig. 6**).
2. The constructed lip-like labia minora have double surfaces with different color and texture on either surface, with the length running each side posteriorly from the clitoral region toward the bottom of the vagina. The labia minora is clearly differentiated from labia majora by the constructed interlabial sulcus. The inner surface of the constructed labia minora in type A is thin, pink color, and hairless, which closely

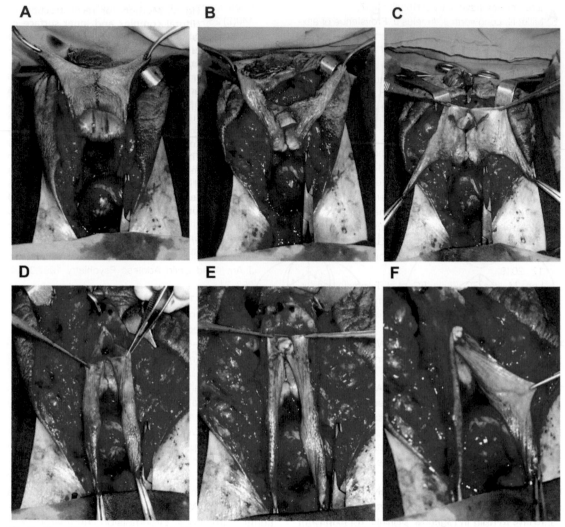

Fig. 3. The clitoral complex and labia minora reconstruction. (*A*) Markings on the glans penis and prepuce for division. (*B*) The middle part of glans penis is for sensate clitoris reconstruction. The lateral parts are sutured together and fixed to the corpus cavernosum stump to become the secondary sensate organ. (*C*) Incision on either side of the upper third part of preputial flap laterally to the constructed clitoris. (*D*) Suturing the preputial flaps to attach the lateral and volar part of the clitoris. (*E, F*) The constructed clitoris, clitoral hood, clitoral frenulum, secondary sensate organ, and inner surface of labia minora, front and lateral views.

simulates the characteristics found in the genetic female (**Fig. 7**).

3. The aesthetic result of the constructed labia minora in type B may be less natural than type A depending on the existing prepuce of penis, the circumcision scar, and the quality and quantity of the donor penile and scrotal tissue (**Fig. 8**).

4. The constructed clitoris, clitoral hood, clitoral frenulum, labia minora, labia majora, urethral orifice, and vaginal introitus are correctly placed relative to each structure in three-dimensional planes. The clitoris is located approximately 3 to 4 cm superior and 0.5 to 1 cm anterior to the urethral orifice. The labia minora and labia majora are anterior to the vaginal introitus. Urethral orifice is located near vaginal entrance with minimum erectile tissue (see **Figs. 7** and **8**).

5. The vaginal wall lining is hairless, thin, and pink color (see **Figs. 7**F and **8**F; **Fig. 9**F).

SEXUAL SENSATION

Sexual sensation is the primary priority requirement for most patients. This is achieved with the dorsal neurovascular whole glans penis preputial island flap. Because the whole sensate glans penis

A

B

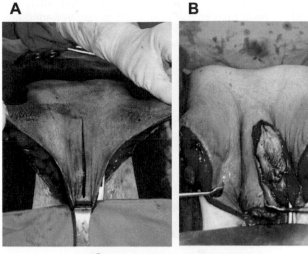

C

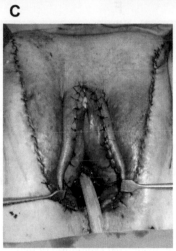

Fig. 4. Type A labia minora reconstruction (adequate donor penile tissue). (*A*) After the clitoral complex and inner surface of labia minora reconstruction, the proximal penile skin flap is pulled down and divided in midline. (*B*) The interlabial sulcus on either side are created to differentiate the labia minora from the labia majora. (*C*) The constructed inner and outer surface of labia minora are sutured together to form the double surfaces of labia minora.

preputial flap is used, patients can have sexual sensation on these constructed structures:

1. The clitoris created from the middle part of glans penis.
2. The secondary sensate organ created from the lateral parts of corona glans penis.
3. The clitoral hood and the inner surface of labia minora created from the prepuce, particularly the part of prepuce close to the corona of penis.

NEOVAGINAL DEPTH

Neovaginal depths were measured with a 32-mm diameter dilator intraoperatively, 1 week, 1 month, and later than 1 year postoperatively as listed in **Table 1**. Using the full-thickness genital skin-mucosal grafts vaginoplasty, adequate neovaginal depth is achieved in almost all cases including those with limited penile skin (**Fig. 9**).

EARLY POSTOPERATIVE COMPLICATIONS

In 580 patients, early postoperative complications noted were as follows:

- 39 patients (6.7%) experienced difficulty with urination after removal of the vaginal packing and urethral catheter on Day 7 and needed further urethral catheterization for 4 to 7 days.
- 8 patients (1.4%) needed additional measures to stop bleeding from the urethra or vaginal canal in operative room.
- There was partial necrosis of clitoris in 96 cases (16.5%).
- 10 patients (1.7%) had significant necrosis of glans penis flap (more than 50% of the constructed secondary sensate organ).
- Partial necrosis of the constructed labia minora with spontaneous healing was seen in 178 cases (30.7%).

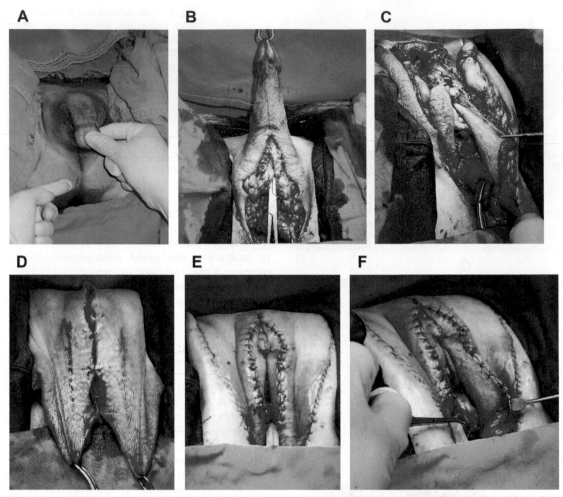

Fig. 5. Type B labia minora reconstruction (limited donor penile tissue). (*A*) Evaluation of penile skin. (*B*) Marking the circumferential incision at 3 to 4 cm from the corona of glans. (*C*) In cases of inadequate penile skin, all or almost existing penile skin is used for construction of clitoral hood, clitoral frenulum, and inner surface of labia minora. (*D*) Marking for dividing the scrotal skin flap into two flaps, medial and lateral scrotal skin flap. The medial scrotal flap is used for outer surface of labia minora reconstruction and lateral scrotal flap is used for labia majora reconstruction, which are separated by the deep interlabial sulcus. (*E, F*) The constructed inner and outer surface of labia minora are sutured together to form the double surfaces of labia minora, front and lateral views.

- 32 patients (5.5%) had significant necrosis of labia minora with detachment requiring immediate minor revision.
- No rectovaginal fistula occurred during the study period.

SECONDARY AESTHETIC IMPROVEMENT SURGERY

One hundred and sixty-two patients (27.9%) subsequently requested further minor aesthetic vulvar improvement surgery later than a year postoperative. Typical aesthetic improvement surgery requested were as follows:

- Posterior commissure reconstruction in 33 cases (5.7%) to narrow the exposure of the vaginal entrance. If the labia minora are long and have adequate tissue, the lower part of both labia minora are mobilized and joined together to form the posterior fourchette.
- Labia minora revision in 95 cases (16.4%) to improve asymmetrical shape and size of either labia minora.
- Revision of clitoris, clitoral hood, and clitoral frenulum in 58 cases (10%) to improve the clitoris complex appearance. In case of clitoris loss, secondary sensate clitoris reconstruction is performed using the secondary sensate organ.
- Urethral orifice revision in 95 cases (16.4%) to reduce prominent erectile tissue.

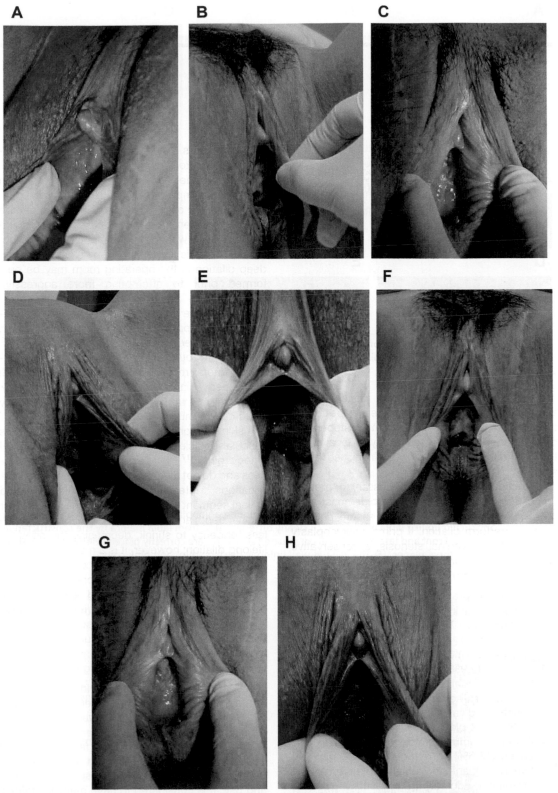

Fig. 6. The clitoris complex appearance. The round projection shape of the clitoris with the clitoral hood superiorly and clitoral frenulum inferior-laterally. (*A, B, C, D*) Lateral view. (*E, F, G, H*) Front view.

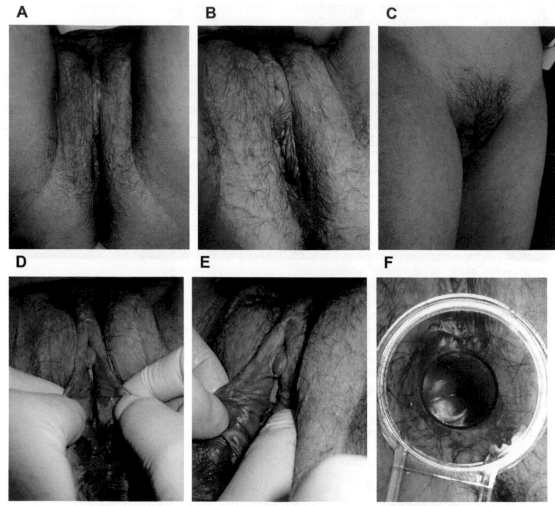

Fig. 7. Vulvar aesthetic appearance of type A Suporn technique vaginoplasty. (*A, B, C*) Front, lateral and top views. The constructed lip-like labia minora which clearly differentiated from labia majora by the constructed interlabial sulcus. (*D, E*) Front and lateral views. All constructed structures are correctly placed relative to each structure in three dimensional planes. (*F*) The vaginal wall lining is hairless, thin, and pink color.

- Removal of granulation on vaginal entrance or vaginal canal in 30 cases (5.2%) by electrical cauterization. Three patients (0.5%) needed full-thickness skin graft coverage of the wound after the granulation removal.
- 17 cases (2.9%) had narrow vaginal entrance from scar contraction on the junction of the skin-mucosal grafts and the skin flap of the constructed vaginal introitus, which were corrected by Z-plasty.
- Anterior commissure reconstruction in 108 cases (18.6%) to reduce the wide gap between the anterior labial commissure. The prominent dorsal neurovascular pedicle bundle is set backward to the deep plane tissue by mobilizing the subcutaneous fat of anterior labia majora on either side to midline

and suturing together. Loose skin on the gap is excised and closed to form the anterior commissure (**Fig. 10**).

DISCUSSION

Most MTF GCS conducted world-wide are performed by using PIV, in which generally satisfactory neovaginal depth is achieved, but there is usually insufficient surplus material to create a realistic facsimile of external female genitalia because most penile tissue is consumed for vaginal lining. Despite its widespread adoption and use, it is considered to have many limitations toward achieving a satisfactory vulvar aesthetic outcome, particularly natural appearance of the constructed labia minora.

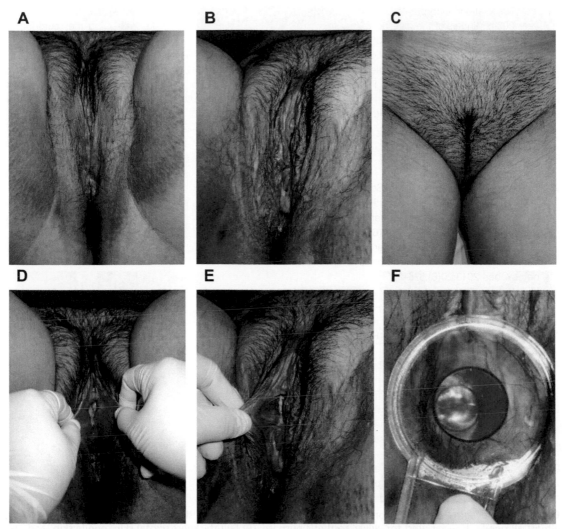

Fig. 8. Vulvar aesthetic appearance of type B Suporn technique vaginoplasty. (*A, B, C*) Front, lateral and top views. The external appearance. (*D, E*) Front and lateral view. All constructed structures are correctly placed relative to each structure in three dimensional planes. (*F*) The vaginal wall lining is hairless, thin, and pink color.

Development of the clitoroplasty technique using the dorsal portion of glans penis with dorsal neurovascular pedicle island flap is the gold standard for providing satisfactory sexual sensation and was the first significant step for vulvar aesthetic improvement.[7,8] Various techniques exist to construct the clitoral hood and labia minora reconstruction by using the glans penis preputial flap and yield varied aesthetic results.[9–11]

Vulvar aesthetic expectation is much more important than neovaginal depth in most of our patients. The inner layer of prepuce is the only tissue of male genitalia that has the same texture, color, and quality as the inner surface of labia minora. The prepuce and penile shaft skin are the most appropriate donor tissue used by the author to construct the double surface of labia minora for the vulvar aesthetics purpose.

By using the dorsal neurovascular whole glans penis preputial island flap to reconstruct the sensate clitoris, clitoral hood, clitoral frenulum, secondary sensate organ, and inner surface of labia minora, vulvar aesthetics have been improved significantly. It allows sexual sensitivity to be preserved located on the constructed sensate clitoris, clitoral hood, secondary sensate organ, and the inner surface of labia minora.

Two types of labia minora reconstruction procedures were developed to allow for variances in quantity and quality of donor genital tissue. Ideal aesthetic labia minora is created by using two pairs of different matching donor tissue. Type A labia minora reconstruction is used where

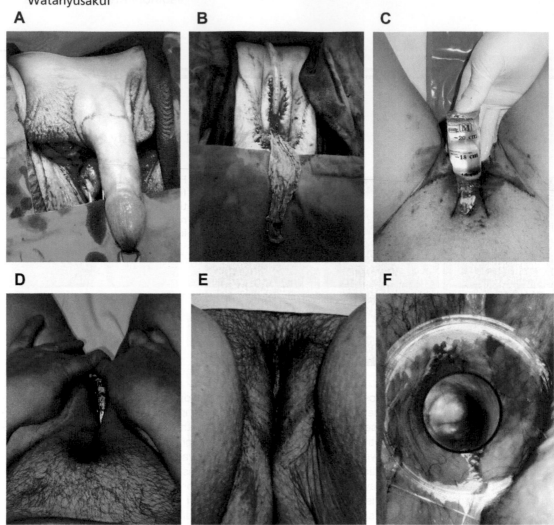

Fig. 9. The neovaginal depth outcome in cases of limited donor penile skin. (*A*) Limited donor penile tissue, almost all penile skin was used for vulvar aesthetic purpose. (*B*) Full-thickness scrotal skin, penile skin, and urethral mucosal graft vaginoplasty for neovaginal wall lining. (*C*) Neovaginal depth of 16 cm on the 7th day postoperatively. (*D*) Neovaginal depth of 17 cm in the 16th month postoperatively. (*E*) Vulvar aesthetic appearance. (*F*) Aesthetic outcome of the neovaginal canal.

adequate length of penile skin exists, whether circumcised or not. The inner surface of labia minora is reconstructed from the preputial skin flap in noncircumcised cases, or from the distal penile skin flap in circumcised cases. The outer surface of labia minora is reconstructed from the proximal penile skin flap. Where there is inadequate penile skin, an alternative type B labia minora reconstruction is used. The inner surface of labia minora is reconstructed from existing penile skin and the outer surface of labia minora is reconstructed from the medial part of scrotal skin flap.

The labia minora constructed by both methods have double surface with different color and texture on each surface. Particularly in type A, the inner surface of the constructed labia minora is thin, pink color, and hairless skin matching to biologic females.

Table 1
Neovaginal depth measurement immediately, 1 week, 1 month, and later than 1 year postoperatively compared with patients' preoperative depth expectation

	Neovaginal Depth (cm)		
	Minimum	Maximum	Average
Preoperative expectation	10.2	22.9	16.6
Intraoperative	10.2[a]	17.8	15.8
Day 7	12.7	20.0	17.2
Week 4	12.0	20.3	16.3
>1 y	6.0[b]	21.6	16.0

[a] By patient's request.
[b] 3 in 162 patients who returned for aesthetic improvement surgery had neovaginal depth less than 12 cm.

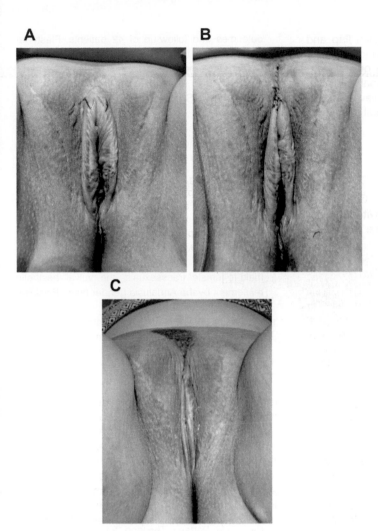

Fig. 10. Anterior commissure reconstruction. (*A*) The wide gap between the anterior labial commissure. (*B*) The skin on the gap was excised then the subcutaneous fat of anterior labia majora was undermined and sutured together in midline. (*C*) Aesthetic improvement seen after the anterior commissure reconstruction.

The constructed labia minora have adequate length running each side posteriorly from the clitoral region toward the bottom of the vagina.

By carefully selecting the most appropriate donor tissue, the ideal aesthetic clitoris, clitoral hood, clitoral frenulum, and labia minora are created. The constructed clitoral complex, labia minora, labia majora, urethral orifice, and vaginal introitus all must be realistically placed in the correct three-dimensional planes to achieve ideal vulvar aesthetics.

Because all or almost all penile skin is used for aesthetic purposes, adequate neovaginal depth by PIV is usually not possible. Instead, full-thickness genital skin-mucosal graft vaginoplasty harvested from the excess scrotal skin, penile skin, and urethral mucosa is the author's choice because of the simplicity of the technique, minimum complications, and no additional donor scar. This enables reconstructing an adequate vaginal cavity in every case. Long-term (>1 year)

average vaginal depth is 16 cm with maximum depth of 21.6 cm. Only 3 out of 162 patients (1.8%) had neovaginal depth less than 12 cm.

Because of the skin graft technique used, vaginal prolapse is not possible. Primary colon vaginoplasty is never necessary.

SUMMARY

Based on the author's previous personal experience of gaining satisfactory neovaginal depth results by the scrotal skin graft addition with the traditional PIV, a modified non-PIV technique, the Suporn technique for MTF GCS, was originated in September 2000 to provide enhancement of vulvar aesthetics without detriment to neovaginal depth. The technique uses the dorsal neurovascular whole glans penis preputial island flap for the sensate clitoris, clitoral hood, clitoral frenulum, and inner surface of labia minora reconstruction. It offers two different techniques (type A using preputial flap and penile skin flap, and type B using penile skin flap and scrotal skin flap) for the double surface of labia minora reconstruction. Full-thickness genital skin-mucosal graft is the choice for neovaginal wall lining. The technique has been proven to achieve satisfactory results of vulvar aesthetics, sexual sensation, and neovaginal depth in most cases.

ACKNOWLEDGMENTS

The author sincerely" thanks colleagues Dr Poonpissamai Suwajo and Dr Chayamote Chayangsu for their invaluable help with supportive medical information, and to Sophie Taylor, executive coordinator.

REFERENCES

1. Abraham F. Genitalumwandlung an zwei maennlichen Transvestiten. Z Sexualwiss 1931;18:223.
2. Hage JJ, Karim RB, Laub DR Sr. On the origin of pedicled skin inversion vaginoplasty: life and work of Dr Georges Burou of Casablanca. Ann Plast Surg 2007;59(6):723–9.
3. Pandya NJ, Stuteville OH. A one-stage technique for constructing female external genitalia in male transsexuals. Br J Plast Surg 1973;26(3):277–82.
4. Meyer R, Kesselring UK. One-stage reconstruction of the vagina with penile skin as an island flap in male transsexuals. Plast Reconstr Surg 1980; 66(3):401.
5. Selvaggi G, Ceulemans P, De Cuypere G, et al. Gender identity disorder: general overview and surgical treatment for vaginoplasty in male-to-female transsexuals. Plast Reconstr Surg 2005;116(6): 135e–45e.
6. Bouman MB, van der Sluis WB, Buncamper ME, et al. Primary total laparoscopic sigmoid vaginoplasty in transgender women with penoscrotal hypoplasia: a prospective cohort study of surgical outcomes and follow-up of 42 patients. Plast Reconstr Surg 2016;138(4):614e–23e.
7. Rubin SO. A method of preserving the glans penis as a clitoris in sex conversion operations in male transsexuals. Scand J Urol Nephrol 1980;14(3): 215–7.
8. Fang RH, Chen CF, Ma S. A new method for clitoroplasty in male-to-female sex reassignment surgery. Plast Reconstr Surg 1992;89(4):679–82 [discussion: 683].
9. Wangjiraniran B, Selvaggi G, Chokrungvaranont P, et al. Male-to-female vaginoplasty: Preecha's surgical technique. J Plast Surg Hand Surg 2015;49: 153–9.
10. Giraldo F, Esteva I, Bergero T, et al. Corona glans clitoroplasty and urethropreputial vestibuloplasty in male-to-female transsexuals: the vulval aesthetic refinement by the Andalusia gender team. Plast Reconstr Surg 2004;14:1543–50.
11. Mañero Vazquez I, García-Senosiain O, Labanca T, et al. Aesthetic refinement in the creation of the clitoris, its preputial hood, and labia minora in male-to female transsexual patients. Ann Plast Surg 2018;81(4):393–7.
12. Buncamper ME, van der Sluis WB, de Vries M, et al. Penile inversion vaginoplasty with or without additional full-thickness skin graft: to graft or not to graft? Plast Reconstr Surg 2017;139(3):649e–56e.
13. Watanyusakul S. A new method for sensate clitoris and labia minora reconstruction in male-to-female sex reassignment surgery. Paper Presented at the 27th Annual Scientific Meeting of The Royal College of Surgeons of Thailand, The Ambassador City Hotel, Pattaya, Thailand, 24-27 Dec 2002.
14. Watanyusakul S. The effectiveness of full thickness scrotal and groin skin graft vaginoplasty in MTF sex reassignment surgery. Paper presented at the 9th oriental society of aesthetic plastic surgery (OSAPS). The Shangri-La Hotel, Bangkok, 6–10 Dec 2004.

Metoidioplasty

Marta R. Bizic, MD, PhD[a,b,*], Borko Stojanovic, MD[a,c], Ivana Joksic, MD, PhD[a,d], Miroslav L. Djordjevic, MD, PhD[a,c]

KEYWORDS

• Clitoris • Transmen • Transmale • Metodioplasty • Urethroplasty • Neophallus • Reconstruction

KEY POINTS

- Metoidioplasty is a time-saving procedure that offers masculine external genitals.
- Metoidioplasty can be combined with the removal of female reproductive organs and vaginectomy as a one-stage procedure.
- Metoidioplasty, combined with urethral reconstruction using vascularized hairless skin flaps and mucosal grafts, provides standing micturition to the patients.
- Neophallus created by metoidioplasty has full erogenous sensation and provides erection and orgasm during sexual intercourse.
- Belgrade metoidioplasty presents an excellent solution with maximal lengthening, voiding while standing, and satisfying esthetic appearance in one-stage repair.

INTRODUCTION

Creation of a phallus in transmen still poses great challenges for surgeons performing these surgeries even after more than 50 years of using different surgical approaches to satisfy patients' needs for functionality and esthetics of their new male genitals.[1] Unfortunately, there are still no optimal replacements for erectile, fascial, and urethral tissue that would provide ideal male genitals.[2] Preferably, creation of a neophallus should be performed as a single-stage procedure, providing tactile and erogenous sensation and functional neourethra that will enable voiding while standing and causing minor morbidity and scarring of the donor site.[3] Patients' wishes regarding neophallus length and urinary and sexual function should be considered when proposing a surgical approach, because an ideal procedure does not exist.[4] There are 2 main surgical approaches for genital reconstruction for transmale patients: phalloplasty and metoidioplasty. Phalloplasty involves creation of the neophallus from extragenital tissue and is usually performed as a multistage procedure. Phalloplasty involves the use of pedicled or free flaps with neurovascular anastomosis. One of the main advantages of phalloplasty is the creation of an adult-sized phallus that will allow the patient to engage in penetrative intercourse once a penile prosthesis has been implanted. Metoidioplasty includes creation of a small phallus from a hormonally enlarged clitoris in transmen, with or without urethral reconstruction and scrotoplasty with testicular prostheses implantation. It is sometimes combined with hysterectomy with bilateral salpingo-oophorectomy (BSO) and colpectomy or performed as a second-stage surgery after bilateral mastectomy ("top surgery") and hysterectomy with BSO.[5] Metoidioplasty provides "male-looking genitalia" to the patient, as is

Disclosure Statement: The authors have no disclosures to identify.

This work is supported by Ministry of Education, Science and Technological Development, Republic of Serbia, Projects No. 175048 and 173046.

[a] Belgrade Center for Genitourinary Reconstructive Surgery, Kumodraska 241v, Belgrade 11000, Serbia; [b] Department of Urology, Faculty of Medicine, University of Belgrade, Tirsova 10, Belgrade 11000, Serbia; [c] Faculty of Medicine, University of Belgrade, Belgrade, Serbia; [d] Clinic for Gynecology and Obstetrics "Narodni Front", Kraljice Natalije 62, Belgrade 11000, Serbia

* Corresponding author. Department of Urology, Faculty of Medicine, University of Belgrade, Tirsova 10, Belgrade 11000, Serbia.

E-mail address: martabizic@uromiros.com

Urol Clin N Am 46 (2019) 555–566
https://doi.org/10.1016/j.ucl.2019.07.009
0094-0143/19/© 2019 Elsevier Inc. All rights reserved.

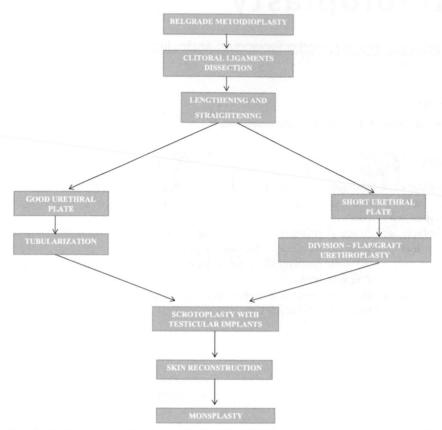

```
                    BELGRADE METOIDIOPLASTY

                    CLITORAL LIGAMENTS
                        DISSECTION

                    LENGTHENING AND
                      STRAIGHTENING


   GOOD URETHRAL                          SHORT URETHRAL
      PLATE                                    PLATE

   TUBULARIZATION                        DIVISION – FLAP/GRAFT
                                            URETHROPLASTY


                    SCROTOPLASTY WITH
                   TESTICULAR IMPLANTS

                    SKIN RECONSTRUCTION

                       MONSPLASTY
```

Fig. 1. Algorithm for Belgrade metoidioplasty. Maximal lengthening and straightening of the clitoris with urethral reconstruction and scrotoplasty in one-stage surgery.

suggested by its name, from the Greek words "meta" meaning toward and "oidion" meaning male genitalia.[6] Metoidioplasty can be considered for patients who do not wish to have multiple surgical interventions in order to complete their transition or for those who do not wish to have visible scars outside of the genital area.

This article presents the most recent updates of surgical techniques for metoidioplasty as well as outcomes and complications.

METOIDIOPLASTY

Metoidioplasty, as a less invasive variant of phalloplasty, is one of the most popular surgical approaches in male genitalia creation for transmen. Familiarity with female and male anatomy and embryology is essential in gender-affirmation surgeries (GAS). Embryologically, penis and clitoris develop from the same ambisexual tubercle, depending on the presence/absence of the androgens. One of the most important differences is that in women, the urethra becomes separated from the clitoris. Recent studies on human cadavers and magnetic resonance studies brought into light

new knowledge about the clitoris and its innervation and role in female sexual response.[7–9]

The main goal of metoidioplasty is to give the patient male-looking genitalia and the possibility to void in standing position.[10] The neophallus created by metoidioplasty is sensate and can achieve an erection during arousal, although less rigid than in cis-males, while penetration during sexual intercourse is impossible for most of the patients.[11] Metoidioplasty is ideal for thin- to medium-built transmen without mons pubis adiposity. Mons pubis adiposity with poor clitoral growth after hormonal therapy can be a limiting factor for standing micturition.[12]

PREOPERATIVE ASSESSMENT

Patients undergoing GAS are required to have spent at least 12 months on hormonal substitution therapy according to the Standards of Care of World Professional Association for Transgender Health.[13] Local use of a dihydrotestosterone gel in combination with a vacuum pump for a period of 3 months before metoidioplasty is recommended to secure better postoperative results.[11]

Before proceeding with metoidioplasty, the operating surgeon must have a detailed knowledge of the clitoral and vulvar anatomy. The clitoris is a female erectile organ that projects from the pubic bones into the mons fatty tissue, then descends and folds back, creating a boomerang-like shape.[7] The clitoral glans and prepuce are the only visible parts of the clitoris that lie on the upper apex of the vestibule. The prepuce is formed from the fused labia minora anterior borders at the level of the clitoral glans. In transmen, clitoris is enlarged due to hormonal therapy, so one part of the clitoral body becomes visible as well. According to different studies, preoperative size of the hypertrophied clitoris may vary from 2.5 to 4.6 cm.[4,14] There are 2 corpora cavernosa that diverge and form 2 crura, which are attached to the pubic bones. The clitoral body measures 1 to 2 cm in width and 0.5 to 3.5 cm in length, whereas the crura, the internal and hidden parts of the corpora, measure 5 to 9 cm in length.[15] Suspensory ligaments with their superficial and deep portion hold the clitoris firmly attached to the pubic symphysis and fascia of the mons pubis, keeping it curved and preventing its straightening during arousal.[7] Clitoral innervation is mainly based on the dorsal clitoral nerve as the final branch of the pudendal nerve, which plays an important role in sexual response.[15,16] The cavernous nerves supply the clitoral erectile tissue; signaling between dorsal clitoral nerve and cavernous nerves, through the communicating branches, results in clitoral swelling.[15] These findings point out the importance of cautious dissection of these nerves during clitoral surgery in order to prevent their intraoperative injury as well as postoperative consequences.[7] Vascularization of the clitoris originates from the branches of the pudendal artery.

Labia minora are paired, hairless mucocutaneous folds, rich in nerve endings and sensory receptors. Their dermis is rich in elastic fibers and small blood vessels, making it similar to the corpus spongiosum of the penis. Vascularization of labia minora originates from internal and external pudendal arteries, which provide very good vascularization to the tissue when there is a need to mobilize the flap for urethral and neophallic skin reconstruction.[14] Labia minora are innervated along their edge and inner side, with branches originating from internal pudendal nerve, ilioinguinal and genitofemoral nerves.[17] Awareness of these structural features of the clitoris and labia minora is of paramount significance in female to male GAS for preservation of sensation and sexual stimuli in the neophallus created by metoidioplasty. Labia majora are homologous to the scrotum in men; that is why they are used in scrotum reconstruction in masculinizing GAS.[7]

OPERATIVE TECHNIQUES

Durfee and Rowland were the first to report surgical penile substitution using a hypertrophied clitoris in transmale patients.[18,19] However, because the urethral plate was left intact, according to clitoral anatomy, the neophallus remained small and curved without the ability to allow for voiding in standing position. The original technique has been refined by Lebovic and Laub, releasing the ventral chordee of the clitoris and creating the neourethra out of the inner portion of labia minora starting from the tip of the clitoral glans but ending as a cul-de-sac at the base of the neophallus, which did not contribute to standing micturition to the patients.[6,18,20] Bouman's modification of the original technique included lengthening of the urethra to the tip of the clitoris using an anterior vaginal flap, but without clitoral release.[4,18] According to Hage and colleagues,[21] 99% of the patients from their study considered standing micturition as a priority after female-to-male genital reconstructive surgery.[4] Hage reported a modification of the original technique, characterized by urethral lengthening using urethral plate and labia minora skin flap.[18] In a long-term follow-up study on a sample of 70 patients, Hage and Turnhout concluded that an average 2.6 procedures were needed to achieve the ideal result in metoidoplasty.[22] In the light of continuous improvement of surgical techniques, Perovic and Djordjevic reported their first results on 22 transmen, with 77.27% success after their modification of the metoidioplasty procedure.[1] The surgical approach was based on the experience and good results in cases of severe hypospadias and differences of sexual development with penoscrotal transposition.[10,23]

Because urethral fistula is the most common postoperative complication in masculinizing genitoplasty by metoidioplasty, some patients do not wish to have several surgical procedures and decide to undergo simple metoidioplasty, which involves clitoral release and male-like appearance of external genitals without urethral reconstruction.[12] On the other hand, the patients who desire the urethral extension can choose metoidioplasty with urethral reconstruction. Ring metoidioplasty provides clitoral lengthening and straightening by suspensory ligaments dissection and urethral reconstruction using labia minora flaps and a long flap originating from the anterior vaginal wall.[24] Relatively high percentage of postoperative urethral complications (range from 10% to 26%) led to improvement of urethral reconstruction in transmen undergoing metoidioplasty, with the use of vascularized hairless skin flaps, free skin/mucosal grafts, and periurethral vaginal tissue.[4,10,25] In the last decade, several papers from Belgrade Team for Transgender Surgery were published related to advances of the original metoidioplasty technique. The latest iteration of the Belgrade metoidioplasty consists of maximal clitoral lengthening and straightening with complete urethral reconstruction and scrotoplasty with testicular prostheses insertion in one-stage surgery. This novel approach offers a neophallus of adequate length, ability of standing micturition, and an acceptable esthetic appearance of external male genitalia (**Fig. 1**).[5,10,12,25–27]

BELGRADE METOIDIOPLASTY
Clitoral Lengthening and Straightening

Clitoral lengthening and straightening are mostly performed as previously described. The patient is positioned in lithotomy position. Elasticated thigh-height stockings and low-molecular-weight heparin are used to minimize the risk of deep vein thrombosis. Antibiotic prophylaxis (vancomycin) is administered after anesthesia is introduced. A stay suture is placed through the clitoral glans and a circular incision is made between the outer and inner layer of clitoral prepuce, continuing downwards around the urethral plate and the urethral orifice. After clitoral degloving, the superficial and deep portion of the suspensory clitoral ligaments is dissected to enable clitoral straightening. In cases where the urethral plate is a limiting factor for complete clitoral straightening, additional lengthening and straightening is completed by dissection of the urethral plate, with careful dissection to prevent the injury of spongy tissue with subsequent bleeding.[26] Because of this radical dissection from the dorsal and ventral aspect of the clitoris, complete straightening and maximal lengthening of the clitoris are achieved. After this radical lengthening and straightening procedure, the potential gain in length ranges from 3 to 6 cm, depending on clitoral size before surgery.

Urethral Reconstruction

Urethral reconstruction is the key step in male genitalia reconstruction for transmen who pursue voiding while standing as a major goal. Urethroplasty modifications have resulted in decreased complication rates and increased patients' satisfaction after one-stage metoidioplasty with urethroplasty.[4,11,25,27] The reconstruction of the bulbar neourethra is very important, as the strongest urinary stream is at the point of the junction of the native urethral orifice and reconstructed neourethra. The novel technique includes the use of periurethral vaginal tissue for the bulbar urethra reconstruction. All suture lines are covered with bulbar muscles and surrounding vascularized tissue, as support and to prevent fistula formation. In lie with literature data and the authors' own experience, we do not use a long vaginal flap for urethral reconstruction, because the characteristics of vaginal mucosa (natural folds) can lead to higher postoperative complications.[10,24] Their refinements in urethroplasty in transmen offered several different techniques for the neophallic urethra reconstruction, and the choice is usually made during the dissection according to the patient's anatomy:

- *Urethral plate tubularization*: this is a simple technique that includes tubularization of the well-developed and elastic urethral plate over a silicone Foley catheter. All suture lines must be covered with vascularized tissue to prevent postoperative complications. Contraindication for this procedure could be short clitoral length after ligaments dissection (**Fig. 2**).
- *Flap urethroplasty*: this surgical approach includes urethral plate dissection at the glanular corona level and harvesting of the island dorsal clitoral skin flap that is transposed ventrally using a "buttonhole" maneuver and its tubularization over a silicone Foley catheter.[1] In cases where labia minora are very developed, the skin flap for the neophallic urethra reconstruction can be harvested also from the inner hairless side of the labia minora. Remaining genital skin is used for the neophallic shaft reconstruction.
- *Graft/flap urethroplasty*: this surgical procedure also includes dissection of the urethral plate to obtain maximum length of the neophallus. The "gap" after urethral plate dissection is usually filled using an oral mucosa graft, as a gold standard in urethral reconstruction.[4,10] Oral mucosa is tough, elastic, and resistant to many microorganisms, always available for harvesting in adequate length, and with minimal morbidity and scarring of the donor site. Oral mucosa has thin lamina propria and thick squamous epithelium that makes it very good grafting material for urethral reconstruction with insignificant retraction.[10,28] In patients with well-developed labia minora, a free skin graft can be harvested from the outer layer of labia minora, to lessen the morbidity of an additional donor site, with satisfying postoperative results (**Fig. 3**). The

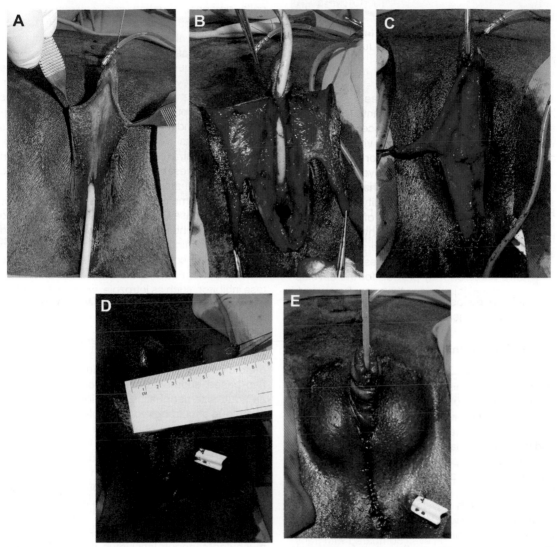

Fig. 2. (*A*) Preoperative appearance. Wide and well-developed urethral plate. (*B*) Urethral plate of adequate width is dissected and tubularized over a Foley catheter. (*C*) Vascularized subcutaneous flap is mobilized from the left labia minora to cover all suture lines to prevent urethral fistula. (*D*) Maximal length of the neophallus is achieved. (*E*) Appearance at the end of surgery with 2 testicular implants inserted into scrotum created out of both labia majora.

size of the graft depends on the size of the gap left by urethral plate dissection and usually varies from 3 to 6 cm. The graft is positioned on the corporal bodies and quilted to ensure its survival and to prevent hematoma formation and graft disruption. In this fashion, the dorsal wall of the urethra is formed. The ventral wall of the neourethra can be obtained using either longitudinal dorsal clitoral skin flap transposed ventrally by the buttonhole maneuver or by harvesting the inner hairless skin flap from the labia minora over a silicone urethral stent of 12-14 Ch. The decision is usually made according to the anatomy of the patient

and abundancy of the available skin. Whenever possible, it is recommended to use the inner surface of labia minora, because it is elastic and hairless, and is proved to have a very low complication rate. All suture lines are covered with well-vascularized tissue to prevent fistula formation[25] (**Fig. 4**).

Glans and Skin Reconstruction

Glanular urethra is reconstructed by formation of 2 parallel glans wings and their tubularization. The neophallic shaft reconstruction is performed using the available clitoral and labial skin to make a

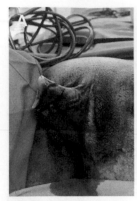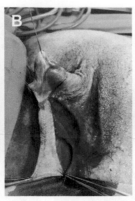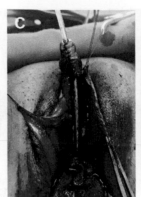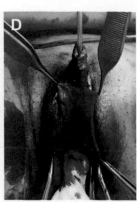

Fig. 3. (*A*) Preoperative appearance. Design for skin graft harvesting from the outer layer of left labia minora. (*B*) Harvested hairless skin graft. (*C*) Neourethra is reconstructed up to the clitoral tip by glans tubularization and labia minora skin graft, together with the labia minora skin flap, over a silicone catheter. (*D*) All suture lines are covered with vascularized tissue to prevent fistula formation.

well-defined penoscrotal angle to provide male-looking external genitals.[10]

Scrotoplasty with Testicular Prostheses Implantation

Because colpocleisis is performed, and vaginal vault completely obliterated with circular resorbable stitches, perineum is created as in men. Scrotoplasty is performed by joining labia majora in the midline and implantation of silicone testicular prostheses of appropriate size for the patients' anatomy using 2 symmetric incisions above the labia majora.[10]

In patients with developed mons pubis, additional monsplasty with the resection of the adipose tissue can be important to secure voiding in standing position by bringing up the newly formed male genitals.

Postoperative Care

A suprapubic cystostomy tube is introduced to the bladder, and broad-spectrum antibiotics (ceftriaxone and metronidazole) and anticholinergic drugs are administered while the catheter is in place. A self-adherent dressing is used for the neophallus for 10 days. Urethral stent is removed 10 days after the surgery, whereas suprapubic catheter is removed 3 weeks after the surgery. Whenever possible and when patients are available for a control examination, the voiding cystourethrogram is performed before removal of suprapubic catheter. Postoperatively, patients are advised to continue the use of vacuum pump for a period of 6 months postoperatively in combination with phosphodiesterase type-5 inhibitors to prevent retraction of the neophallus.[29]

METOIDIOPLASTY COMBINED/FOLLOWED BY TOTAL PHALLOPLASTY

According to the available literature data, between 1% and 24% of patients who underwent metoidioplasty as GAS, continue on to have a flap-based augmentation phalloplasty to obtain an adult-size neophallus.[4] The ideal phalloplasty technique should be reproducible and performed in one stage, with a phallus of a size adequate to engage in penetrative sexual intercourse, with preserved tactile and erogenous sensation and ability of standing micturition. So far, none of the described techniques could satisfy all the requirements for an ideal phallus. There are different techniques available now; the most commonly used are radial forearm free flap and musculocutaneous latissimus dorsi (MLD) flap.[2] The authors' Center prefers the use of the MLD flap, because its anatomy can be relied on to meet the esthetic and functional requirements of neophallus reconstruction.[10,30]

In patients who previously underwent the metoidioplasty procedure, a neophallus of adequate dimensions for the patient's anatomy is fashioned from the nondominant side of the body, with its pedicle, and transposed to the infrapubic region where the microvascular anastomosis is performed between the thoracodorsal artery and superficial femoral artery and thoracodorsal vein and saphenous vein.[10,31,32] At the end of the first stage of the surgery, the small phallus created by metoidioplasty remains at the base of the MLD neophallus.

The second stage of phalloplasty is usually performed after 6 to 9 months after the first stage. During the second stage, the small neophallus is incorporated and further urethral reconstruction

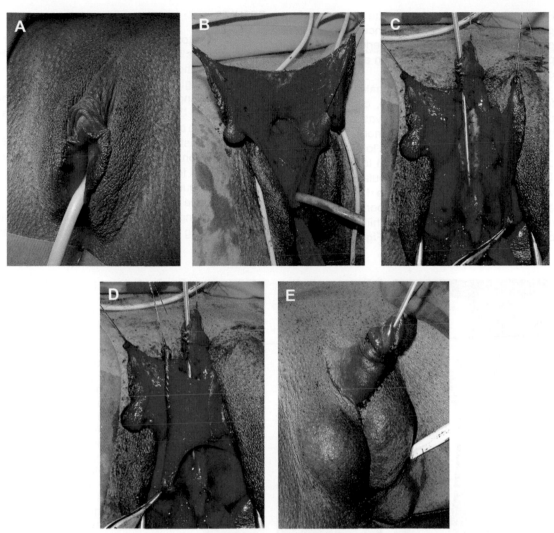

Fig. 4. (*A*) Preoperative appearance. The Foley catheter is introduced into the bladder. (*B*) After clitoral degloving, clitoral suspensory ligaments are dissected to lengthen the clitoris. Labia minora are mobilized. (*C*) Urethral plate is dissected at the level of glanular corona, to lengthen and straighten the clitoris. The gap is filled with oral mucosa graft quilted to the clitoral body by interrupted monofilament resorbable sutures. (*D*) Labia minora flap is mobilized with abundant vascular pedicle. (*E*) Outcome at the end of surgery. Neophallic shaft is reconstructed using available genital skin. Two testicular prostheses are inserted into the scrotum created from both labia majora.

is performed using oral mucosa grafts harvested from both inner cheeks and lower lip to obtain a suitable size neourethral plate. Previously, the ventral side of the neophallus is opened in the midline to create the "bed" for oral mucosa placement. The grafts are then quilted to the ventral side of the neophallus by interrupted resorbable monofilament sutures starting from the small phallus to the tip of the glans. In postoperative recovery, patients are instructed to treat oral mucosa grafts with moisturizing creams to prevent shrinkage and scarring. Tubularization of the neourethral plate is usually performed 3 to 6 months later to

form the phallic urethra, according to the Johanson principle of staged urethroplasty.[10,33]

The third stage of phalloplasty includes insertion of a penile prosthesis to enable the rigidity necessary for penetrative sexual intercourse. There are 2 types of penile prostheses that are available on the market: semirigid and inflatable. Because the girth of the neophallus created from MLD is sufficient to accept 2 penile prosthesis cylinders, it allows better rigidity and stability of the neophallus. The approach for the prostheses insertion is usually infrapubic using a semilunar incision at the dorsal side of the neophallus.

Hegar dilators are used to create the space for penile prosthesis cylinders. Once placed, the prosthesis is anchored to the periosteum of the pubic bone to prevent protrusion and movement of the cylinders.[10]

In cases where the MLD flap phalloplasty is performed as a primary procedure, clitoral urethral plate is left intact, whereas all vascularized and hairless tissues (both labia minora and dorsal clitoral skin) are used to create a long neourethral channel starting from the natural female meatus. The neourethra is formed by tubularization of the vascularized flaps over a silicone 12-14 Ch Foley catheter, which is then incorporated into the neophallus.[10,32] Second and third stages are performed as described earlier (**Fig. 5**).

RESULTS

The gain in clitoral length under testosterone therapy in patients undergoing metoidioplasty can be between 2.5 and 4.6 cm, adding up to the average neophallic length of 4 to 10 cm in maximal extension, depending on the initial measurements of the clitoris.[2,4,10,30,34] Dissection of the urethral plate plays the crucial role in clitoral lengthening.[25] Urethral reconstruction using an oral mucosa graft in combination with vascularized hairless skin flaps provides for upright voiding, which is one of the main requirements of patients undergoing female-to-male GAS.[21,25] Creation of a normal penoscrotal angle is another prerequisite that will enable voiding while standing in patients after

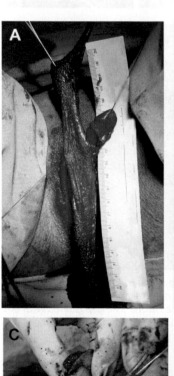
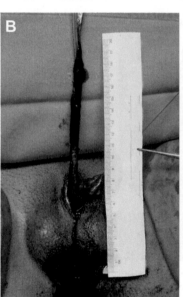
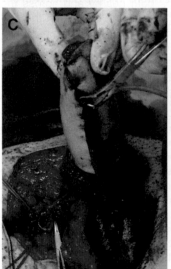
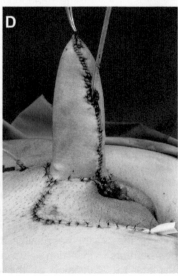

Fig. 5. (*A*) Long pedicled flap from both labia minora and dorsal clitoral skin is harvested for urethral reconstruction. (*B*) Vascularized labia minora and clitoral skin flap is tubularized over the silicone Foley catheter for additional urethroplasty. Silicone testicular prostheses are implanted in scrotums created out of labia majora. (*C*) Placement of the neophallus in the genital region and microvascular anastomosis with recipient blood vessels of the right leg. Neocreated urethra is long enough to reach distal third of the neophallus. (*D*) Outcome at the end of surgery: neophallus is fixed in the anatomically adequate position after microvascular anastomosis. Clitoris is fixed at the base of the neophallus. Urethral opening is at the distal third of the neophallus facilitating upright voiding.

one-stage metoidioplasty[10] (**Fig. 6**). Additional monsplasty provides better visibility of the neophallus and secures the standing micturition.

According to the literature data, metoidioplasty is performed as a single-stage procedure in more than 80% of the studies, with a high satisfaction rate regarding esthetic appearance of the new male genitalia (77.3%–100%).[35] Most patients succeed to void while standing (87%–100%) after metoidioplasty with urethral reconstruction. Compared with flap-based phalloplasty techniques, metoidioplasty can be considered as a less technically demanding and time-saving procedure, with shorter hospital stay and subsequent treatment expenses.[4]

COMPLICATIONS

Overall complication rates after metoidioplasty vary from 10% to 37% according to different literature data and are mainly related to the urethra.[4] Complications after metoidioplasty can be divided into minor (no need for surgical repair) and major (require surgical repair). Minor complications such as urinary tract infection (UTI) and burning during voiding can be treated with antibiotics. Temporary spraying and dribbling usually stops spontaneously after internal sutures dissolve. In most cases, urethral fistula can close spontaneously, without the need for surgical correction.

Major complications can be divided into urethral (more common) and nonurethral. The most common urethral complications are urethral fistula and urethral stricture. According to literature data, urethral fistula has a higher rate when compared with urethral strictures. The most common site for urethral fistula formation is at the junction of the native and reconstructed urethra, because urinary stream is the strongest there and because of possible diminished vascular perfusion of the flaps used in urethral reconstruction.[36] Also, the reconstructed urethra is of a smaller lumen than the native female urethra, which can cause relative obstruction of the urinary stream and subsequent leaking of urine through the suture lines.[37] Urethral stricture is a less common complication, and depending on the localization, meatoplasty or urethroplasty can be performed. Persistent vaginal cavity, as a less common complication, usually presents with prolonged urine dribbling and UTI. It is mainly associated with a small internal fistula and can be solved by perineal approach and complete vaginal cavity removal and obliteration with urethroplasty.[37] Nonurethral complications that require surgical repair are testicular prostheses displacement or testicular prosthesis rejection, when a new implant can be reinserted and fixed in the right position. In some cases with a lack of genital skin, the neophallic shaft remains short, so shaft reconstruction can be performed to obtain a better result using VY or Z plasty.

PERSONAL EXPERIENCE

Between April 2002 and August 2018, 793 patients underwent one-stage metoidioplasty in the authors' Center with the mean age of 33 years (range: 18–62 years). Vaginectomy was not performed in 2 patients, per their request. After clitoral degloving, metoidioplasty was performed by completely lengthening and straightening the clitoris by division of clitoral ligaments on the dorsal side. Urethral plate had to be dissected in 89.16% patients to provide complete straightening of the clitoris. Urethral reconstruction was performed in all patients using different operative techniques, according to the patients' anatomy, to obtain the best possible result (**Table 1**).

Median neophallic length in maximal extension was 5.6 cm (range: 4–10 cm) in the series. Erection of the neophallus was present in all the patients with completely preserved sensation and sexual stimulation. Urethroplasty was successful for 89.79% of the patients and did not require any additional surgeries. Buccal mucosa graft in combination with labia minora flap was the most commonly used technique, with a success rate of 90.82% in the series. The urethroplasty technique with the highest success rate was the labia minora graft and flap technique, with a success rate of 92.31%, and was performed in 52 patients (see **Table 1**).

Overall complications occurred in 46.8% of patients in the authors' sample. Minor complications

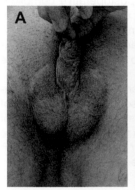 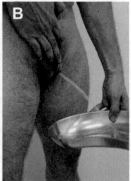

Fig. 6. (*A*) Outcome 2 years after the surgery. Adequate position of the testicular prostheses and satisfying appearance of the male external genitalia with normal penoscrotal angle. (*B*) The goal of metoidioplasty achieved: micturition in standing position.

Table 1
Belgrade urethroplasty results

Type of Urethroplasty	No of Cases/%	Fistula, No/%	Stricture, No/%	Success Rate, No/%
Tubularization urethroplasty	86/10.84	8/9.3%	1/1.16%	77/89.53%
Onlay flap urethroplasty	42/5.30	6/14.29%	2/4.76%	34/80.95%
BMG with clitoral skin flap	79/9.96	9/11.39%	2/2.53%	68/86.08%
BMG with labia minora flap	534/67.34	43/8.05%	6/1.12%	485/90.82%
Labia minora graft/flap	52/6.56	4/7.69%	0/0%	48/92.31%
Total	793/100	70/8.83%	11/1.39%	712/89.79%

Abbreviation: BMG, buccal mucosa graft.

occurred in 17.7% of patients, such as dribbling and spraying after voiding, and resolved spontaneously, whereas UTI required prolonged antibiotic administration. Complications that required surgical repair occurred in 29.1% of the patients and were solved by minor surgical revisions, 6 to 12 months after primary surgery. The most common complication requiring surgical repair was the vaginal remnant that occurred in 98 patients (**Table 2**).

Most of the patients (94.7%) were satisfied with the appearance of their new male genitals. All patients from the authors' sample were able to void while standing, which was the main goal of one-stage metoidioplasty with urethral extension (see **Fig. 6**B). The real percentage of the patients experiencing postoperative complications might be higher, as some patients could have been referred to other centers. In 14% of the patients who required further neophalloplasty, one of the available phalloplasty techniques was used.

SUMMARY

The need for GAS is increasing. The ideal technique that will encompass all characteristics for a perfect genitalia reconstruction is still missing. There are gold standards, but still all features are not achieved.

Metoidioplasty, as a variant of phalloplasty, can be a method of choice for male genitalia reconstruction in patients who require male-like genitalia and adequately enlarged clitoris after hormonal therapy and desire to void while standing and to obtain satisfactory esthetic appearance and sexual function in a one-stage surgery and in whom vaginal penetration is not of the utmost importance. Metoidioplasty is a safe and time-saving procedure with minimal hospitalization and low postoperative complications rate. Advanced urethral reconstruction with oral mucosa graft and labia minora flap provides excellent results and enables real lengthening of the urethra to provide voiding while standing.

One of the main advantages of the metoidioplasty is minimal local scarring and absence of the stigma to the patients. The main drawback of the metoidioplasty is the neophallus of small size and girth, inadequate for the vaginal penetration during sexual intercourse.

Table 2
Complication rate after metoidioplasty with urethral reconstruction

Complication	Number of Cases/%	Treatment
Dribbling/ Spraying	109/13.7%	No
Urinary tract infection	32/4%	Antibiotic therapy
Urethral stricture	11/1.4%	Stricture repair
Urethral fistula	70/8.8%	Fistula closure
Testicular implant rejection	14/1.8%	New insertion
Testicular implant displacement	37/4.7%	Replacement
Perineal cyst/ vaginal remnant	98/12.4%	Excision and obliteration with urethroplasty

REFERENCES

1. Perovic SV, Djordjevic ML. Metoidioplasty: a variant of phalloplasty in female transsexuals. BJU Int 2003;92(9):981–5.

2. Morrison SD, Chen ML, Crane CN. An overview of female-to-male gender-confirming surgery. Nat Rev Urol 2017;14(8):486–500.

3. Hage JJ, De Graaf FH. Addressing the ideal requirements by free flap phalloplasty: some reflections on refinements of technique. Microsurgery 1993;14(9): 592–8.

4. Hadj-Moussa M, Agarwal S, Ohl DA, et al. Masculinizing genital gender confirmation surgery. Sex Med Rev 2019;7(1):141–55.

5. Stojanovic B, Bizic M, Bencic M, et al. One-stage gender-confirmation surgery as a viable surgical procedure for female-to-male transsexuals. J Sex Med 2017;14(5):741–6.

6. Lebovic GS, Laub DR. Metoidioplasty. In: Ehrlich RM, Alter GJ, editors. Reconstructive and plastic surgery of the external genitalia. Philadelphia: WB Saunders; 1999. p. 355–60.

7. Stojanovic B, Djordjevic ML. Anatomy of the clitoris and its impact on neophalloplasty (metoidioplasty) in female transgenders. Clin Anat 2015;28(3): 368–75.

8. Baskin L, Shen J, Sinclair A, et al. Development of the human penis and clitoris. Differentiation 2018; 103:74–85.

9. Agarwal MD, Resnick EL, Mhuircheartaigh JN, et al. MR Imaging of the female perineum: clitoris, labia, and introitus. Magn Reson Imaging Clin N Am 2017;25(3):435–55.

10. Djordjevic ML. Novel surgical techniques in female to male gender confirming surgery. Transl Androl Urol 2018;7(4):628–38.

11. Djordjevic ML, Stanojevic D, Bizic M, et al. Metoidioplasty as a single stage sex reassignment surgery in female transsexuals: Belgrade experience. J Sex Med 2009;6(5):1306–13.

12. Bowers ML, Stojanovic B, Bizic M. Female-to-male gender affirmation metoidioplasty. In: Salgado CJ, Monstrey SJ, Djordjevic ML, editors. Gender affirmation: medical and surgical perspectives. New York: Thieme Medical Publishers Inc; 2017. p. 109–18.

13. The World Professional Association for Transgender Health. Standards of Care for the health of transsexual, transgender and gender non-conforming people. 7th version. 2011. Available at: http://www.wpath.org. Accessed October 30, 2018.

14. Vukadinovic V, Stojanovic B, Majstorovic M, et al. The role of clitoral anatomy in female to male sex reassignment surgery. ScientificWorldJournal 2014; 2014:437378.

15. Mazloomdoost D, Pauls RN. A comprehensive review of the clitoris and its role in female sexual function. Sex Med Rev 2015;3(4):245–63.

16. Baskin LS, Erol A, Li YW, et al. Anatomical studies of the human clitoris. J Urol 1999;162(3 Pt 2): 1015–20.

17. Clerico C, Lari A, Mojallal A, et al. Anatomy and aesthetics of the labia minora: the ideal vulva? Aesthetic Plast Surg 2017;41(3):714–9.

18. Hage JJ. Metaidoioplasty: an alternative phalloplasty technique in transsexuals. Plast Reconstr Surg 1996;97(1):161–7.

19. Durfee R, Rowland W. Penile substitution with clitoral enlargement and urethral transfer. In: Laub DR, Gandy P, editors. Proceedings of the second interdisciplinary symposium on gender dysphoria syndrome. Palo Alto (CA): Stanford University Press; 1973. p. 181–3.

20. Laub DR, Eicher W, Laub DR, et al. Penis construction in female-to-male transsexuals. In: Eicher W, Kubli F, Herms V, editors. Plastic surgery in the sexually handicapped. Berlin: Springer; 1989. p. 113–28.

21. Hage JJ, Bout CA, Bloem JJ, et al. Phalloplasty in female-to-male transsexuals: what do our patients ask for? Ann Plast Surg 1993;30(4): 323–6.

22. Hage JJ, van Turnhout AA. Long-term outcome of metaidoioplasty in 70 female-to-male transsexuals. Ann Plast Surg 2006;57(3):312–6.

23. Djordjevic ML, Majstorovic M, Stanojevic D, et al. Combined buccal mucosa graft and dorsal penile skin flap for repair of severe hypospadias. Urology 2008;71(5):821–5.

24. Takamatsu A, Harashina T. Labial ring flap: a new flap for metaidoioplasty in female-to-male transsexuals. J Plast Reconstr Aesthet Surg 2009;62: 318–25.

25. Djordjevic ML, Bizic MR. Comparison of two different methods for urethral lengthening in female to male (metoidioplasty) surgery. J Sex Med 2013;10: 1431–8.

26. Djordjevic ML, Stojanovic B. Metoidioplasty. In: Tran TA, Panthaki ZJ, Hoballah JJ, et al, editors. Operative dictations in plastic and reconstructive surgery. Cham (Switzerland): Springer International Publishing AG; 2017. p. 573–7.

27. Djordjevic ML, Bizic M, Stanojevic D, et al. Urethral Lengthening in metoidioplasty (female-to-male sex reassignment surgery) by combined buccal mucosa graft and labia minora flap. Urology 2009;74(2): 349–53.

28. Markiewicz MR, Lukose MA, Margarone JE 3rd, et al. The oral mucosa graft: a systematic review. J Urol 2007;178(2):387–94.

29. Djordjevic ML, Bizic MR, Stanojevic D. Phalloplasty in female-to-male transsexuals. In: Djordjevic M, Santucci R, editors. Penile reconstructive surgery. Saarbrucken (Germany): LAP Lambert Academic Publishing; 2012. p. 279–304.

30. Bizic MR, Stojanovic B, Djordjevic ML. Genital reconstruction for the transgendered individual. J Pediatr Urol 2017;13(5):446–52.

31. Djordjevic ML, Bumbasirevic MZ, Krstic Z, et al. Severe penile injuries in children and adolescents: reconstruction modalities and outcomes. Urology 2014;83:465–70.

32. Djordjevic ML, Bencic M, Kojovic V, et al. Musculocutaneous latissimus dorsi flap for phalloplasty in female to male gender affirmation surgery. World J Urol 2019. https://doi.org/10.1007/s00345-019-02641-w.

33. Johanson B. Reconstruction of the male urethra in strictures. Application of the buried intact epithelium technic. Acta Chir Scand 1953;176(Suppl 176):1–89.

34. Morrison SD, Shakir A, Vyas KS, et al. Phalloplasty: a review of techniques and outcomes. Plast Reconstr Surg 2016;138(3):594–615.

35. Frey JD, Poudrier G, Chiodo MV, et al. An update on genital reconstruction options for the female-to-male transgender patient: a review of the literature. Plast Reconstr Surg 2017;139(3):728–37.

36. Rohrmann D, Jakse G. Urethroplasty in female-to-male transsexuals. Eur Urol 2003;44(5):611–4.

37. Nikolavsky D, Hughes M, Zhao LC. Urologic complications after phalloplasty or metoidioplasty. Clin Plast Surg 2018;45(3):425–35.

Single-Stage Phalloplasty

Mang L. Chen, MD[a],*, Bauback Safa, MD[b]

KEYWORDS

- Single stage • Phalloplasty • Gender-affirming surgery • Scrotoplasty • Urethroplasty

KEY POINTS

- Single-stage phalloplasty with urethral lengthening can be reliably and expeditiously performed by microsurgeons and a reconstructive urologist working simultaneously.
- Understanding the techniques used during phalloplasty enhances the surgeon's ability to recognize and repair complications that arise, the most common of which are urethral fistulas and strictures.
- Fistulas will often heal spontaneously. Strictures almost always require surgery.

INTRODUCTION

Transmasculine individuals seeking genitourinary gender-affirming surgery (GUGAS) as treatment of gender dysphoria frequently desire phalloplasty, arguably "the most complete genitoperineal transformation."[1] Phalloplasty may be modified by individualized surgical goals but often includes vaginectomy, full-length urethroplasty, and scrotoplasty. Staging of these surgeries varies from surgeon to surgeon. Despite the moniker "single-stage phalloplasty," the operation typically involves 2 stages: phalloplasty with vaginectomy, scrotoplasty, and urethral lengthening, with their associated procedures, followed by penile and/or testicular prostheses roughly 9 to 12 months later. Some surgeons will further "stage" phalloplasty by dividing the urologic portions (vaginectomy, scrotoplasty, urethroplasty) from the microsurgical portions (neophallus creation) of the procedure. The first stage of phalloplasty may therefore be the urologic components followed later by the phalloplasty, or vice versa. With multiple variations in staging definitions, single-stage phalloplasty is generally defined as the combined urologic and microsurgical portions of the procedure (glansplasty, phalloplasty, full-length urethroplasty, vaginectomy, scrotoplasty, and perineal reconstruction), without implant insertion.

Phalloplasty involves a microsurgical team and the reconstructive urologist. Both teams work simultaneously: the microsurgeons harvest the flap, dissect the cutaneous nerve or nerves and vascular pedicle, and create the pars pendulans (PP) urethra, neophallus, and glans. The urologist simultaneously performs the vaginectomy, pars fixa (PF) urethroplasty, dorsal nerve dissection, and scrotoplasty with perineal reconstruction. A recent metaanalysis of single-stage phalloplasty studies with full-length urethroplasty demonstrates a complication rate of approximately 90% with a urethral complication rate of roughly 50%.[2] Monstrey and colleagues[3] performed 287 single-stage phalloplasties and had an overall complication rate of 77% and a urethral complication rate of 43%, indicating that lower complication rates are achievable in high-volume, specialized centers. Given the urologic complications associated with full-length urethroplasty in patients desiring phalloplasty, some patients are not candidates for, or choose not to undergo, urethroplasty. Most, however, have the primary surgical goal of standing micturition. In this review, the authors describe single-stage phalloplasty from initial consultation to the postoperative setting, followed by analysis and discussion of the urologic complications.

Disclosures: None.
[a] 45 Castro Street, Suite 111, San Francisco, CA 94114, USA; [b] The Buncke Clinic, 45 Castro Street, Suite 121, San Francisco, CA 94114, USA
* Corresponding author.
E-mail address: mang@gurecon.com

Urol Clin N Am 46 (2019) 567–580
https://doi.org/10.1016/j.ucl.2019.07.010
0094-0143/19/© 2019 Elsevier Inc. All rights reserved.

INITIAL CONSULTATION

Most patients will have already established hormonal and mental health care and will likely have undergone mastectomy and hysterectomy by the time they seek genitourinary GUGAS. The World Professional Association for Transgender Health Standards of Care outlines the prerequisites for GUGAS that are followed and tailored for each potential phalloplasty patient.[4] During the phalloplasty consultation, the patient's surgical goals are assessed; flap and urologic options are discussed, including their associated risks and benefits, and the postoperative course is reviewed. Many patients desire physiologic-appearing and functional male external genitalia with an average-sized phallus, a pouchlike scrotum, the ability to void while standing, and the future ability to achieve penetrative intercourse. In the authors' experience, the radial forearm (RF) free flap is most likely to help patients achieve these goals. Sensation is an important surgical goal, the quality of which depends on the flap chosen, in general resulting in tactile and/or erogenous sensation in more than 90% of patients.[5] Microsurgeons therefore favor flaps like the anterolateral thigh (ALT) and RF because they have distinct sensory nerves (lateral femoral cutaneous nerve; lateral and medial antebrachial cutaneous nerves) that can be coapted to the dorsal nerve of the clitoris and/or the ilioinguinal nerve. Patients who do not care about standing micturition may forego urethroplasty altogether, and some may or may not desire vaginectomy. The RF free flap phalloplasty, with glansplasty, full-length urethroplasty, neuroplasty, vaginectomy, scrotoplasty, and perineal reconstruction all done in a single stage, is the most commonly desired surgical combination.

It is important for the surgeons to thoroughly review the past medical and surgical history, as well as a past urologic history, in addition to assessing the surgical goals. Patients who have a history of kidney stones may benefit from preoperative imaging to determine the status of their disease. It is easier and safer to surgically treat stones through a short native urethra than a long neourethra. Patients with a hematologic history may have an increased risk of flap failure or surgical site bleeding or hematoma. Patients with autoimmune diseases requiring chronic immunosuppression may not be candidates for GUGAS altogether, because these medications have an adverse effect on wound healing. A thorough review of the patient's social history is also vital because inhalational drugs like cigarettes and marijuana can be detrimental to flap healing.[6] The authors require patients to stop inhalation products as soon as possible and for a minimum of 3 months before any surgical procedures.

The urologic portion of the physical examination involves assessment of the mons pubis, the labia minora and majora, the clitoris, and any abdominal scars. Patients with lower abdominal scars may make placing a suprapubic (SP) tube difficult, and patients with a ptotic mons may require monsplasty before phalloplasty. The microsurgical component of the examination involves a thorough assessment of the donor site (RF and the ALT). An Allen's test helps confirm collateral blood flow to the hand via the ulnar artery, and thigh thickness assessment can determine the feasibility of its use as a flap. Thick thighs are less favorable because they preclude the ability to create a PP urethra at the time of phalloplasty, necessitating possible staged urethral reconstruction with its associated problems. Some thighs are too thick altogether, even for a single tube phalloplasty. Also, the microsurgeon should avoid acute thinning of the ALT flap because the lateral femoral cutaneous nerve travels on the deep aspect of the flap; acute thinning therefore potentially denervates some or the entire flap. On rare occasion, patients may be candidates for a combined ALT and RF flap phalloplasty, whereby the ALT flap forms the neophallus and the RF free flap forms the urethra.[7,8] A suggested body mass index (BMI) for patients seeking phalloplasty is less than 35 kg/m^2, although the authors do not have a strict BMI cutoff. A single-stage ALT phalloplasty with urethroplasty is usually only considered for patients with minimal fat on their donor site thigh.[9]

With multiple options to choose from, determining the correct donor site for phalloplasty and the associated procedures is very much a shared decision. This decision is based on the patient's goals, medical comorbidities, anatomy, socioeconomic circumstances, and other individualized factors. For example, some patients interested in phalloplasty with full-length urethroplasty may not desire vaginectomy. These patients should therefore be counseled about the higher risk of urethrocutaneous and urethrovaginal fistulas with this specific combination.[10] Phalloplasty with individualized desires for vaginectomy, urethroplasty, and scrotoplasty is scheduled only after thorough evaluation, examination, and counseling. Once the donor site is confirmed, patients are instructed to begin hair removal and complete their hysterectomy if they have not yet done so.

PHALLOPLASTY

The most common surgical goals for phalloplasty are the creation of an aesthetic and sensate phallus with a full-length urethra, a pouchlike ante-riorly positioned scrotum, vaginectomy, and an anatomically male perineum.[11] Phalloplasty per-formed by microsurgeons and a reconstructive urologist in a single stage meets these goals. The current gold standard for neophallus creation is the RF free flap.[11] It is well vascularized and inner-vated and allows for concomitant urethroplasty and glansplasty, with lower complication rates than other neophallus flaps that include PP ure-throplasty.[3,12] An alternative flap is the ALT pedi-cled (or free) flap. ALT phalloplasty is desired by about 10% to 30% of patients. The complication rates are higher given the inferior vascularity, higher fat content, and lower skin pliability.[9,12] Despite these facts, some patients are not candi-dates for RF phalloplasty because of anatomic, surgical, and personal reasons, specifically the strong desire to avoid an obvious donor site scar.[1] Because of the predictably larger girth of the ALT neophallus, complication rates and the need for surgical revisions are higher.[9,12] Occa-sionally, staged urethroplasty and phallus girth reduction procedures are required for 1 to 3 years after initial ALT phalloplasty. D'Arpa and col-leagues[8] evaluated 86 ALT flap phalloplasties with urethroplasty. Five patients had a tube-in-tube design, 8 had a prelaminated ALT flap with skin graft, 29 had a combination flap with RF free flap urethroplasty, 38 has a pedicled superficial circumflex iliac artery perforator flap urethroplasty, and 6 had a skin flap from previous phalloplasty. The urethral complication rate ranged from 16.7% to 87.5%. Patients are made aware that ALT phalloplasty complications are generally dou-ble that of the RF phalloplasty.[12]

Other examples of neophallus flaps include the musculocutaneous latissimus dorsi (MLD) and fib-ula free flaps, and the groin/abdomen local/regional flaps.[1,5,13] Some centers give preference to MLD flaps, and in expert hands, the urethro-plasty has the potential to reach the proximal or mid phallus.[14] It should be noted that some of these flap options do not have defined cutaneous nerves to coapt with the dorsal nerve, and rarely do they offer the ability to create a full-length PP urethra at time of phalloplasty. Because of these limitations, these flaps are not offered in the au-thors' practice.

The reconstructive urologist's operative role for the flap portion of phalloplasty is minimal. As the microsurgeons harvest and shape the flap, the urologist concomitantly performs the SP tube placement, vaginectomy, PF urethroplasty, dorsal nerve dissection, clitoral neurovascular transposi-tion with ventral chordee release, and scrotal and perineal reconstruction. The total operative time is approximately 6 to 8 hours with this team approach to single-stage phalloplasty.

Operative Details

The urologic component begins with SP tube insertion. Subsequent vaginectomy involves sharp excision and fulguration of the vaginal mucosa, fol-lowed by purse-string closure of the canal with thick polydioxanone suture (**Fig. 1**). The labia minora is marked, and local flaps are created around the native urethral meatus to lengthen the urethra to the glans clitoris. Depending on the pa-tient's anatomy, a U-shaped or a ring-flap[15] PF urethroplasty is performed. Patients with a large clitoris and plentiful labia minora tissue undergo U-shaped urethroplasty (**Fig. 2**); smaller clitorises with deficient labia minora and/or a prominent mons pubis may benefit from the recruitment of hairless labia minora tissue around the vaginal introitus–the ring-flap urethroplasty (**Fig. 3**). In addition, the authors develop vascular subepithe-lial flaps proximal to the labia minora flaps to cover the urethral suture line (**Fig. 4**) and deepithelialize the periurethral fornices (**Fig. 5**) that make catheter placement difficult, closing the indentations to create a cylindrical PF urethra (**Fig. 6**). These ma-neuvers allow for urethral catheter placement without cystoscopic guidance.

The clitoris is subsequently deepithelialized, and the suspensory ligament is transected. One of the 2 dorsal nerve bundles is then iso-lated, which is identified between the corpora cavernosa and Buck's fascia (**Fig. 7**); the bundle is later coapted to the sensory nerve of the flap. An opening is made overlying the inferior aspect of the pubic symphysis, and the extended ure-thra and deepithelialized clitoris are then translo-cated to the infrapubic position to allow for later placement of the neophallus and neourethra (**Fig. 8**).

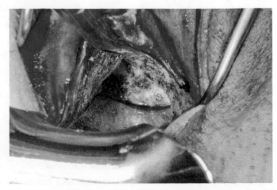

Fig. 1. Vaginectomy. Mucosa is sharply excised and cauterized, followed by purse-string closure of the canal.

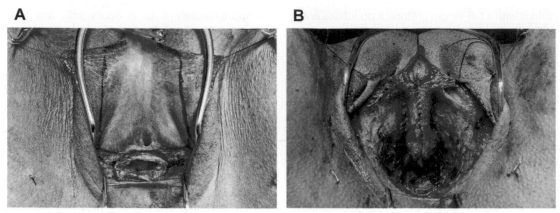

Fig. 2. (*A*) U-shaped PF urethroplasty. Patients with plentiful labial minora tissue and an enlarged clitoris are candidates for this type of urethroplasty. (*B*) U-shaped PF urethroplasty. Ventral closure is completed with monofilament absorbable suture.

Scrotoplasty is performed by dissecting the labia majora flaps based on the superior blood supply (external pudendal artery) (**Fig. 9**). The flaps are subsequently elevated, rotated, and advanced to create an anteriorly positioned pouchlike scrotum (**Fig. 10**). The perineum is then reconstructed: deep layer closure focuses on additional urethral suture line coverage with bulbospongiosus muscle, followed by adipofascial and skin closure (**Fig. 11**).

Concomitantly, the RF free flap or ALT pedicled flap is harvested and fashioned into the neophallus and PP urethra. The microsurgeons elevate a rectangular flap that is separated into a urethral component and phallus component (**Fig. 12**) via deepithelialization of a strip of skin. In RF patients, the strip of skin is used for glansplasty. The urethral component of the flap is rolled into the PP urethra; the remainder of the flap is wrapped around the urethra to create the neophallus (**Fig. 13**). Glansplasty is possible in many RF neophalluses and is carried out by measuring approximately 3 cm proximal from the tip of the neophallus; this line is curved ventrally toward the meatus. The skin is incised circumferentially roughly 1 cm proximal to this line, undermined,

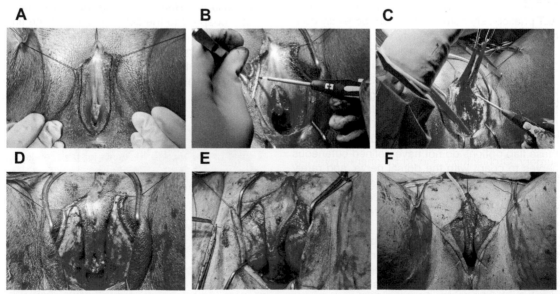

Fig. 3. (*A*) Ring-flap markings. Labia minora tissue flanking the vaginal introitus is included in the urethroplasty. (*B*) Ring-flap dissection. The ring is transected in the midline, and bilateral flaps are created with eventual chordee release. (*C*) Ring-flap elevation with chordee release. (*D*) Ring-flap urethroplasty dorsal closure. (*E*) Ring-flap urethroplasty ventral closure. (*F*) Ring-flap urethroplasty complete.

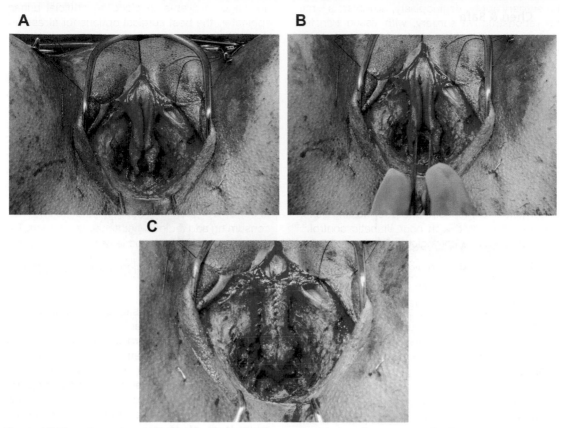

Fig. 4. (*A*) Flaps for native urethral meatus to PF anastomosis. (*B*) Flaps for native urethral meatus to PF anastomosis coverage with urethral meatus exposed. (*C*) Flaps for meatus to PF coverage secured.

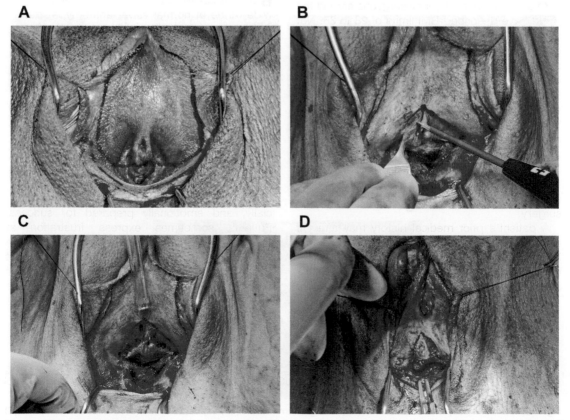

Fig. 5. (*A*) Periurethral fornices marked as triangles. (*B*) Periurethral forniceal epithelium excised. (*C*) Periurethral fornices excised. (*D*) Periurethral fornices excised and closed.

A
B

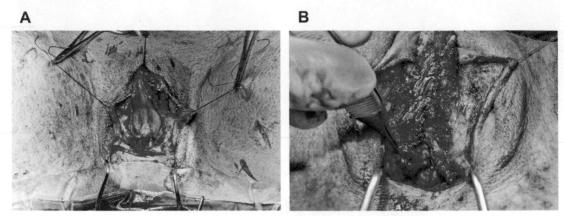

Fig. 6. (*A*) Periurethral fornices excised and closed. (*B*) Meatus to PF anastomotic closure coverage with local flaps.

and then rolled distally to create a corona. The previously deepithelialized skin graft is then used to cover the adipofascial tissue proximal to the corona (**Fig. 14**). Glansplasty is delayed in ALT neophalluses owing to a higher risk of distal flap necrosis.

An incision is then made in the groin to expose the femoral vessels and the saphenous vein along with its branches at the saphenofemoral junction. The flap vessels are then divided, and the neophallus is brought toward the midline infrapubic position. The urologist performs the urethral anastomosis after placing a urethral catheter retrograde through the PP and PF urethra (**Fig. 15**). Using an operative microscope, the microsurgeons complete the coaptation between the

A
B
C

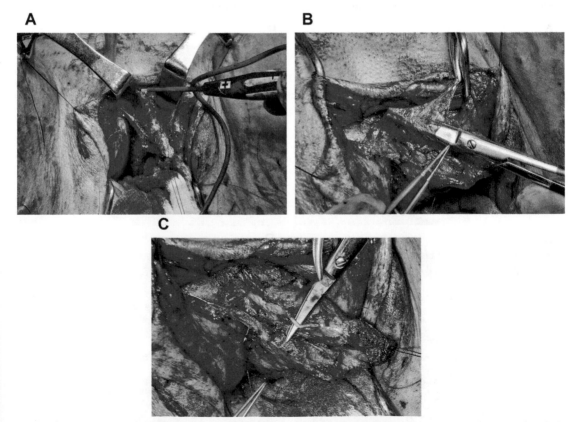

Fig. 7. (*A*) Clitoris deepithelialization and dorsal ligament release. (*B*) Exposure and dissection of Buck's fascia. (*C*) Dorsal nerve isolated.

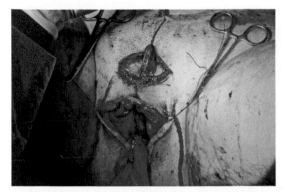

Fig. 8. Translocation of distal urethra and clitoris.

dorsal nerve and antebrachial or lateral femoral cutaneous nerve; if additional nerve branches are present, a second coaptation to the ilioinguinal nerve can also be performed. Once the nerves are coapted, an additional adipofascial layer that is typically harvested with the flap is advanced to provide an additional layer of closure over the urethral anastomosis. The vascular anastomoses of the RF flap are then performed after insetting of the phallus in the midline position. The radial

artery is typically anastomosed in an end-to-side fashion to either the common femoral artery or the superficial femoral artery (depending on the location of takeoff of the profunda femoris) using a 2.4-mm vascular punch, after first obtaining proximal and distal control of the femoral system. The cephalic vein is then anastomosed to either the saphenous vein or a large branch. The profunda cubitalis vein connecting the venae comitantes of the radial artery to the cephalic is typically preserved in order to maximize venous drainage of the flap. The authors prefer to perform an additional venous anastomosis that drains, specifically, the urethral component of the flap. This vein is typically anastomosed to either the superficial inferior epigastric vein or another small branch off the saphenous vein. An implantable venous Doppler is placed on the cephalic vein; the groin incision is closed over a Penrose drain, and the neophallus is fully inset (**Fig. 16**). The donor site is covered with split-thickness sheet grafts (STSG) harvested from the thigh (**Fig. 17**) and secured using negative pressure wound therapy. Patients are admitted for an average of 5 days with 4 days of bed rest.

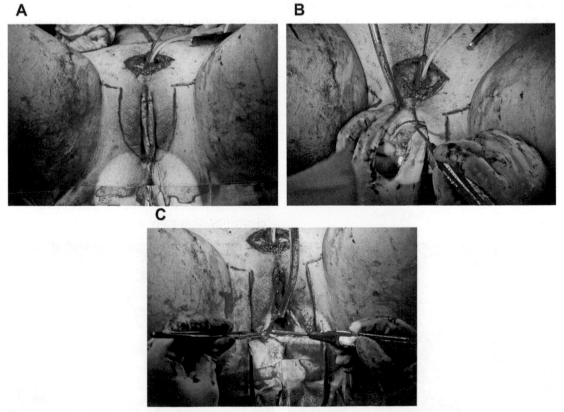

Fig. 9. (*A*) Scrotoplasty markings. (*B*) Labia minora and clitoral excess skin deepithelialization. (*C*) Scrotoplasty labia majora flap development.

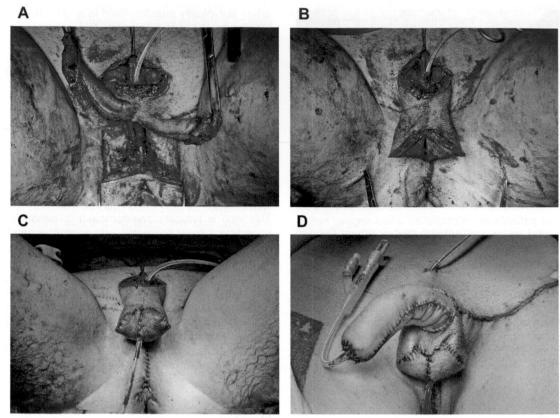

Fig. 10. (*A*) Scrotoplasty labia majora flaps elevated. (*B*) Scrotoplasty labia majora flaps folded. (*C*) Scrotoplasty completed and drain placed. (*D*) Scrotoplasty completed with inset RF phallus with no glans.

Nearly all ALT flaps are performed in a pedicled fashion, with adequate mobilization of the pedicle. The flap is shaped on the thigh and then tunneled under the rectus femoris and sartorius muscles into the midline. The ALT flap may need to be converted to a free flap if pedicle mobilization alone is insufficient to deliver the flap to the midline position.

POSTOPERATIVE FOLLOW-UP

Patients are followed weekly for about 1 month after surgery. At the first postoperative visit, the urethral catheter is removed, and the donor site dressings are changed and evaluated. If patients are healing as expected by the second postoperative visit, a voiding trial is conducted whereby the

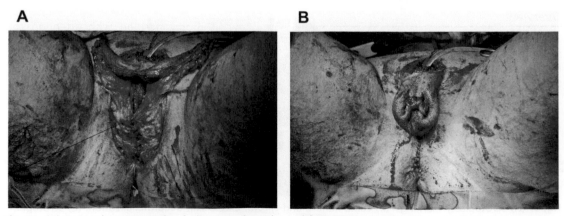

Fig. 11. (*A*) Perineal reconstruction bulbospongiosus layer. (*B*) Perineal reconstruction complete.

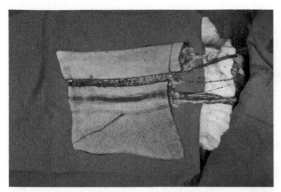

Fig. 12. RF flap has been elevated, and the urethral and phallus component is separated by a deepithelialization segment.

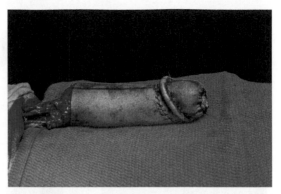

Fig. 14. Glansplasty with coronal slant ventrally and skin graft.

SP tube is clamped and patients are instructed to void through the urethra. If patients are able to void well for several days, the SP tube is removed. Some urologists will wait 4 to 6 weeks, after radiographic evaluation with a retrograde urethrogram or voiding cystourethrogram, before instructing patients to urinate through the neophallus.[9]

Patients who have a urethrocutaneous fistula are instructed to delay voiding until the fistula heals. Low-output fistulas will often heal spontaneously; higher-output fistulas may require prolonged drainage and/or surgical correction. Phallus edema, especially of the tip, can cause compression of the distal PP urethra. Phallus elevation and rest can help minimize this edema. Strictures rarely occur during the first month of recovery. When they do develop, they are usually of the distal PP urethra or the PP-PF anastomosis.

UROLOGIC COMPLICATIONS

Patients who undergo single-stage phalloplasty with full-length urethroplasty, vaginectomy,

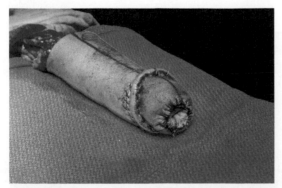

Fig. 13. Phallus component of the flap has been wrapped around the urethra, and the glansplasty with meatoplasty has been completed.

scrotoplasty, and perineal reconstruction may develop urinary tract infections (UTIs), fistulas, strictures, and diverticula.[2,10] Patients are more prone to UTIs because of the need for prolonged catheterization and the neourethral anatomy. UTIs in these patients are treated as complex UTIs, and 7 days of culture-directed antibiotic therapy are prescribed. Patients with recurrent UTIs beyond the first 6-week recovery period may have urethral hair (Fig. 18), urethral pseudodiverticula (Fig. 19), incomplete bladder emptying, stricture, and/or urolithiasis (Fig. 20). Small amounts of thin hair in the PP urethra are inconsequential, but longer, dense, and thick hairs, more commonly seen in ALT neophalluses, may lead to obstruction, bothersome postvoid leakage, debris buildup, stones, fistulas, and recurrent UTIs. Conservative management includes a combination of endoscopic removal and topical therapy. However, these methods are rarely successful, and patients may often desire and require more invasive management, including the complete removal of hair-bearing PP urethral tissue followed by staged urethroplasty using hairless epidermal autografts. Perineal urethrostomy creation with PP urethrectomy is also a reliable option.

The risk of urethral complications for phalloplasty with full-length urethroplasty is estimated at 20% to 50%,[2,3,16] although this number is likely an underestimate. For urethral strictures alone, the risk is 20% to 50%,[17] and the estimated risk does not take into account the fact that most phalloplasty centers are a national and international draw for patients, making urologic follow-up unreliable and difficult. Urethrocutaneous fistulas are more common than strictures, and both occur at predictable locations.[12] The distal PP urethra and neourethral meatus are at risk for stricture, especially if distal necrosis is noted during the postoperative visits. The PP and PF urethral anastomosis

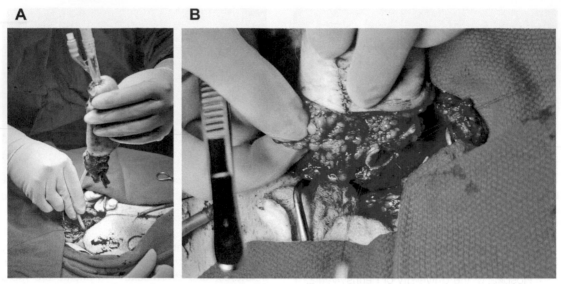

Fig. 15. (*A*) PF PP urethral catheterization. (*B*) PF PP anastomotic urethroplasty.

is prone to both strictures and fistulas. The PF urethra fistulizes and/or strictures less frequently.

Fistulas rarely occur after 3 months unless there is prolonged phallus edema or distal urethral strictures. Fistulas in this setting are frequently located on the ventrum of the neophallus incision line. Strictures typically occur after 3 months, and patients are at risk of stricture development for about 2 years after phalloplasty.[3] Urethral diverticula are more common when a stricture is present, which may be explained by the upstream urethral dilation from increased intraurethral voiding pressures. Patients are therefore instructed to have regular follow-up. For local patients, the authors recommend office visits every 3 months for the first year and less frequently thereafter. Out-of-town patients are encouraged to establish local urologic care, but are also encouraged to continue care with their phalloplasty surgeons should additional surgical procedures be required.

Urethrocutaneous fistulas that are small and low output will often heal spontaneously.[3,15] Some urologists will leave the SP tube until the fistula has completely healed. The authors have found that these fistulas will heal with or without a catheter. Therefore, patients who have intolerable catheter-related symptoms frequently want earlier catheter removal and prefer voiding through their phallus despite having a small fistula. If repair is required, flexible cystoscopy is performed to verify that there is no other urethral pathologic condition (like stricture) and to confirm the location of the urethral fistula or fistulas. Granulation tissue is sometimes seen within the neoscrotum and urethra at the fistula site; if so, it will require excision followed by urethroplasty to repair the defect.

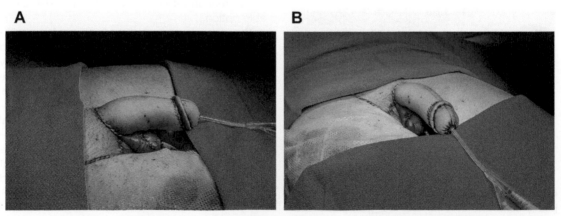

Fig. 16. (*A*) RF phallus completely inset. (*B*) RF phallus completely inset from a second angle.

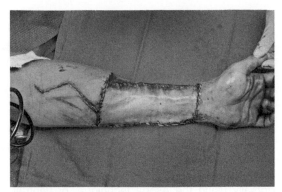

Fig. 17. Donor site closure with STSG.

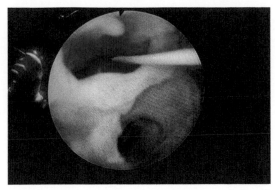

Fig. 19. Cystoscopic view of proximal PF urethra with wire through native urethra and a ventral pseudodiverticulum.

Layered vascular tissue coverage over the urethral suture line will help decrease the risk of fistula recurrence. Occasionally, a dermal interposition graft is harvested to cover the suture line, separating the urethral closure from the skin closure.

Strictures associated with ALT and RF phalloplasty with full-length urethroplasty are most frequently at the watershed areas of the neophallus, namely the distal and proximal PP urethra. The PF-PP urethral anastomotic strictures are more likely caused by neophallus base compression and resultant tissue ischemia.[3] Isolated PF urethral strictures are less common. Treatment of urethral strictures varies depending on the stricture location, length, and neighboring tissue quality.

Distal strictures are managed with temporizing dilation followed by urethroplasty when the tissues are softer and more vascularized (typically 3 months or more after phalloplasty). If strictures are less than 2 cm, many patients tolerate a ventral stricturotomy or meatoplasty with a resultant hypospadiac meatus. Longer strictures may require a dorsal onlay first-stage Johanson urethroplasty followed 6 months later by a second-stage urethroplasty. Most strictures of the PP urethra will require a staged approach. Skin and buccal epidermal autografts often take well on neophallus adipose tissue.

Anastomotic strictures at the PF-PP junction are frequently short (2 cm or less) and can be managed with periodic endoscopic dilation or single-stage anastomotic urethroplasty. During urethroplasty, the surgeon must take into account the proximity of the glans clitoris, which is located

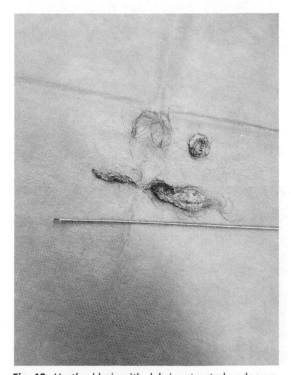

Fig. 18. Urethral hair with debris extracted endoscopically with flexible stent graspers.

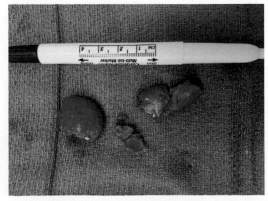

Fig. 20. Bladder stone after phalloplasty with PF PP urethroplasty.

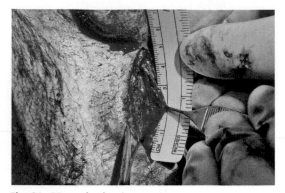

Fig. 21. PF urethral stricture, 4cm.

immediately dorsal to the urethra. A Heineke-Mikulicz (HM) repair of a ventral stricturotomy at this location will minimize the risk of glans clitoris injury. HM urethroplasty is feasible when the stricture is nonobliterative and less than 2 cm long. In addition, with these strictures, there is often ample PF urethral tissue available, facilitating the HM or anastomotic urethroplasty. The abundance of PF urethral tissue is likely due to proximal PF urethral dilation caused by the stricture. Urethral strictures that are longer than 2 cm may require substitution urethroplasty with an epidermal autograft (buccal or skin). The graft can be placed dorsally via the Asopa technique (ventral stricturotomy and urethrotomy with a dorsal graft inlay)[18] or ventrally when neighboring vascular tissue is present. Staged urethroplasties are rarely required for PF-PP anastomotic strictures.

For isolated PF strictures, short strictures are amenable to anastomotic or HM urethroplasty; substitution urethroplasty is a good option for longer strictures (**Fig. 21**). The graft may be placed dorsally using the Asopa technique, or ventrally given the reliable presence of neighboring vascularized bulpospongiosus tissue (**Fig. 22**). Staged urethroplasty may be required if there is inadequate tissue for single-stage repair.

Urethral diverticula are occasionally seen ventral to the native urethral meatus and are commonly associated with strictures. Distal obstruction leads to proximal urethral dilation and disruption of the reconstructed urethra, leading to opening of the closed vaginal canal followed by epithelialization. Inadvertent retention of remnant vaginal mucosa may also produce mucous, which can contribute

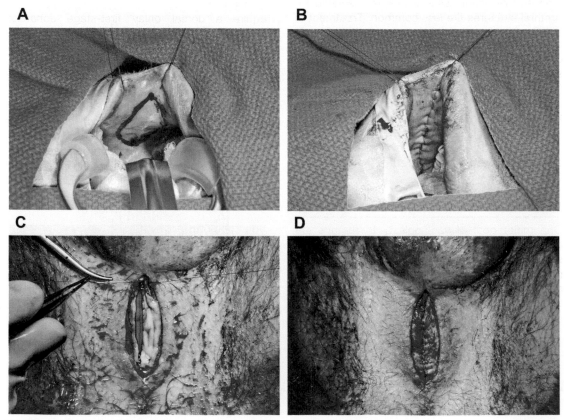

Fig. 22. (*A*) Buccal graft site marked. (*B*) Buccal graft donor site closed. (*C*) Buccal graft quilted to neighboring vascular tissue. (*D*) Buccal graft urethroplasty complete.

to diverticulum development. Patients may complain of postvoid urinary leakage of large amounts of urine, perineal pain, and/or recurrent UTIs. After treatment of the stricture, the first step in management is postvoid diverticulum, PF urethra, and PP urethra external compression from proximal to distal (compression of the perineum, then scrotum, then base of phallus to the tip, in that order). Manual compression will often resolve the leakage symptoms. When conservative management fails, or if a patient has perineal pain, persistent urinary leakage, and/or recurrent UTIs from the diverticula, diverticulectomy is indicated. Diverticulectomy involves a perineal incision with exposure of the diverticulum. It is then resected and the PF urethra is reconstructed.

Catheter management after urethroplasty is highly variable. The authors prefer using a urethral catheter because it is generally better tolerated. SP catheterization is used when patients request it or if they already have one placed previously. Rarely are both a urethral and SP catheter placed. For urethroplasties not needing grafts, the authors leave the catheter in for 1 week; for substitution urethroplasties, the catheter is left in 2 to 3 weeks depending on stricture length and severity. Longer durations of urethral catheterization do not improve outcomes and may lead to new PP urethral fistulas owing to local inflammatory reactions of the PP skin urethra to the catheter.

SUMMARY

Phalloplasty with urethral lengthening involves complex procedures performed at an increasing rate. As a result, more patients are seeking urologic care. Understanding the techniques used during phalloplasty enhances the surgeon's ability to recognize and repair complications that arise, the most common of which are urethral fistulas and strictures. Fistulas will often heal spontaneously. Strictures almost always require surgery. Diverticula occur occasionally with strictures and may be managed conservatively. Urethral hair is usually inconsequential unless there is a high density. Transmasculine patients will benefit greatly from surgeons who are able to perform single-stage phalloplasty reliably and manage the complications associated with it.

REFERENCES

1. Schechter LS, Safa B. Introduction to phalloplasty. Clin Plast Surg 2018;45(3):387–9.
2. Frey JD, Poudrier G, Chiodo MV, et al. A systematic review of metoidioplasty and radial forearm flap phalloplasty in female-to-male transgender genital reconstruction: is the "ideal" neophallus an achievable goal? Plast Reconstr Surg Glob Open 2016; 4(12):e1131.
3. Monstrey S, Hoebeke P, Selvaggi G, et al. Penile reconstruction: is the radial forearm flap really the standard technique? Plast Reconstr Surg 2009; 124(2):510–8.
4. Selvaggi G, Dhejne C, Landen M, et al. The 2011 WPATH standards of care and penile reconstruction in female-to-male transsexual individuals. Adv Urol 2012;2012:581712.
5. Morrison SD, Shakir A, Vyas KS, et al. Phalloplasty: a review of techniques and outcomes. Plast Reconstr Surg 2016;138(3):594–615.
6. Timmermans FW, Westland PB, Hummelink S, et al. A retrospective investigation of abdominal visceral fat, body mass index (BMI), and active smoking as risk factors for donor site wound healing complications after free DIEP flap breast reconstructions. J Plast Reconstr Aesthet Surg 2018;71(6):827–32.
7. van der Sluis WB. Double flap phalloplasty in transgender men: surgical technique and outcome of pedicled anterolateral thigh flap phalloplasty combined with radial forearm free flap urethral reconstruction 2017;37(8):917–23.
8. D'Arpa S, Claes K, Lumen N, et al. Urethral reconstruction in anterolateral thigh flap phalloplasty: a 93-case experience. Plast Reconstr Surg 2019; 143(2):382e–92e.
9. Xu KY, Watt AJ. The pedicled anterolateral thigh phalloplasty. Clin Plast Surg 2018;45(3): 399–406.
10. Massie JP, Morrison SD, Wilson SC, et al. Phalloplasty with urethral lengthening: addition of a vascularized bulbospongiosus flap from vaginectomy reduces postoperative urethral complications. Plast Reconstr Surg 2017;140(4):551e–8e.
11. Monstrey SJ, Ceulemans P, Hoebeke P. Sex reassignment surgery in the female-to-male transsexual. Semin Plast Surg 2011;25(3):229–44.
12. Ascha M, Massie JP, Morrison SD, et al. Outcomes of single stage phalloplasty by pedicled anterolateral thigh flap versus radial forearm free flap in gender confirming surgery. J Urol 2018;199(1): 206–14.
13. Schaff J, Papadopulos NA. A new protocol for complete phalloplasty with free sensate and prelaminated osteofasciocutaneous flaps: experience in 37 patients. Microsurgery 2009;29(5):413–9.
14. Djordjevic ML, Bencic M, Kojovic V, et al. Musculocutaneous latissimus dorsi flap for phalloplasty in female to male gender affirmation surgery. World J Urol 2019;37(4):631–7.
15. Takamatsu A, Harashina T. Labial ring flap: a new flap for metaidoioplasty in female-to-male

transsexuals. J Plast Reconstr Aesthet Surg 2009; 62(3):318–25.

16. Remington AC, Morrison SD, Massie JP, et al. Outcomes after phalloplasty: do transgender patients and multiple urethral procedures carry a higher rate of complication? Plast Reconstr Surg 2018; 141(2):220e–9e.

17. Santucci RA. Urethral complications after transgender phalloplasty: strategies to treat them and minimize their occurrence. Clin Anat 2018;31(2):187–90.

18. Pisapati VL, Paturi S, Bethu S, et al. Dorsal buccal mucosal graft urethroplasty for anterior urethral stricture by Asopa technique. Eur Urol 2009;56(1): 201–5.

"Staging" in Phalloplasty

Sara Danker, MD, Nick Esmonde, MD, MPH, Jens Urs Berli, MD*

KEYWORDS

- Phalloplasty • Phalloplasty staging • Phalloplasty complications • Urethral reconstruction

KEY POINTS

- Phalloplasty surgery for gender dysphoria is an amalgam of procedures that can be sequenced and staged differently and practices are largely dependent on surgeon preference.
- The risks and benefits of single versus multistage phalloplasty is debated by gender surgeons and there is no consensus as to which approach is superior.
- A staged approach allows for any complications to be compartmentalized and managed piecemeal, potentially minimizing their impact on the functional outcome.

INTRODUCTION

Although most surgeons agree that the overall goal of phalloplasty is to mirror the form and function of cis-male genitalia,[1] there is less agreement about the means of obtaining this goal. Similar to breast reconstruction, a number of techniques and staging methods have evolved over the past several decades.[2] Educational exposure to this type of surgery is currently limited in the United States, and the published literature often falls short in explaining the technical intricacies and management of complications specific to any given technique.[3]

There are overarching principles that apply to phalloplasty and knowledge of these will lay the foundation upon which the surgeon can select his or her preferred techniques. Surgeon preference may be limited by resources, availability of colleagues in associated specialties, training background, institutional constraints, and clinical variables. Regardless of the selected technique, the gender surgeon should be familiar with the various options and their respective advantages and disadvantages to provide a true informed consent to the patient.

The creation of a neo-phallus has to achieve aesthetic ideals, be neurotized, allow for insertion of a multipart foreign body (erectile device), and serve as a patent urinary conduit. Its recipient site also differs from traditional tissue transfers in that advanced local tissue rearrangement, extirpative surgery, and pelvic floor reconstruction are needed to create a suitable site for urinary diversion and perineal masculinization. When deconstructed into its various subprocedures, phalloplasty is not one but a multitude of operations (**Table 1**).

The procedures necessary for a comprehensive phalloplasty include:

Removal of reproductive organs and tissues
- Hysterectomy (with or without oophorectomy)
- Colpectomy and colpoclesis
Perineal masculinization
- Perineal urethra (ie, urethral lengthening or pars fixa)
- Scrotoplasty
- Perineoplasty
Creation of the phallus
- Shaft
- Shaft urethra (ie, pars pendula or neo-urethra)
- Glansplasty

Disclosure Statement: The collective authorship would like to report that we have no financial, commercial, or other conflicts of interest that would potentially influence the content of this article, nor do we have any past or current relationships or affiliations relevant to the subject of this article to disclose. This endeavor received no funding.
Division of Plastic and Reconstructive Surgery, Oregon Health & Science University, Mail Code L352A. 3181 Southwest Sam Jackson Park Road, Portland, OR 97239, USA
* Corresponding author.
E-mail address: Jens.berli@gmail.com

Urol Clin N Am 46 (2019) 581–590
https://doi.org/10.1016/j.ucl.2019.07.011
0094-0143/19/
© 2019 Elsevier Inc. All rights reserved.

Table 1
Options for staging and sequencing phalloplasty procedures

First Stage	Second Stage	Third Stage	Fourth Stage
Perineal masculinization, shaft, neo-urethra, urethral lengthening, glansplasty	Testicular implants, erectile device	*	*
Shaft	Perineal masculinization, perineal urostomy, glansplasty	Testicular implants, erectile device	*
Shaft with or without neo-urethra	Urethral lengthening, perineal masculinization, glansplasty	Testicular implants, erectile device	*
Metoidioplasty	Shaft, neourethra, urethral lengthening	Testicular implants, erectile device	*
Metoidioplasty	Shaft, neourethra	Urethral lengthening	Testicular implants, erectile device
Shaft	Perineal masculinization, urethral graft-1	Urethral graft-2	Testicular implants, erectile device

Urethral graft-1, first urethral grafting; urethral graft-2, second stage urethral grafting.
* There are no procedures for those stages.

Implants
- Testicular implants
- Erectile implants

Each of these procedures comes with its own risk and complication profile. It is no surprise that there are many different approaches and philosophies around staging of this procedure. Here, we outline the principles underlying staging of phalloplasty and the associated benefits and pitfalls. The word "staging" itself is a source of significant confusion for patients and surgeons alike, because phalloplasty, unless performed as an osteocutaneous flap, is always performed in stages when considering each element listed.[4,5] It is also important to note that not all patients desire a comprehensive phalloplasty, but may opt for only some of the components (eg, shaft-only phalloplasty) (**Fig. 1**).

The single-stage versus 2-stage approach refers specifically to the 2 parts of the urethroplasty. This is a topic of debate among experts in the field.[6–8] The crux of the decision to stage or not to stage is whether creation of the perineal urethra and the shaft urethra should happen at the same time or at 2 time points. Another area of debate is whether the urethra should be constructed with vascularized or grafted tissue. These authors believe in the benefits of a staged approach using a vascularized urethroplasty, but recognize that current evidence remains at the level of expert opinion.

The current literature offers no definitive answer on the best staging method. The outcomes presented in retrospective studies of individual centers vary widely in the techniques used (eg, grafted urethra vs vascularized urethra) and may not account for inadequate follow-up owing to a geographically mobile patient population. A systematic review on staging has been published, but the limitations of these reviews on such heterogenous data do not allow for meaningful conclusions.[9,10] In addition to variations in technique, individual surgeon mastery increases with any given technique and early outcomes may be more reflective of the steep slope of the learning curve rather than the superiority of one technique over the other.

This article outlines the most commonly practiced staged approaches and their proposed advantages. There are countless ways to perform phalloplasty and any article will inevitably fall short in describing every iteration. Because the senior author is a proponent of the Big Ben method (coined after the city of its inventors, Dr Ralph and Dr Nim), there is a more detailed focus on this approach.

PROPOSED ADVANTAGES OF A SINGLE-STAGE APPROACH

It is easy to understand why a patient might prefer to have the majority of the reconstruction completed during one operation with a single hospital stay. It simplifies the process logistically and may give the impression of fewer opportunities for surgical complications. The desire to consolidate the procedures may be

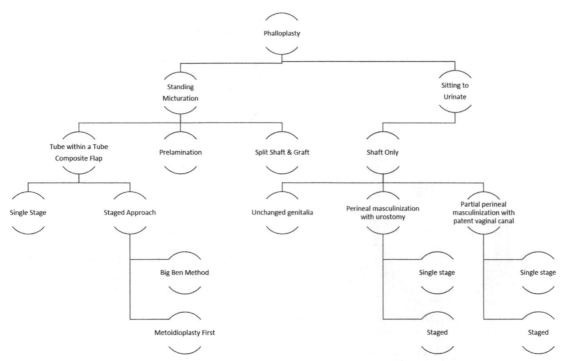

Fig. 1. Phalloplasty options.

especially attractive for patients who travel long distance—sometimes transoceanic—to undergo their operation. In the absence of complications, this technique comes with a significantly lesser financial burden to the patient and insurance carrier.

PROPOSED ADVANTAGES OF THE STAGED APPROACH

Each subprocedure comes with its own complication profile and any event, regardless of magnitude, may affect the outcome of the entire reconstruction (eg, infection leading to urethral stenosis). The separation of stages may allow for isolation of complications and management thereof. This strategy, in theory, minimizes the potential negative downstream effects on the final outcome. Also, the management of complications may be simplified (eg, partial flap loss without need for urinary diversion). Logistically, a staged approach omits the absolute need for a 2-team approach and, depending on the practice set up, allows the plastic surgery and urology team to perform each stage independently. Furthermore, the case length for each surgery is decreased, with benefits for the surgeon and the patient.

The surgeon and patient may choose between 2 basic sequences of this staged approach: (1)

Creation of the phallus and shaft urethra first, followed at the subsequent procedure by creation of the perineal urethra, colpectomy/colpoclesis, and scrotoplasty (ie, the Big Ben method); and (2) Urethral lengthening akin to a metoidioplasty at the first surgery followed by tissue transfer and connection of the shaft urethra at the second surgery.

Both the flap transfer and the creation of the perineal urethra come with the potential for relative tissue ischemia at the site of urethral repair. After wound closure in a single-stage approach, there is no way to assess this area short of urethroscopy. By separating the 2 surgical incidents temporally, it allows for assured healing of one of the components before the introduction of a new tissue. The scars will have matured, absorbable sutures should be dissolved, and the conduit established with adequate caliber. Minor incidences of delayed wound healing, spitting sutures, or necrosis of wound edges that in a single stage would lead to areas of weakness and potential fistula are prevented in at least one part of the urethral reconstruction (**Fig. 2**). If larger issues arise, those can be tackled independently while minimizing risk to the already healed segment.

Important: With this technique, flap-related and urologic complications can be managed separately in most cases.

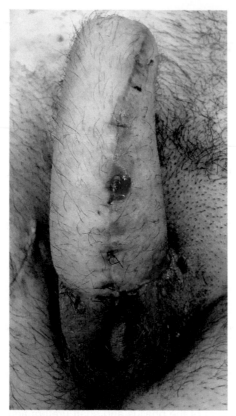

Fig. 2. Shaft with suture abscess in setting of "Big Ben" method.

FREE OR REGIONAL TISSUE TRANSFER FIRST; THAT IS, THE BIG BEN METHOD
Surgical Technique: First Stage

In this method (practiced by the senior author [JUB]), the tissue of choice is transferred at the first operation[8] (**Fig. 3**). The flap design is similar to previous descriptions. Both the clitoral and ilioinguinal nerve as well as the recipient vessels of choice are accessed through a suprapubic approach. The urethral extension is approximately 1 cm longer than in other approaches because it is not anastomosed to the perineal urethra. Rather, it is marsupialized lateral to the clitoral shaft and medial to the labia majora on either side. The extension is routed through the same access as the clitoral nerve dissection. In preparation for the next stage, the ipsilateral labia minora is resected and oversewn to create a smooth surface. The intervening area between the marsupialized orifice of the shaft urethra and the native urethra will become the posterior wall of the future perineal urethra.

Postoperative Management

At our center, we hospitalize the patient postoperatively for an average of 7 days. The phallus is kept at 90° for 4 weeks, during which time the patient is encouraged to mainly lay supine or stand. We limit the amount of walking to the absolute minimum during the same time period. After the fourth week, a catheter is passed daily through the shaft urethra to monitor patency and assess occurrence of strictures. However, in our experience, stricture has not been an issue for the shaft urethra. Any meatal stenosis can be addressed at the next stage. We have observed suture abscesses and wound separations, which, except for one case, all were addressed or resolved before the next stage.[6]

Flap-Related Complications After the First Stage

The demands that are placed on this type of flap are greater than for the typical free or regional tissue transfer owing to the large size as well as the folding of the tissue. Partial flap loss in the literature is reported to be between 4% and 8%, depending on the technique used.[11,12] If this complication occurs, there is ample opportunity to address it with either debridement and grafting, transfer of new tissue, or abandonment of the reconstruction altogether before any irreversible manipulation of the urinary tract (**Fig. 4**). Even in the case of total flap loss, the patient would not be in a dire situation with need for prolonged urinary diversion or genital disfigurement.

The same is true for hematomas, infections, and wound separations. If any of these entities lead to the formation of a fistula, then this can be addressed directly at the second operation. If a stricture is identified, then a 2-stage stricture repair can be initiated at the time of the second procedure. Meatal stricture can be problematic because it can increase backstream pressure and possibly lead to fistula formation. However, in this staging scenario, a meatal stricture is easily repaired at the time of the second surgery with a slit meatoplasty.

Surgical Technique: Second Stage

The patient returns for their next operation a few months later, with the exact timing depending on the surgeon's preference. In the senior author's opinion, after 5 months the scar tissue has remodeled sufficiently, the genital tissue is supple, and most buried suture material has been absorbed. At our institution, a urologist with a focus on urogynecology performs a formal colpectomy and colpoclesis as well as suprapubic catheter placement. The remainder of the operation is performed either by the plastic surgeon or by reconstructive urologic colleagues. Both parties perform a variation of the technique described by Dr Ralph and Dr Nim (**Fig. 5**). A 16F catheter is

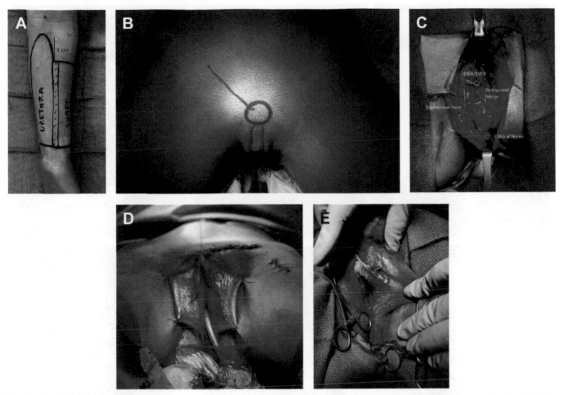

Fig. 3. The Big Ben method as performed at Oregon Health & Science University. (*A*) Flap design with longer urethral extension compared with other techniques (4 cm). (*B*) Incision markings. (*C*) Recipient site (lower retractor in space where urethral extension will be routed). (*D*) Status after unilateral labia minora resection. Circle marks the inset of proximal shaft urethra. (*E*) Postoperative appearance after inset of phallus and neo-urethra. DIEA/DIEV, deep inferior epigastric artery/deep inferior epigastric vein.

passed through the shaft urethra and then into the bladder. The genital skin surrounding the catheter is elliptically incised with a width of at least 25 mm. The predominant tissues included in the urethroplasty are: urethral plate, clitoral shaft skin, and vulvar skin. In the most proximal portion, an anterior vaginal wall flap is incorporated into the reconstruction. The area around the external urethral meatus presents the most difficult area to close because the Skene's glands are adjacent to the

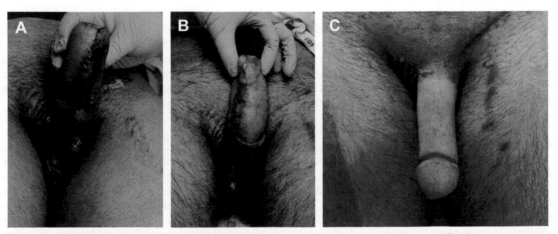

Fig. 4. Example of partial flap loss management. (*A*) Patient with previous simple metoidioplasty – status post first stage Big Ben method, complicated by increased phallic pressure necessitating release of ventral seam and associated partial flap loss. (*B*) Healed appearance before second stage. (*C*) Final appearance after second stage. No fistula or stricture formation and awaiting erectile implant.

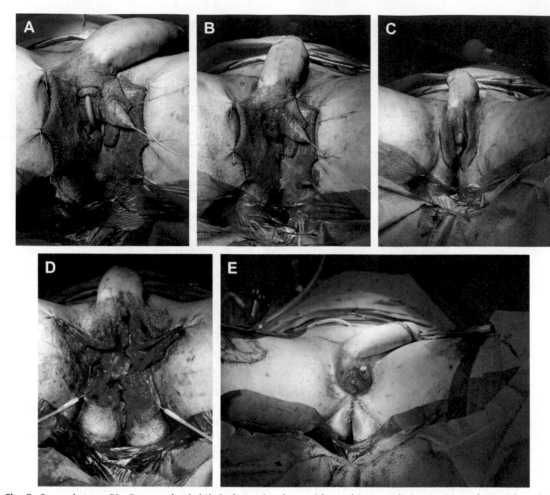

Fig. 5. Second stage Big Ben method. (*A*) Catheter in place with markings outlining incisions for urethroplasty. Vaginectomy has been performed and an anterior vaginal flap created. (*B*) Completed urethroplasty (except most proximal portion). (*C*) Labia majora flaps outlined for creation of the neoscrotum. (*D*) Layered closure of the urethral reconstruction including vascularized contralateral labia minora flap. The clitoris has been denuded and secured to the pubic symphysis thereby pulling the urethroplasty toward the midline. (*E*) Final appearance after perineoplasty and closure of neoscrotum.

meatus and the vaginal mucosa is rugged and bulky. Closure occurs on both sides from posterior to anterior with meticulous placement of 4-0 polyglactin sutures. The inverted V-shaped vaginal flap meets the linear closure superiorly, which will allow the urinary stream from the native urethra to hit the vaginal flap rather than a suture line.

Important: This technique allows the urethroplasty suture line to be an inverted Y rather than a circular or spatulated design, thereby decreasing the risk for circular stenosis (**Fig. 6**).

The remaining labia minora and clitoral skin is deepithelialized. Bilateral, superiorly based labia majora flaps are raised and fashioned into the neoscrotum. The perineum is closed in a V-Y fashion with the scrotoplasty inset into the saddle of the Y. There is an abundance of vascularized genital tissue, which is used to bolster the closure of

the perineal urethra with as many layers as possible—ideally, at least five. The layers are overlapped and any dead space obliterated. The final layers of the perineoplasty include Cooper's fascia, deep dermis, and skin. Glansplasty is also performed during this second stage.

Postoperative Management

The patient is admitted for 2 to 3 days postoperatively and is discharged with 2 catheters. The phallic catheter remains until postoperative day 10. The suprapubic catheter remains until week 4, at which time a retrograde urethrogram is performed. If there are any wound healing complications or minor areas of contrast extravasation, the catheter is kept another 2 weeks, after which time a capping trial is initiated and, if successful,

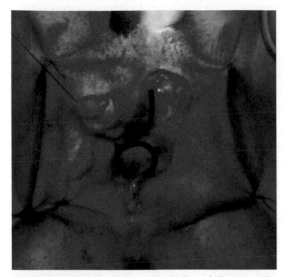

Fig. 6. Demonstration of suture line following the inset of the vaginal flap.

the catheter removed. The patient is again instructed to limit walking as much as possible during the healing period.

Complications After the Second Stage

Wound healing complications around the area of the scrotoplasty occur frequently, but typically only affect the most superficial layers of the closure. It is in the interest of the aesthetic appearance and patient comfort to reconstruct a high-riding scrotum. However, this comes with an increase in tension in the area of the Y closure and risk for dehiscence. In the author's experience, minor wound dehiscences do not correlate with fistula formation. Fistula and stricture management is no different than it would be in a single-stage phalloplasty. The authors routinely perform a simple slit meatoplasty during the second stage to avoid subsequent meatal stenosis.

Important: The only complication requiring prolonged urinary diversion in this technique is a stricture.

PERINEAL URETHRA FIRST

In contrast with the Big Ben method, this method is not one defined technique, but has more potential variety. The overarching principle is that the perineal urethra is created at the first operation leaving the patient to heal this aspect of the phallic reconstruction before tissue transfer. Technical details may vary widely among surgeons, but in its simplest form it is the creation of a metoidioplasty-like phallus at the first operation. An advantage of this sequence is that it allows for immediate relief from the dysphoria associated

with the presence of female genitalia. Similarly, if a patient loses insurance or has other reasons why reconstruction cannot proceed, the absence of female genitalia may provide some relief. At the second operation, the urethra is separated from the glans and the shaft urethra anastomosed. Metoidioplasty can also be viewed as an intermediary procedure for patients who are undecided about phalloplasty, because it can later be converted into a phallus. At our center, we offer this staging option for patients with previous metoidioplasty who regret not having had a phalloplasty. We do not, however, routinely offer it owing to the inability to separate the flap-related complications from the urologic complications. This factor, in our opinion, is the greatest drawback of this approach.

The use of a permutation of this approach is also suitable for surgeons who opt for one of the prelamination techniques, which are outlined elsewhere in this article.

SHAFT-ONLY AND STAGING OPTIONS

Patients undergoing shaft-only phalloplasty have various options, some of which may be considered atypical requests and fall outside the current World Professional Association for Transgender Health Standards of Care[13] (**Fig. 7**).

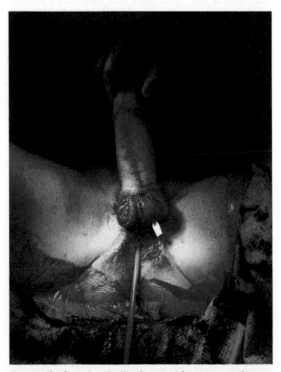

Fig. 7. Shaft only phalloplasty with neoscrotal creation. Labia minora, vaginal canal, and native urethra are left in their native position. A superior commisuroplasty was performed.

- Shaft only without genital modification
- Shaft only with scrotoplasty but without vaginectomy
- Shaft only with vaginectomy, scrotoplasty, and perineal urostomy
- Shaft only cranial to a previous metoidioplasty

In the opinion of the authors, any of these are safe and reliable to be performed in a single stage. However, we currently still separate the shaft creation from any genital modification owing to concern for an increase in wound healing complications.

MISCELLANEOUS PHALLOPLASTY OPTIONS AND CURRENT METHODS OF STAGING

Here we discuss phalloplasty variations that are less widely performed and how staging applies to these flaps and techniques. This section is included for comprehensiveness but, given the lack of personal experience of the senior author, we cannot comment on the nuances and philosophy that are involved in performing these reconstructions.

Prelamination

Prelamination of an osteofasciocutaneous fibular flap with a skin graft was first described in 1997 by Capelouto and colleagues[14] and later applied by Papadopulos and colleagues.[15] The fibula flap is prelaminated 6 months before transfer, at which time the perineal urethra is lengthened similar to the technique described previously. In 2011, Song and colleagues[16] published their series of prelaminated radial forearm free flaps (RFFFPs) using skin graft for the urethra. More recently, a modification using mucosal grafts in the RFFFP has been popularized at the University of Miami. Capitalizing on the principle of homology, vaginal, or uterine mucosa— which better resemble urothelium—are used to prelaminate the RFFFP around a catheter. The flap transfer is performed in a staged manner after the graft has healed.[17] The obvious downside is the high degree of postoperative care required. The primary benefit is having actual mucosa lining the urethra, although we do not yet know the clinical implications of the cellular composition of the neourethra.

Dancing Phallus

In 1972, Orticochea[18] described the use of innervated myocutaneous gracilis flaps for phallic reconstruction with the proposed benefit of a natural erection. The group at the Helsinki Hospital in Finland have rediscovered this technique, as has Koshima, and modified it to include a superficial circumflex iliac perforator flap for urethral reconstruction and a split-thickness skin graft for the shaft skin. Koshima and colleagues[19] have also published on their technique for bilateral superficial circumflex iliac perforator flaps, to avoid the radial forearm donor. These techniques are most often performed in a single stage.

Secondary Grafting of the Urethra

An alternative to a vascularized urethral flap is a skin or buccal graft to line the shaft urethra. Perovic and colleagues[20] provided one of the earliest descriptions of a grafted urethra. The group in Serbia performs a latissimus dorsi myocutaneous free flap and perineal masculinization during a single operation. The urethra is lengthened using the urethral plate, labia minora, and dorsal clitoral skin and is marsupialized through the ventral surface of the shaft, in essence creating a hypospadias at the proximal or middle third of the shaft. A 2-stage buccal graft urethroplasty is then subsequently performed to lengthen the urethra to the tip of the phallus. In the first stage, the buccal graft is placed on the ventral surface of the distal half of the phallus; this will be the new urethral plate. Three months later it is tubularized to create the new urethra.[21,22]

Another approach that has been performed but not published is lining of the entire shaft urethra with full-thickness skin graft and tubularization at the next procedure (**Fig. 8**).

The authors of this article, however, believe in the superiority of vascularized flap tissue over grafted tissue to fabricate the new urethra.

STAGING OF ADJUNCT PROCEDURES
Glansplasty

The glansplasty is a somewhat neglected, but important, component of phalloplasty. A strategy around the ideal timing is important. Although it is not the favored approach of the authors, it is considered safe to perform glansplasty in an RFFFP at the time of shaft creation. Most surgeons will refrain from doing so with the Anterolateral thigh because the perforator(s) enter on the more proximal aspect of the flap in contrast with the RFFFP, where perforators enter distally.

There are 4 general options in glansplasty timing:

1. Immediate at the time of shaft creation in a single-stage approach
2. Delayed during the second stage of the Big Ben sequence (there is no surgical benefit for immediate glansplasty in this sequence, although it

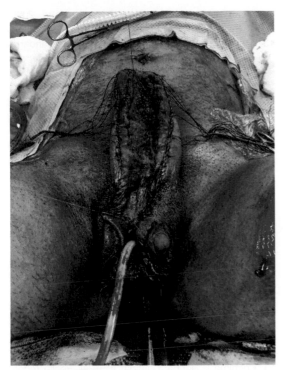

Fig. 8. Anterolateral thigh phalloplasty was performed at an earlier stage. In the second stage this is split and lined with a full-thickness skin graft. Tubularization will occur at a separate surgery.

may delay patient satisfaction with aesthetic result)
3. Immediate at the time of flap transfer in the perineal urethra first sequence
4. Delayed as a separate stage in the perineal urethra first sequence

Because it is not advised to perform a glansplasty during the placement of an erectile device for obvious reasons, it is therefore only the Big Ben method that allows to perform the glansplasty in a delayed fashion without adding an additional stage before placement of an erectile device.

It is ill-advised to place the erectile implant at the time of glansplasty because it will compromise the aesthetic outcome and the vascularity of the flap. Of note, the Big Ben technique omits the need for an isolated glansplasty stage.

The authors are proponents of delayed glansplasty for all flaps, because it allows for phallic healing and resolution of edema, which can be significant after flap transfer. Shaping the glans when the phallus has reached a stable circumference may result in a more permanent coronal ridge.

Testicular Implants

Based on the experience of immediate implant insertion in breast cancer reconstruction,

surgeons may be inclined to add testicular implants at the time of scrotoplasty. However, we strongly advise against performing testicular implants at the time of scrotoplasty. An infection of the implants can affect the adjacent neourethra and lead to fistula and/or stricture formation. Any measure to decrease the risk for infection ought to be taken with placement of implants. Testicular implant placement can be performed at the same time as erectile devices.

Erectile Devices

Erectile devices come in 2 types: semimalleable and inflatable devices. Before insertion, the phallic construct has to be in a steady state and all components of the reconstruction fully healed without any potential nidus for infection. One or 2 testicular implants can be placed at this stage if the scrotal size allows. Although lore teaches that protective sensation is a prerequisite for the implantation of erectile devices, this has never been formally examined and practices around this vary. The inflatable device, in these authors' opinion, can be inserted even in the absence of meaningful sensation.

SUMMARY

Phalloplasty consists of several components, each of which comes with its own set of potential complications. The ideal sequence and staging protocol is neither agreed upon by experts nor is it elucidated in the available literature. In these authors' opinion, staging allows for management of complications stepwise, minimizing the downstream effects of any one issue on the functional and aesthetic outcome. We advocate for taking advantage of the tried-and-true principles of delay and conservative staging whenever possible in this complex, multipart reconstruction, which is prone to high-stakes complications.

ACKNOWLEDGMENTS

The authors would like to thank the urologists with whom we work: Dr Daniel Dugi, Dr Jon Witten, and Dr Kamran Sajadi, as well as Dr Lishiana Shaffer from Obstetrics and Gynecology, for their invaluable participation in the care of our patients.

REFERENCES

1. Hage JJ, Bout CA, Bloem JJ, et al. Phalloplasty in female-to-male transsexuals- What do our patients ask for? Ann Plast Surg 1993;30:323–6.

2. Morrison SD, Shakir A, Vyas KS, et al. Phalloplasty: a review of techniques and outcomes. Plast Reconstr Surg 2016;138(3):594–615.

3. Morrison SD, Dy GW, Chong HJ, et al. Transgender-related education in plastic surgery and urology residency programs. J Grad Med Educ 2017;9(2):178–83.

4. Kim S, Dennis M, Holland J, et al. The anatomy of forearm free flap phalloplasty for transgender surgery. Clin Anat 2018;31(2):145–51.

5. Schechter LS, Safa B. Introduction to phalloplasty. Clin Plast Surg 2018;45(3):387–9.

6. Esmonde N, Bluebond-Langner R, Berli JU. Phalloplasty flap-related complication. Clin Plast Surg 2018;45(3):415–24.

7. Garaffa G, Christopher NA, Ralph DJ. Total phallic reconstruction in female-to-male transsexuals. Eur Urol 2010;57(4):715–22.

8. Garcia MM, Christopher NA, De Luca F, et al. Overall satisfaction, sexual function, and the durability of neophallus dimensions following staged female to male genital gender confirming surgery: the Institute of Urology, London U.K. experience. Transl Androl Urol 2014;3(2):156–62.

9. Kuzon WM Jr. Discussion: outcomes after phalloplasty: do transgender patients and multiple urethral procedures carry a higher rate of complication? Plast Reconstr Surg 2018;141(2):230e–1e.

10. Remington AC, Morrison SD, Massie JP, et al. Outcomes after phalloplasty: do transgender patients and multiple urethral procedures carry a higher rate of complication? Plast Reconstr Surg 2018;141(2):220e–9e.

11. Leriche A, Timsit MO, Morel-Journel N, et al. Long-term outcome of forearm flee-flap phalloplasty in the treatment of transsexualism. BJU Int 2008;101(10):1297–300.

12. Monstrey S, Hoebeke P, Selvaggi G, et al. Penile reconstruction: is the radial forearm flap really the standard technique? Plast Reconstr Surg 2009;124(2):510–8.

13. Coleman E, Bockting W, Botzer M, et al. Standards of care for the health of transsexual, transgender, and gender-nonconforming people, version 7. Int J Transgend 2012;13(4):165–232.

14. Capelouto CC, Orgill DP, Loughlin KR. Complete phalloplasty with a prelaminated osteocutaneous fibula flap. J Urol 1997;158(6):2238–9.

15. Papadopulos NA, Schaff J, Biemer E. The use of free prelaminated and sensate osteofasciocutaneous fibular flap in phalloplasty. Injury 2008;39(Suppl 3):S62–7.

16. Song C, Wong M, Wong CH, et al. Modifications of the radial forearm flap phalloplasty for female-to-male gender reassignment. J Reconstr Microsurg 2011;27(2):115–20.

17. Salgado CJ, Fein LA, Chim J, et al. Prelamination of neourethra with uterine mucosa in radial forearm osteocutaneous free flap phalloplasty in the female-to-male transgender patient. Case Rep Urol 2016;2016:8742531.

18. Orticochea M. A new method of total reconstruction of the penis. Br J Plast Surg 1972;25(4):347–66.

19. Koshima I, Nanba Y, Nagai A, et al. Penile reconstruction with bilateral superficial circumflex iliac artery perforator (SCIP) flaps. J Reconstr Microsurg 2006;22(3):137–42.

20. Perovic SV, Djinovic R, Bumbasirevic M, et al. Total phalloplasty using a musculocutaneous latissimus dorsi flap. BJU Int 2007;100(4):899–905 [discussion: 905].

21. Djordjevic ML, Bencic M, Kojovic V, et al. Musculocutaneous latissimus dorsi flap for phalloplasty in female to male gender affirmation surgery. World J Urol 2019;37(4):631–7.

22. Djordjevic ML, Bumbasirevic MZ, Vukovic PM, et al. Musculocutaneous latissimus dorsi free transfer flap for total phalloplasty in children. J Pediatr Urol 2006;2(4):333–9.

Prosthetic Placement After Phalloplasty

Gideon A. Blecher, MBBS, FRACS (Urol)[a,b,*], Nim Christopher, MPhil, FRCS (Urol)[c],
David J. Ralph, BSc, MS, FRCS (Urol)[c]

KEYWORDS

- Gender-affirming surgery • Transgender persons • Penile prosthesis • Penis • Phalloplasty
- Genital • Reconstruction

KEY POINTS

- Although significant developments have occurred over the last century, the inflatable hydraulic prosthesis remains the best tool in aiming for the ideal phalloplasty erectile device.
- Penile implantation should occur as a last stage of phalloplasty, once other complications of surgery have been dealt with and stabilized.
- Key differences in surgical placement include absence of corpora, scarring within the shaft, proximal pubic fixation and distal sock formation, scarring, and vascular pedicle considerations for incision and reservoir placement.
- Prosthesis options include semirigid devices and inflatable 2-piece or 3-piece devices.
- Complication rates are higher in phalloplasty cohorts, including infection, mechanical failure, erosion, and malposition/migration.

RATIONALE FOR PROSTHESIS

Trans men opting for phalloplasty undergo many surgeries before this final step and although relatively straightforward, the insertion of a prosthetic device for stiffness develops what was previously an appendage into a functional anatomic unit. Although some trans men choose not to undergo this step, it allows for phallic rigidity for sexual purposes and can often be one of the most fulfilling and exciting steps for them.

The ideal phalloplasty erectile prosthesis should be soft during detumescence and functionally firm enough for penetration while erect. It should be easily inserted, activated, deactivated, and replaceable, and inert with minimal infection risk, as well as affordable. To date, no perfect device exists, although much progress has been made over the past century.

EVOLUTION OF PROSTHESIS IN PHALLOPLASTY

The notion of a penile stiffener has existed for many years; texts refer to the baculum of animals,[1] a cartilaginous structure that aids in mammalian erection. Although no such structure exists in humans, it forms the inspiration for obtaining rigidity in phalloplasty. Although attempts have been made to find the ideal stiffener, some investigators suggest that dependent edema and fibrosis of the phallus alone may suffice for some clients.[2,3] Bogoras[4] described the first successful penile reconstruction, with a tubularized local skin flap, using rib cartilage as a stiffener. However, rib

Disclosure: G.A. Blecher, consultant for Advisory Board for Coloplast; N. Christopher, consultant for Innovations Advisory Board for Coloplast; D.J. Ralph, consultant for Coloplast, Advisory Board for Boston Scientific.
[a] Department of Urology, The Alfred Hospital, 55 Commercial Road, Melbourne 3004, Australia; [b] Monash Health, 823-865 Centre Road, Bentleigh East, Australia; [c] University College London Hospitals & St Peter's Andrology, 145 Harley Street, London W1G 6BJ, UK
* Corresponding author. Department of Urology, The Alfred Hospital, 55 Commercial Road, Melbourne 3004, Australia.
E-mail address: info@drblecher.com

Urol Clin N Am 46 (2019) 591–603
https://doi.org/10.1016/j.ucl.2019.07.013
0094-0143/19/© 2019 Elsevier Inc. All rights reserved.

cartilage may be curved, become distorted, or be of insufficient length. Furthermore, it is rigid and does not allow for flaccidity. Bone with periosteum has been used, although resorption over time seems to be a drawback.[5] In the late 1940s, an acrylic rigid prosthesis was used in several patients; however, some developed a significant tissue response.[6] A skin-lined pocket within the phallus has been described, into which a removable penile prosthesis may be placed, thus potentially reducing the risk of infection and erosion.[7] A major step forward for the use of stiffeners in phalloplasty was the development of sensate flaps, which, although the overall publication numbers are low, seemed to reduce the complication rates in terms of erosion. Orticochea[8] in 1972 described the gracilis flap phalloplasty with a silicone elastomer supportive rod, which rests against the pubis. A phallus with incorporated vascularized bone stiffener was described in 1999 by Fang and colleagues,[9] using the free radial osteocutaneous flap; radial bone forearm fracture occurred in 1 of 22 patients at 1 month. Although the free osteocutaneous radius or free osteocutaneous fibula flaps may not be complicated by bone resorption, issues with permanent erectile state remain.[10] Recently Selvaggi and colleagues[11] reported their use of titanium bone anchoring to the pubis for a penile episthesis. Although this option may not appeal to most clients, the avoidance of multiple surgeries (for either free, pedicled, or local flaps) with their inherent risks and complications may be a viable future alternative for selected individuals.

In 1978, Puckett and Montie[12] described the first use of a hydraulic Brantley-Scott prosthesis into a transgender phallus, which was associated with high failure rates. More successful, albeit small, series were subsequently published by Levine and colleagues[13] and Jordan and colleagues.[14] Since then, larger series of phalloplasty erectile prostheses have been published, but complication rates remain high.[15,16] A 1-piece hydraulic device, which is no longer manufactured, as well as more modern 2-piece and 3-piece hydraulic devices have emerged. Despite the complication rate, it seems the inflatable hydraulic device remains the best tool yet, in aiming for the ideal phalloplasty erectile device.

TIMING OF PLACEMENT

Phalloplasty techniques such as osteocutaneous flaps inherently contain their erectile component. It is logical that the phallus be created first, in as many stages as each takes. A myriad of complications may occur along the way, including phallus ischemia or necrosis, urethral fistula or stricture, vaginectomy-related fluid collections, and phallus scar contracture; these need to be dealt with before penile implant. A reasonably capacious scrotoplasty needs to be created to house the pump of the inflatable erectile device. Glans sculpting should also ideally be performed before erectile device insertion, because any surgical wound may increase the risk of penile prosthesis infection. Hence typically in the case of a radial artery forearm flap phallus, the erectile device can be placed as a last step, 12 to 16 months from the first stage, which also allows the phallus to develop some protective tactile sensitivity.

SURGICAL TECHNIQUE

For the final stage of the reconstructive process, following phallus formation, urethral join-up, hysterectomy, oophorectomy, vaginectomy, clitoral burying, scrotoplasty, and glans sculpting, an inflatable or semirigid penile prosthesis is inserted into the phallus, providing rigidity for penetrative sexual intercourse.

Initial Steps

The procedure is performed under general anesthetic with prophylactic intravenous antibiotics. The patient is prepped and draped in the supine position with the legs separated on a vein board, to enable easier access to the groins. A 14-F urethral catheter is placed with the assistance of an introducer. This step is often one of the most challenging. If required, a flexible cystoscope should be on standby to enable a guided catheter placement over a wire. For overweight patients, those with unfavorable body habitus, and sometimes for double-cylinder penile prosthesis, surgical access may be easier in the lithotomy position.

Surgical Approach

There are various incisions used to gain access. If the vascular pedicle of the phalloplasty is inferolateral to the phallus (eg, pedicled anterolateral thigh flap phalloplasty or any free flap phalloplasty connected to the superficial femoral artery), then some surgeons open the cephalad part of the phalloplasty base scar similar to an infrapubic approach. This approach allows easy dilation of the phallus and easy placement of the reservoir and the pump can be dropped into the scrotum. There is good access to the superior part of the pubis but not the inferior pubis.

Care must be taken to not disrupt any nerve anastomoses. For superolateral vascular pedicles such as from the inferior epigastric artery, it is easier to make a groin crease incision between lateral edge of scrotum and medial border of thigh. This approach allows good access the whole anterior face of the pubis. As long as the incision is deepened close to the pubic bone surface, any clitoral nerve connections should not be disrupted. In some cases the phallus/scrotum can be opened ventrally to access the anterior pubic bone surface. This approach is only practical for a phallus without an urethra. Our preference is for the lateral groin approach.

Pubis Dissection and Proximal Fixation

An incision is made in the groin crease down to fat (**Fig. 1**). A small self-retaining retractor, along with a Langenbeck retractor, facilitates the view and dissection just superficial to the periosteum of the pubis. A useful landmark is the adductor longus tendon, which inserts to the side of the pubis. Care should be taken not to breach the muscle fascia over the adductor tendon to prevent bleeding and pain. The dissection plane should be carried just over the midline, evident by the median groove of the pubis and as low as the lower third of the pubis. It is important

not to dissect below the inferior pubic ramus because there are large venous plexuses in that area that would cause bleeding. Also this avoids potential disruption of any clitoral nerve connections and avoid damage to the native urethra.

There are multiple options for proximal fixation. The cylinders can just be placed in the phallus and against the pubic bone and a natural fibrous capsule allowed to form. This method theoretically has the least risk of infection but often results in cylinder dislocation and instability during sexual intercourse because the cylinder is not firmly anchored. The rear tip or rear tip extender of the cylinder can be sutured to the pubic bone, which provides better cylinder stability for penetration but the cylinder can hinge at the attachment point with some instability. The third option is to use a nonabsorbable sock, which is firmly sutured to the anterior surface of the pubic bone. The cylinder is placed within the sock and has very good penetration stability and little hinge effect when erect. A fourth option is to drill holes in the superior surface of the pubic bone, which seats the rear tip of the cylinder.[17] Our preference is for the cap and sock approach.

For option 3, a minimum of 3 heavy, nonabsorbable anchoring sutures, or wires are secured in a triangular fashion across the midline for a single cylinder, and to each side of the pubis for double cylinders (**Figs. 2** and **3**). The longer the distance between the upper and lower sutures, the better the stability of the erect device will be. The lower lateral suture ensures stability and the angle of the erect phallus, and the upper lateral and medial sutures determine the overall length of the prosthesis within the phallus.

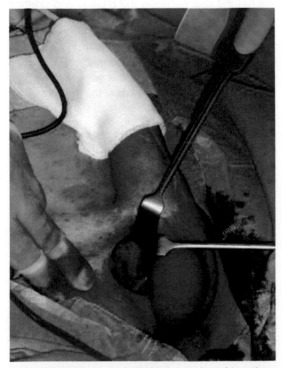

Fig. 1. Lateral scrotal incision and pubis plane development.

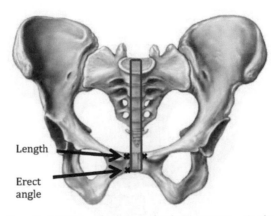

Length

Erect angle

Fig. 2. Actions of the anchoring sutures, single cylinder.

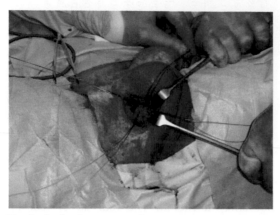

Fig. 3. Anchoring suture placement.

Anchoring has the potential for bone pain, infection, and prominence of the proximal sock causing discomfort. To minimize prominence, ensuring a medial location of the sock when securing the anchoring sutures may be of benefit. It is important not to inadvertently anchor the device to the adductor tendon because this will cause a lot of pain.

Preparation of the Corporal Space

A combination of blunt dissection with a finger, as well as scissors, helps initiate the dilatation within the phallus. There are commonly 2 locations where scarring is more prominent: at the phalloscrotal junction, as well as at the site of the glans sculpting. If 1 cylinder is to be used, dilatation should be performed in the midline, dorsal to the urethra, Otherwise, 2 separate dilatations are needed, dorsolateral to the urethra (**Fig. 4**). The dilatation should extend all the way to the tip of the phallus leaving 1 cm of fat and subcutaneous tissue to prevent erosion and prominence of the prosthetic

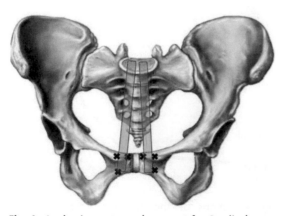

Fig. 4. Anchoring suture placement for 2 cylinders.

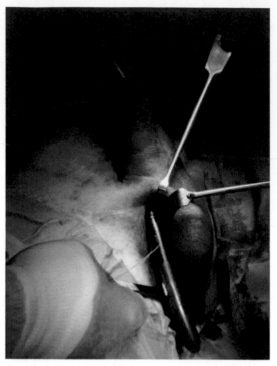

Fig. 5. Phallus space dilatation with Hegar dilator.

tips. Following the use of scissors, Hegar dilators are used to dilate the space for the cylinders (**Fig. 5**). If done carefully, the space created is the natural gap between the phallus and urethral parts of the flap and avoids the blood vessels. There is still the possibility of damage to the vascular pedicle within the phallus. If a nonabsorbable cap is planned, then the dilation needs to be at least 1 size bigger than the cap diameter; for example, for 16-mm wide caps, the authors dilate to Hegar 18. If no cap is planned, then dilation to slightly bigger that the cylinder is appropriate; for example, Hegar 12 for AMS 700CX, Hegar 14 for Coloplast Titan, and smaller for the narrow-base devices. Irrigation of this pseudocorporal space with antibiotic solution is used to confirm urethral integrity (**Fig. 6**). If a urethral injury is confirmed, then the prosthesis insertion should be abandoned because there is a high rate of prosthesis infection. The urethra should be repaired and the prosthesis inserted at a later date when the urethra has healed. The Hegar dilator can be left in place while the contralateral side is prepared to prevent crossover.

Once both corporal spaces are defined, length measurement is made from the lowest anchoring suture point to the tip of the dilated space. In our experience, the most reliable method is to use a straight measuring tool (the blue measuring tool from the AMS accessory kit is ideal for this) from

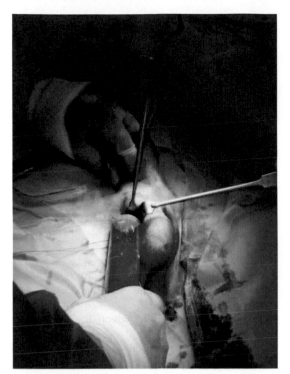

Fig. 6. Irrigation of dilated corporal space to check for urethral injury.

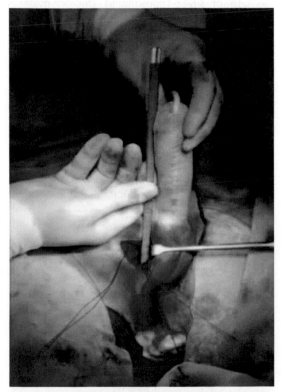

Fig. 7. Length measurement from inferior pubic fixation suture to midglans using the AMS measuring tool (Boston Scientific Corporation, Marlborough, MA).

the lowest anchor suture to the midglans of the partially stretched phallus in the proposed erect position on the outside of the phallus (**Fig. 7**). This method ensures there is less likelihood of erosion or floppy glans syndrome.

Prosthesis Type and Number of Cylinders

This decision depends on the length and girth of the phallus, as well as the size of the glans. The patient may also have a particular preference for both the bulk of the phallus and the implant characteristics. Although 2 cylinders provide maximal axial rigidity, some patients' phalluses do not accommodate the bulk. In our experience about two-thirds of patients fit a single cylinder device and one-third accommodate double cylinders. It is the authors' opinion that the Coloplast Titan inflatable device is slightly more palpable when deflated, but gives a more rigid feel to the erection compared with a Boston Scientific AMS 700CX. If more than 21 cm of cylinder is needed, then the Coloplast Titan has extralong cylinders available. The erection is more rigid and stable if rear tip extenders can be avoided. One of the problems that can arise from using rear tip extenders is that the exit tubing of the cylinder becomes more palpable in the phallus base and can be uncomfortable. The semirigid implants (Coloplast Genesis and Boston Scientific Spectra) are less complicated to insert, but the impression of a permanent erection, plus slightly less axial rigidity (size for size), is a consideration. Although Boston Scientific AMS 700 series implants are precoated with Inhibizone and thus should not be placed into antibiotic solution, Coloplast implants have a hydrophilic surface and should be dipped in an appropriate antibiotic solution before placement. The exact antibiotic solution used depends on local microbiology advice. The authors use rifampicin 600 mg with 160 mg of gentamicin in 100 mL of normal saline as our dipping solution.

Sock and Cap Formation

Although not all surgeons use a distal cap, it is the author's preference to do so as per Jordan and colleagues,[14] in order to minimize the risk of distal erosion. Vascular prosthetic grafts such as Dacron, Gore-Tex, or polytetrafluoroethylene (PTFE)[18] can be used; a 3-cm to 4-cm section is fashioned and the 2 corners are trimmed to create a rounded end. The cap is closed at the rounded end with continuous 2-0 polypropylene or nylon suture, to ensure the prosthesis does not herniate through. A nonabsorbable 2-0 suture is brought from outside to inside the distal cap, through the distal tip of the implant, and back through the cap, mimicking the traction suture for standard implant placement. The suture ends will later be loaded onto a Keith needle. It is important to securely knot the suture over the cap to ensure the cylinder tip is firmly anchored to the cap. Once the cap has formed enough fibrosis to the phallus fat, the anchoring suture prevents the cylinder tip from being displaced and migrating elsewhere.

Unlike genetic males, whereby the corpora albuginea facilitate proximal fixation of the implant (**Fig. 8**), an anchoring sock is required in gender cases. The proximal end of the sock can be folded over itself by 4 mm and secured with interrupted nonabsorbable sutures. A small incision can be made in the anteromedial aspect of the sock to enable the tubing to exit. By making the exit tubing come out slightly medial, it will be less palpable to the patient. Just distal to the tubing, the sock defect can then be repaired with nonabsorbable sutures. The implant together with socks and caps is now ready for placement.

The point of using a synthetic sock is to create enough fibrosis so that the cylinder base is firmly seated on the pubis. Dacron causes a lot of fibrosis and is ideally suited for this application. Hernia mesh material has also successfully been used; for example, Prolene Mesh and Vypro II Mesh. A potential disadvantage is that the infection rate is probably higher with the use of synthetic socks and is likely to be higher the more synthetic material is used. The original description by Hage and colleagues[19] was to use a full synthetic sheath to simulate the corpora cavernosa. However, the authors have found that, by using less synthetic material (ie, only cap and sock), the surgery is easier to

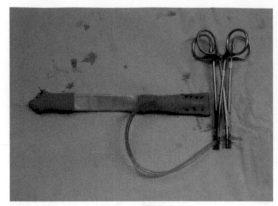

Fig. 9. Dacron cap and sock with AMS 700CX cylinder (Boston Scientific Corporation, Marlborough, MA).

perform (**Fig. 9**). The phallus is also much softer in the flaccid state because of the reduction in synthetic material. Distal caps are not required in revision procedures in which the capsule is well placed and formed.

Regarding sheaths, the authors have also found that, when using malleable devices (eg, AMS Spectra or Coloplast Genesis), it is necessary to use a full synthetic sheath, to prevent the rigid prosthesis from being displaced. Theoretically, the use of silver-impregnated Dacron material should reduce the infection risk. This method is commonly used in revisions of infected aortic vascular grafts.

Placement

The device is threaded into the dilated space in the standard fashion using a Furlow instrument and inflated to check its position. Once the cylinder tip is in a satisfactory position, the preplaced pubic anchoring sutures are each placed through the sock and sequentially tied in place (**Fig. 10**). In cases of 2-piece or 3-piece inflatable devices,

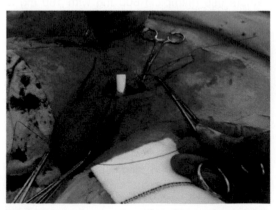

Fig. 8. Corporal spacer insertion during genetic male phalloplasty.

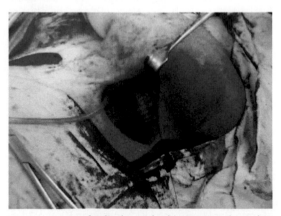

Fig. 10. Proximal cylinder tucked in against the pubis.

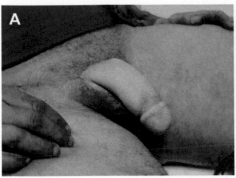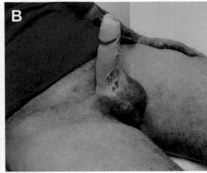

Fig. 11. Final result in (*A*) flaccid and (*B*) erect positions (transgender).

the pump is placed into the neoscrotum. The location of the reservoir depends on the presence and location of a vascular pedicle as well as the surgeon's preference. The ipsilateral space of Retzius should be avoided when the pedicle arises from the ipsilateral femoral artery or inferior epigastric vessels. There is potential for the reservoir to erode into the bladder when placed in the space of Retzius, particularly if the patient has had pelvic surgery and/or multiple suprapubic catheters. Instead, a high appendix type incision for retroperitoneal access to the iliac fossa/paracolic gutter can be made; the tubing is easily tunneled just deep to the rectus sheath and exits lateral to the superficial inguinal ring, avoiding any vascular pedicles and the ilioinguinal nerve. The reservoir is then far away from the bladder. If there is considerable subcutaneous fat, then the tubing can be placed subcutaneously. As far as the authors are aware, high submuscular reservoir placement under the rectus muscle has not been described in phalloplasty penile prosthesis to date. If this method is chosen, then the reservoir should be placed on the contralateral side of the vascular pedicle. The pump is placed within the neoscrotum and the neck closed to prevent retraction. It is recommended to fixate at least 2 of the tubings from the pump to prevent rotation of the pump in order to keep the deflate mechanism in an anterior position for ease of use.

The device is closed over in multiple layers. Although some clinicians argue for the use of drains to reduce infection,[14] the authors think it is necessary only in cases when clinically required. For revision surgery when a new space is not dilated, drains are often not required.

Postoperative Management

The device is left 50% inflated for 7 days to allow the formation of a pseudocapsule around the cylinders. If there are signs of skin bruising or skin ischemia, then the device should be deflated to prevent skin necrosis and tissue loss. Postoperative prophylactic antibiotics are prescribed for 5 to 7 days. Note that there is no published evidence on the optimal length of postoperative antibiotic therapy, but this regime has served us well for the last 20 years. The catheter is removed the following day and clients can be taught to cycle their device at 2 weeks or when comfortable. Use of the device for sex should not occur before 6 weeks, by which time the bone sutures will have healed. The authors recommend that patients inflate their devices daily for 20 to 30 minutes for at least 4 weeks so that the cylinder capsule matures in a straight position (**Fig. 11**) rather than curved if left deflated for a few weeks over the scrotum (**Table 1**).

PATIENT SATISFACTION

Although most of the literature regarding implants in phalloplasty pertains to nongender patients, there are several studies with heterogeneous outcome measurements, focusing on this specific cohort. It should be noted that, overall, there is a paucity of rigorous outcome data regarding penile prostheses in phalloplasty.

Regarding satisfaction outcomes, Falcone and colleagues[16] have the largest series, of 104 transgender patients. This study involved an in-house nonvalidated questionnaire. All patients underwent placement of a 3-piece inflatable penile prosthesis with median 20 months of follow-up. They surmised that penetrative sex was possible in 77%, whereas functional and cosmetic satisfaction rates were 88%. Several other smaller studies using either in-house questionnaires or retrospective note reviews show sexual penetration ability rates of 51% to 81%.[20,21]

Table 1
Studies of penile prostheses in transgender phalloplasty

Author, Year	Number of Transgender Clients (Total in Study)	Implant Type (Number Cylinders)	Duration of Follow-up	Complication					Sexual Function
				Infection	Erosion	Mechanical Failure	Malposition/ Migration	Other	
Jordan et al,[14] 1994	3 (8)	Duraphase (1) Uniflate 1000 (1) ×3	Up to 3 y	2/4	—	—	—	—	Sexually active: synergist device ×1 Difficult sexual activity ×2
Krueger et al,[2] 2007	105	AMS 650 malleable (1) AMS Dynaflex (1) AMS 700CXM (2)	—	2/105	2/105	7/105	3/105	3/105	—
Leriche et al,[20] 2008	38	Prototype Ambicor AMS 600 AMS 700S	Mean 110 mo	11(29%) (some were mechanical failure)	—	—	—	Exchange 8 (21%) Explant 3(8%)	18 (51%) Satisfactory sexual function
Hoebeke et al,[30] 2010	129 (189 implants)	15 Dynaflex (1)	Mean 56 mo	1 (6.7%)	0 (0%)	8 (6%)	2 (13%)	2 (13%) leakage	—
		69 AMS CX/CXM (1) ×37 (2) ×13	Mean 42 mo	9 (13%)	7 (10%)	11 (8.5%)	14 (20%)	12 (17.6%) leakage 1 (1.4%) other	
		47 Ambicor (1) ×22 (2) ×25	Mean 12 mo	9 (15%)	5 (8.5%)	0 (0%)	7 (11.9%)	1 (12.5%) leakage	
		8 Coloplast (2)	Mean 22 mo	1 (12.5%)	0 (0%)	2 (1.6%)	1 (12.5%)	1 (12.5%) other	
		AMS CX Inhibizone (1) ×13 (2) ×4	Mean 28 mo	2 (5.9%)	3 (8.8%)	4 (3.1%)	3 (8.8%)	3 (8.8%) leakage	
		—	—	—	—	—	—	Overall Infection/ erosion 18 (13.8%) Mechanical failure 40 (30.8%)	

Study	N	Device	Follow-up					
Terrier,[36] 2014	14	—	—	1/14	1/14	21% (includes malposition)	—	79% satisfied with current sexual life (includes all aspects of phalloplasty)
Segal,[37] 2015	2 (9 total)	AMS 700CX (—) Semirigid (—) AMS 700CXR (—)	Mean 9.6 mo	1 (33%)	2 (66%) erosion	—	—	—
Zuckerman et al,[21] 2015	15 (31 total)	Semirigid (—) ×21 AMS 700CX/CXR Coloplast Titan (1) 5% (2) 95%	Mean 59.7 mo	3 (9.7%)	2 (6%)	1 (3%)	1 (3%)	Sexually active 81%
Neuville et al,[31] 2016	62 (95 total)	Ambicor (—) Ambicor with graft (—)	Mean 4 y	8 (8.4%)	4 (4.2%) erosion	10 (10.5%)	12 (12.6%) malposition	—
Falcone et al,[16] 2018	247	AMS 700 CX/CXM/R Coloplast Titan Ambicor (1) ×39 (2) ×208	Median 20 mo	21 (8.5%)	38 (15.4%)	—	48 (19.4%) dissatisfaction	97 (77%) engaged in penetrative sexual intercourse 97 (88%) fully satisfied with function
Neuville et al,[32] 2019	20	ZSI 475 FtM	Mean 8.9 mo	1 (4.7%)	2 (9.5%)	1 (4.7%)	2 (9.5%)	12 (85.7%) engaged in regular penetrative intercourse

These rates seem comparable with the nontransgender phalloplasty cohort. Callens and colleagues[22] incorporated a novel method of assessment using psychological interview. All 10 patients were having penetrative sex and 80% were able to orgasm during sex. A small study by Young and colleagues[23] using validated questionnaires for nontransgender men (trauma and bladder exstrophy cohort) undergoing phalloplasty and penile prosthesis showed no difference before and after penile prosthesis in terms of sexual quality of life scores. They also showed overall satisfaction scores of 5 out of 10, orgasm 6 out of 10, intercourse satisfaction 10.5 out of 15, and subjective quality of life 60 out of 100.

IMPLANT SURVIVAL

Penile prostheses experience mechanical failure at some point. Several modifications have improved the durability, including multilayer woven fabrics, kink-resistant tubing, and other reinforcements. With the introduction of Parylene coating, designed to reduce silicone friction, 3-year revision-free rates for the AMS 700 series devices improved from 78.6% to 87.4%.[24] Bioflex polyurethane was used instead of silicone for Coloplast Mentor inflatable implants to improve tensile strength.[25] In the nonphalloplasty cohort, prosthesis survival rates at 5, 10, and 15 years of 85%, 68%, and 57%, respectively, were reported for the AMS 700CX device.[26] Contemporary data indicate freedom from mechanical failure rates for AMS 700CX and Coloplast Titan inflatable implants at 87% to 91% at 5 years.[27] Semirigid devices inherently carry a significantly lower risk of failure, with 100% mechanical survival rates at 5.7 and 11.7 years.[28,29] Despite these improvements, the overall survival of prosthesis in phalloplasty is significantly less; with a median follow-up of 20 months in the largest series using AMS 700 devices, mechanical failure rates approximate 15%.[16] The main reasons for failure included cylinder rupture (69%), cylinder aneurysm (19%), and rupture of the tubing between the cylinder and the pump (12%).

Although the overall median survival of implants in phalloplasty range from 4.2 to 4.9 years in some studies, the Falcone and colleagues[16] study showed 5-year survival rates of 78%[16,30,31] (**Fig. 12**).

Despite the developments of InhibiZone and hydrophilic coatings that adsorb antibiotics, infection rates for penile prosthesis in phalloplasty are 8.5% in the largest study (median 20-month follow-up) and up to 9.7% in other studies.[21]

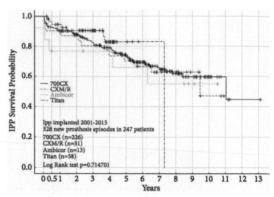

Fig. 12. Kaplan-Meier curves for penile prosthesis survival. (*From* Falcone M, Garaffa G, Gillo A, Dente D, Christopher AN, Ralph DJ. Outcomes of inflatable penile prosthesis insertion in 247 patients completing female to male gender reassignment surgery. BJU international. 2018;121(1):139-44; with permission.)

A complication more specific to phalloplasty implants is that of proximal or distal malposition, caused by excessive mobility or migration of the device. This malposition is caused by the lack of

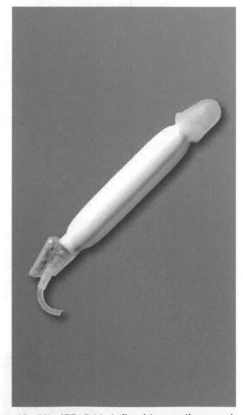

Fig. 13. ZSI 475 FtM inflatable penile prosthesis. (*Courtesy of* Zephyr Surgical Implants, Geneva, Switzerland; with permission.)

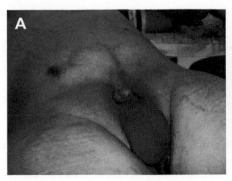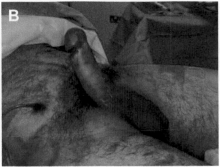

Fig. 14. Final result in (*A*) flaccid and (*B*) erect positions (bladder exstrophy).

secure housing within an anatomic corporal space. Although specific detail is not provided by some studies, proximal migration seems to be an issue in 11.5% in contemporary studies.[21,31] This issue may be improved by new developments such as the ZSI 475 FtM and ZSI 100 FtM (semi-rigid) (Zephyr Surgical Implants, Geneva, Switzerland) penile prosthesis, specifically designed for phalloplasty (**Fig. 13**). These implants incorporate a large base for pubic bone fixation: it is anticipated that this may reduce the specific complication of proximal migration with rates of 4.7% within a small sample size of 20.[32] The single distal "glans" of this device is designed to mimic a natural shape, which may help reduce the distal erosion rates, although this was not specifically commented on in the feasibility and safety article. However, sexual function scores seem similar to other prosthesis studies, with 87.5% of clients engaged in regular penetrative sexual intercourse.[32]

Although erosion occurs in nonphalloplasty contexts, the rates of distal cylinder erosion in phalloplasty are higher because of the lack of natural anatomic corpora. Distal caps help to mitigate this risk, which approaches 4% to 6% at 4 to 5 years.[21,31]

TESTICULAR PROSTHESIS

A variety of manufactured testicular prostheses have been developed since their first description using Vitallium in 1939[33] and may be placed into the neoscrotum. These prostheses should be inserted into the loose areolar tissue of the labia majora. Both silicone-filled and saline-filled options are available. Tissue expanders have been described being placed into the neoscrotum before prosthesis placement.[18] Alternatively, in the case of small or tight labial tissue, a self-expanding ellipsoid tissue expander (Osmed GMBH, Germany) can be used, which osmotically increases its volume from 1.1 to 10 mL, reaching a length of 31 mm. The size is chosen to fit within the neoscrotum and can replicate the size of the penile prosthesis pump, which is situated in the contralateral hemiscrotum. Although there is minimal literature specifically related to the trans population, the risks seem similar for the nontransgender cohort and include infection, hematoma, erosion, discomfort/tethering to skin, and dissatisfaction related to size, texture, or position.[34,35]

NONTRANSGENDER PHALLOPLASTY CONSIDERATIONS

Although this article concerns transgender surgery, the authors thought it important to briefly discuss the main differences to consider for penile implantation in the genetic male population. Clearly, an anatomic corpora cavernosa is usually present. The authors recommend dilatation of the corporal space and preplacement of a spacer (either shortened semirigid prosthesis or rear tip extenders) during the phalloplasty formation stage (see **Fig. 13**). This spacer then assists with identification of the proximal corpora when it comes time for inflatable penile prosthesis (IPP) insertion. During IPP placement, the spacers are retrieved and no anchoring sutures or proximal socks are required. Because of the laterality of the proximal crus, ideally 2 cylinders should be placed to help aid centralization of the erect phallus (**Fig. 14**). Testicular prostheses are general not required; however, in some cases of hypogonadism, testicular atrophy may lead clinicians to consider their use.

SUMMARY

Although the search for the ideal penile prosthesis for phalloplasty continues, it is early in its development. Initial attempts at creating rigidity for phalloplasty used simple technologies and were plagued with drawbacks, including permanent erectile state, resorption of materials, infection, and erosion. A variety of prosthetic implants, including semirigid devices and 1-piece, 2-piece, and 3-piece inflatable devices, have been incorporated into phalloplasty. Although complication rates seem higher compared with nonphalloplasty cohorts, inflatable penile implants seem to enable most to participate in penetrative intercourse. However, infection, erosion, migration, and device failure remain ever-present hurdles. Newer designs of prosthesis, specific to phalloplasty, are emerging and it is hoped they will continue to develop to enable the ideal erectile device for phalloplasty to become reality in the not too distant future.

REFERENCES

1. Theodore Bergman R, Howard AH, Barnes RW. Plastic reconstruction of the penis. J Urol 1948; 59(6):1174–82.
2. Krueger M, Yekani SAH, Hundt GV, et al. Use of erectile prostheses in patients with free forearm flap phalloplasty. Int J Transgend 2007;10(1): 19–22.
3. Morales PA, O'Connor JJ Jr, Hotchkiss RS. Plastic reconstructive surgery after total loss of the penis. Am J Surg 1956;92(3):403–8.
4. Bogoras N. Uber die voile plastische Wiederherstellung eines zum Koitus fahigen Penis (Peniplastica totalis). Zentralbl Chir 1936;22:1271–6.
5. Munawar A. Surgical treatment of the male genitalia. J Int Coll Surg 1957;27:352.
6. Goodwin WE, Scott WW. Phalloplasty. J Urol 1952; 68(6):903–8.
7. Mukherjee GD. Use of groin and mid-thigh flap in reconstruction of penis with penile and perineal urethra and a dorsal skin-lined socket for a removable prosthesis. Ann Plast Surg 1986;16(3):235–41.
8. Orticochea M. A new method of total reconstruction of the penis. Br J Plast Surg 1972;25:347–66.
9. Fang R, Kao Y, Ma S, et al. Phalloplasty in female-to-male transsexuals using free radial osteocutaneous flap: a series of 22 cases. Br J Plast Surg 1999; 52(3):217–22.
10. Sengezer M, Öztürk S, Deveci M. The first use of free fibula flap as an autogenous penile implant. Plast Reconstr Surg 2004;114(1):142–6.
11. Selvaggi G, Branemark R, Elander A, et al. Titanium-bone-anchored penile epithesis: preoperative planning and immediate postoperative results. J Plast Surg Hand Surg 2015;49(1):40–4.
12. Puckett CL, Montie JE. Construction of male genitalia in the transsexual, using a tubed groin flap for the penis and a hydraulic inflation device. Plast Reconstr Surg 1978;61(4):523–30.
13. Levine LA, Zachary LS, Gottlieb LJ. Prosthesis placement after total phallic reconstruction. J Urol 1993;149(3):593–8.
14. Jordan GH, Alter GJ, Gilbert DA, et al. Penile prosthesis implantation in total phalloplasty. J Urol 1994;152(2):410–4.
15. Hoebeke P, De Cuypere G, Ceulemans P, et al. Obtaining rigidity in total phalloplasty: experience with 35 patients. J Urol 2003;169(1):221–3.
16. Falcone M, Garaffa G, Gillo A, et al. Outcomes of inflatable penile prosthesis insertion in 247 patients completing female to male gender reassignment surgery. BJU Int 2018;121(1):139–44.
17. Large MC, Gottlieb LJ, Wille MA, et al. Novel technique for proximal anchoring of penile prostheses in female-to-male transsexual. Urology 2009;74(2): 419–21.
18. Alter GJ, Gilbert DA, Schlossberg SM, et al. Prosthetic implantation after phallic construction. Microsurgery 1995;16(5):322–4.
19. Hage J, Bloem J, Bouman F. Obtaining rigidity in the neophallus of female-to-male transsexuals: a review of the literature. Ann Plast Surg 1993;30(4):327–33.
20. Leriche A, Timsit M-O, Morel-Journel N, et al. Long-term outcome of forearm flee-flap phalloplasty in the treatment of transsexualism. BJU Int 2008;101(10): 1297–300.
21. Zuckerman JM, Smentkowski K, Gilbert D, et al. Penile prosthesis implantation in patients with a history of total phallic construction. J Sex Med 2015; 12(12):2485–91.
22. Callens N, De Cuypere G, T'Sjoen G, et al. Sexual quality of life after total phalloplasty in men with penile deficiency: an exploratory study. World J Urol 2015;33(1):137–43.
23. Young EE, Friedlander D, Lue K, et al. Sexual function and quality of life before and after penile prosthesis implantation following radial forearm flap phalloplasty. Urology 2017;104:204–8.
24. Salem EA, Wilson SK, Neeb A, et al. Mechanical reliability of AMS 700 CX improved by parylene coating. J Sex Med 2009;6(9):2615–20.
25. Merrill DC. Mentor inflatable penile prosthesis: clinical experience in 52 patients. Br J Urol 1984; 56(5):512–5.
26. Wilson SK, Delk JR, Salem EA, et al. Long-term survival of inflatable penile prostheses: single surgical group experience with 2,384 first-time implants spanning two decades. J Sex Med 2007;4(4, Part 1):1074–9.
27. Chung E, Solomon M, DeYoung L, et al. Comparison between AMS 700™ CX and Coloplast™ Titan inflatable penile prosthesis for peyronie's disease treatment and remodeling: clinical outcomes and patient satisfaction. J Sex Med 2013;10(11): 2855–60.
28. Kim YD, Yang SO, Lee JK, et al. Usefulness of a malleable penile prosthesis in patients with

a spinal cord injury. Int J Urol 2008;15(10): 919–23.

29. Ferguson KH, Cespedes RD. Prospective long-term results and quality-of-life assessment after Dura-II penile prosthesis placement. Urology 2003;61(2): 437–41.

30. Hoebeke PB, Decaestecker K, Beysens M, et al. Erectile implants in female-to-male transsexuals: our experience in 129 patients. Eur Urol 2010; 57(2):334–41.

31. Neuville P, Morel-Journel N, Maucourt-Boulch D, et al. Surgical outcomes of erectile implants after phalloplasty: retrospective analysis of 95 procedures. J Sex Med 2016;13(11):1758–64.

32. Neuville P, Morel-Journel N, Cabelguenne D, et al. First outcomes of the ZSI 475 FtM, a specific prosthesis designed for phalloplasty. J Sex Med 2019;16(2):316–22.

33. Girsdansky JNH. Use of a vitallium testicular implant. Am J Surg 1941;53(3):514.

34. Marshall S. Potential problems with testicular prostheses. Urology 1986;28(5):388–90.

35. Turek PJ, Master VA, Testicular Prosthesis Study Group. Safety and effectiveness of a new saline filled testicular prosthesis. J Urol 2004;172(4 Pt 1): 1427–30.

36. Terrier JE, Courtois F, Ruffion A, et al. Surgical outcomes and patients' satisfaction with suprapubic phalloplasty. J Sex Med 2014;11(1):288–98.

37. Segal RL, Massanyi EZ, Gupta AD, et al. Inflatable penile prosthesis technique and outcomes after radial forearm free flap neophalloplasty. Int J Impot Res 2015;27(2):49–53.

Management of Vaginoplasty and Phalloplasty Complications

Jessica N. Scahrdein, MS, MD[a], Lee C. Zhao, MD[b], Dmitriy Nikolavsky, MD[a],*

KEYWORDS

- Transgender • Gender affirmation surgery • Genital reconstructive surgery • Vaginoplasty
- Phalloplasty • Complications

KEY POINTS

- Genital reconstructive surgery is an important part of gender affirmation for many transgender patients.
- The most common complications after vaginoplasty are wound complications, poor cosmesis, pelvic pain, bothersome urinary symptoms, urethral strictures, prolapse, neovaginal stenosis and loss of depth as well as neovaginal fistulas.
- The most common complications after phalloplasty include urethrocutaneous fistulas, persistent vaginal cavities, and neourethral strictures.
- Proper evaluation and management of complications depends on knowledge of the most common complications along with an understanding of the anatomic differences between cisgender patients and transgender patients.
- Gender affirmation surgery is an innovative field and treatment options for genital reconstruction complications are continuously evolving.

INTRODUCTION

Transgender patients are those whose gender identity differs from that associated with the sex they were assigned at birth. Gender dysphoria exists on a spectrum and affects individuals worldwide. In the United States alone, approximately 1.4 million individuals, or 0.6% of the population, identify as transgender.[1] Those who experience significant distress due to gender dysphoria pursue medical and/or surgical treatments, which can substantially improve their quality of life. There is a growing number of patients pursuing gender-affirming genital reconstructive surgery.[2] For those who undergo genital reconstructive surgery, complications are unfortunately common due to the complex nature of the surgeries. A multidisciplinary approach is necessary for the care of transgender patients.[3] This article reviews the most common complications after vaginoplasty and phalloplasty and discusses how to diagnose and manage those commonly encountered complications.

VAGINOPLASTY

Vaginoplasty is a surgical reconstruction of the anatomic structures of the female genitalia. It typically involves orchiectomy, excision of the male corpora cavernosa and corpus spongiosum, and creation of labia along with a neovagina in the majority of cases. The main goal of the surgery is the creation of a genital complex that is feminine in appearance.[4] A shortened urethra that allows the

Disclosure Statement: No disclosures.
a Department of Urology, SUNY Upstate Medical University, Upstate University Hospital, 750 East Adams Street, Syracuse, NY 13210, USA; b Department of Urology, NYU Urology Associates, 305 East 33rd Street, New York, NY 10016, USA
* Corresponding author.
E-mail address: uroreconstruction@gmail.com

Urol Clin N Am 46 (2019) 605–618
https://doi.org/10.1016/j.ucl.2019.07.012
0094-0143/19/© 2019 Elsevier Inc. All rights reserved.

urinary stream to face downward in the seated position is important as well.[2] For some patients, a sensate clitoris as well as a vaginal cavity that is deep and wide enough for receptive intercourse is essential for quality of life. Current literature describes the ideal neovagina as moist, elastic, and hairless, with a depth of at least 10 cm and a diameter of at least 3 cm.[2,5] Neovaginal maintenance requires a lifelong commitment to scheduled douching and consistent dilations.[3]

Currently, there are several different vaginoplasty techniques that exist. A zero-depth vaginoplasty in which there is no canal may be performed for transgender patients who are uninterested in vaginal intercourse and wish to avoid the need for lifelong dilation and cleaning.[3] For those interested in the creation of a neovagina, this may be achieved with free skin grafts, penoscrotal skin flaps, and pedicled small or large bowel segments.[6]

Penile skin inversion vaginoplasty (PSIV), initially described by Gilles and Millard in 1957,[7] remains the most common vaginoplasty technique currently performed.[2,3] This technique is performed in a single stage, with the penile skin, foreskin, and scrotal skin used for the creation of the neovagina in the rectoprostatic space along with the labia minora, labia majora, and the glans penis used for the creation of the neoclitoris.[2] Because the penile skin becomes the lining of neovagina, additional skin graft may be needed to line the neovaginal canal in cases of insufficient penile shaft skin. Resection of the corporal bodies and corpus spongiosum is necessary to prevent occlusion of the neovagina with bulk from these structures.[2] Permanent hair removal via electrolysis or laser prior to surgery is recommended because hair growth within the neovagina can lead to infections, hairballs, and concretions of bodily fluids/lubricants.[3] It also is important that the neurovascular bundle is kept intact to preserve sensitivity and sensation of the neoclitoris.[2]

A modified robotic-assisted approach to PSIV involves a transperitoneal dissection similar to that of a radical prostatectomy. This facilitates a precise dissection between the prostate and rectum to safely create space for the neovaginal cavity while maximizing depth and width with colpopexy to the posterior peritoneum.[2] Another method of robotic-assisted vaginoplasty involves using peritoneal flaps to create the apex of the vaginal canal.[8] This technique is particularly useful in cases of insufficient genital skin because peritoneal flaps are a suitable substitute for skin graft that can line the canal.

Intestinal vaginoplasty typically is reserved for transgender women with inadequate tissue for PSIV or for salvage procedures.[2] Some investigators offer primary intestinal vaginoplasty for patients with a penile skin length less than 7 cm.[9] Various segments of the intestinal tract, as well as the peritoneum, have been described for fabrication of the neovagina.[3] This review focuses on complications after PSIV and discusses intestinal vaginoplasty only in the context of revision.

VAGINOPLASTY COMPLICATIONS

Complications after vaginoplasty can be separated based on early versus delayed presentations. Early postoperative complications include bleeding, tissue necrosis, and wound dehiscence, whereas delayed complications, usually occurring within 4 months of surgery, include poor cosmesis, pelvic pain, granulation tissue, neovaginal hair, bothersome urinary symptoms, meatal or urethral strictures, prolapse, neovaginal stenosis and loss of depth as well as enteric and urinary neovaginal fistulas.[2–6,10,11] A systematic review and meta-analysis by Manrique and colleagues[5] found that the overall reported incidence of complications after PSIV was less than 15%. The complications most associated with negative patient satisfaction included excessive bleeding or hematomas, poor cosmesis, and prolonged pain.[12]

EVALUATION

A thorough history is vital to the evaluation of vaginoplasty complications. Often, the specific complication can be determined solely from the history. For example, a patient who endorses continuous or position-dependent neovaginal urine discharge likely has a urethroneovaginal fistula.[10] In other situations, a patient may endorse symptoms that are suspicious for more than one complication and warrant further evaluation. For example, a patient complaining of splayed urine and recurrent urinary tract infections may have a urethroneovaginal fistula as well as a urethral stricture.

Visual inspection alone during a physical examination may be adequate to diagnose a bulky corpus spongiosum tissue remnant. This diagnosis may be suspected if a patient endorses swelling and narrowing of the neovagina during sexual arousal, but visualization of a narrow neovagina along with protrusion of the insufficiently shortened corpus spongiosum is key to the diagnosis. Insertion of a Q-tip, which is performed by placing a lubricated Q-tip in the urethral meatus, also can confirm the diagnosis of an insufficiently shortened urethra in a patient complaining of upward deviation of urine and vaginal bulge during sexual activity (**Fig. 1**).

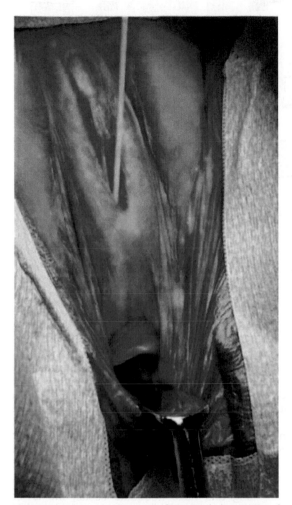

Fig. 1. Patient complaining of upward deviation of urine and vaginal bulging with sexual arousal. Insertion of a Q-tip demonstrates upward direction of the urethra due to insufficient shortening and insufficient debulking of the corpus spongiosum.

Pain can be diagnosed by an internal transvaginal examination of the pelvic floor muscles if there is presence of hypertonicity, spasticity, and tenderness. A complete physical examination should also include an examination with a lighted speculum or a vaginoscopy. This examination can help to diagnose wound complications, neovaginal stenosis and fistulas.

A retrograde urethrogram (RUG), voiding cystourethrogram (VCUG), and urethroscopy can be helpful in the evaluation of suspected fistulas or strictures. Additional imaging, such as a computed tomography (CT) scan or pelvic magnetic resonance imaging (MRI), may be indicated in certain clinical scenarios to evaluate complications and determine the appropriateness of reconstructive surgery.

A successful reconstruction depends on an in-depth preoperative cause-analysis of the complications in order to avoid failure after a revision. Patient selection and thorough preoperative discussions for management of expectations are equally important. Consultation with a pelvic floor physical physiotherapist preoperatively may help to facilitate a successful postoperative dilation regimen. It also has been recommended that psychological assessment is performed prior to revision vaginoplasty to ensure that all of a patient's expectations for revision surgery can be met.[13]

EARLY COMPLICATIONS
Hemorrhage

Surgical bleeding occurs in 3% to 12% of patients postoperatively, with the main source of hemorrhage from the corpus spongiosum surrounding the urethra.[6,14] Bleeding requiring transfusion occurs in less than 1% of patients.[4] In addition, hematomas are seen in up to 10% of patients.[6,12] The formation of hematomas may delay wound healing and can lead to an infection or an abscess.[15]

To prevent bleeding, it is the authors' practice to secure a tie-over bolster or apply negative-pressure wound therapy over the spatulated strip of the remnant corpus spongiosum. This dressing is removed after surgery, either 24 hours for the tie-over bolster or at time of packing removal for the negative-pressure wound therapy sponge. Hematomas can be prevented with a compression dressing or vulvar/labial drains that are removed once sanguineous drainage is determined to be inconsequential.[15] Avoidance of nonsteroidal analgesic medications within the first 48 hours after surgery also may help prevent hematomas.[15] Drainage may be required either at the bedside or in the operating room if the hematoma is large or expanding.[16]

Tissue Necrosis

Partial necrosis of the neovagina ranges from 1% to 4%, and clitoral necrosis ranges from 1% to 3%.[4,6] This complication may be prevented with smoking cessation and cardiovascular optimization.[4] When it occurs, only local wound care and frequent reassessments may be necessary.[4] If there is necrosis of the skin flaps into the canal, strict adherence to the postoperative dilating regimen is needed to prevent this complication from resulting in vaginal shortening or stenosis.

Wound Dehiscence

Wound dehiscence is one of the most common complications within the first postoperative month, with an incidence between 5% and 33%.[6,11] Typically, only local wound care is necessary, although nutritional deficiencies should be treated if present. It is important to instruct patients with this complication to continue scheduled dilations and douching throughout the recovery period.

DELAYED COMPLICATIONS
Cosmesis

Poor cosmesis is the most common reason for reoperation in transgender women.[6,11] Up to 50% of patients pursue secondary cosmetic corrections.[6,11] In one retrospective review, the investigators found that almost 1 in 4 patients requested aesthetic revision surgery with lipofilling, scar revision, and/or removal of excess skin.[16]

Dissatisfaction after PSIV requires management of expectations. The cosmetic outcome should be assessed at least 3 months after surgery to allow for adequate wound healing.[11] When patients remain dissatisfied with the appearance of the genitalia, future surgery may be considered. It is important to stress to patients that the cosmetic result may never be perfect.

Pelvic Pain

Postvaginoplasty pain occurs in up to 20% of patients.[6,12,14] It is attributed to the dissection through the pelvic floor muscles and fascia that is necessary to create the neovaginal cavity.[15] Postoperatively, spasticity of the pelvic diaphragm can result in persistent pain and discomfort because it contains the levator ani muscles.[15] This complication is particularly troublesome because it may interfere with a patient's ability to adequately perform postoperative dilation necessary to maintain a widely patent neovagina.[15] In addition, it can significantly affect a patient's sexual functioning and quality of life.

A referral to physical therapy with dilator therapy is imperative when a patient's pain does not resolve postoperatively. Patients who comply with a rigorous physical therapy routine have significant improvement in their symptoms.[15] When pain is debilitating and challenging to manage, a referral to pain management may be necessary as an adjunct to physical therapy. Although narcotics may help to resolve pain, they should be minimized, and other neuropathic medications, like gabapentin, should be prescribed to avoid the risks associated with narcotic pain medications.[15]

Granulation Tissue

Granulation tissue is one of the most common complications after vaginoplasty, with a reported incidence between 7% and 26%.[11,12] Granulation tissue inside the neovagina is difficult to treat. Because granulation tissue may be associated with infection, antibiotics are a reasonable approach to treatment. Silver nitrate sticks, however, are the mainstay of treatment because they may reduce fibroblast production and lead to resolution of granulation tissue.[17]

Neovaginal Hair

Approximately 29% of patients are concerned about neovaginal hair growth.[18] As previously discussed, hair growth within the neovagina can lead to infections, hairballs, and concretions of bodily fluids and lubricants.[3] To prevent intravaginal hair growth after the use of hair-bearing grafts, patients undergoing vaginoplasty should have electrolysis prior to surgery. When hair is present postoperatively, options include mechanical removal (using a speculum and removing by pulling with sponge forceps) or the use of hair removal creams. Creams should be patch-tested first, then inserted internally, left for the allotted time, and then removed by douching thoroughly. Hair regrowth to the perineum can be removed by repeated electrolysis.[17]

Urinary Complaints

Urinary complaints are not uncommon after vaginoplasty. Up to 20% of transgender women report urination problems postvaginoplasty.[18,19] Urge incontinence, stress incontinence, mixed urinary incontinence, and dribbling are described as the most common urinary complaints.[6,15] An estimated 32% of patients are diagnosed with a urinary tract infection when presenting with bothersome urinary complaints.[19]

Other symptoms may include a weak or deflecting stream, which can be due to urethral stenosis, asymmetrical labia, or an adhesion band.[11] Voiding symptoms also may be the result of bulky residual corpus spongiosum tissue that causes the urethral meatus to protrude forward or point upward.[15] A vaginal bulge that results from inadequate resection of the corpus spongiosum also can cause neovaginal narrowing, which in turn can negatively affect sexual function.[10] This occurs in up to 6% of patients.[4]

Pelvic floor physical therapy may be useful for patients with bothersome urinary complaints postvaginoplasty. Anticholinergics may be helpful for urinary incontinence. Stress urinary incontinence, in particular, may be managed with bulking of the bladder neck and should be considered first-line therapy in symptomatic patients.[15] A biological or autologous sling or a bladder neck artificial urinary sphincter also may be considered for stress urinary incontinence, because after a vaginoplasty patients typically do not have sufficient anterior urethral length for placement of a bulbar artificial urinary sphincter.

Surgery may be necessary to excise excess corpus spongiosum tissue creating a vaginal bulge (**Fig. 2**). The procedure involves removal of the residual erectile tissue of the corpus spongiosum and repositioning of the urethra to a more ventral opening.[17,20] The first step of surgery includes an incision around the urethral meatus that is continued longitudinally in the ventral neovaginal wall running over the urethra.[21] The corpus spongiosum along the urethra then is separated from other surrounding tissues.[21] Finally, the urethral meatus is brought to its new position and sutured in a Y-like fashion to prevent stricture of the meatus.[21]

Meatal or Urethral Stenosis

Meatal stenosis can occur in up to 14% of patients and may account for bothersome urinary complaints, specifically obstructive voiding disorder.[3,4,6] Meatal stenosis, in combination with a more fragile urethral wall, may lead to more proximal dilatation of the urethra, ballooning, and subsequent formation of a urethrovaginal fistula.[10] Urethral strictures more proximal to the meatus also are possible.

For patients in urinary retention, urgent urinary decompression with a suprapubic or urethral catheter is an essential first step in management. A suprapubic catheter allows for proper evaluation of a urethral stricture with a VCUG and RUG

(**Fig. 3**). Further management may include catheter dilation or urethroplasty.[16] Conservative management with dilation is a reasonable initial approach because it is less invasive compared with surgical reconstruction. When meatal stenosis is present, a simple Y-V plastic reconstruction may be performed, although 15% of patients require a second correction due to stricture recurrence.[6] Urethroplasty may involve labiaplasty with lysis of adhesions because the presence of asymmetrical labia or adhesion bands may contribute to a weak or deflecting stream.[11]

Prolapse

The prevalence of neovaginal prolapse is 1% to 2%.[4,6] In a cohort study by Kuhn and colleagues,[22] 7.5% of patients were found on examination to have a stage 2 or greater neovaginal prolapse, and 3.8% required surgery to repair the prolapse (**Fig. 4**). Some surgeons perform a sacrospinous ligament fixation during the initial vaginoplasty to secure the neovagina and prevent prolapse.[4] When prolapse occurs, an abdominal approach for sacrocolpopexy is the most common surgery performed for repair.[4,23,24]

Neovaginal Stenosis and Loss of Depth

The incidence of stenosis of the neovaginal introitus is 12%, with a range from 4% to 15%. The incidence of stenosis of the proximal vaginal canal is less common, at 1% to 12%.[6] Studies have shown that although a majority of transgender women are happy with the neovaginal depth, 12% report inadequate depth.[18,20] This complication accounts for up to 5% of reoperations.[4] Neovaginal stenosis

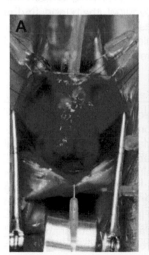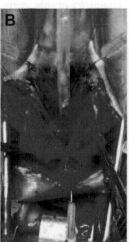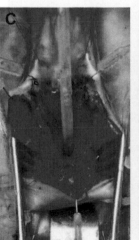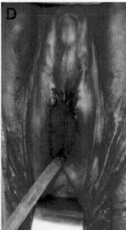

Fig. 2. Revision of excessively long urethra and bulky corpus spongiosum. (*A*) Incised neovaginal epithelium showing remnant corpus spongiosum tissue. (*B*) Proximal advancement of ventral urethrotomy. (*C*) Debulking of corpus spongiosum. (*D*) Repositioning of the urethral meatus to a more ventral opening.

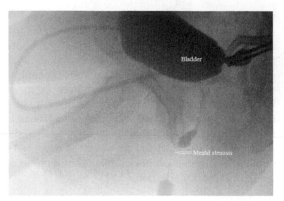

Fig. 3. RUG and cystogram demonstrating severe meatal stenosis and a more proximal urethral distension in a patient after vaginoplasty.

and loss of depth preventing patients from engaging in penetrative intercourse may be consequences of noncompliance with postoperative dilation, although often secondary to local infection and tissue retraction from diminished blood supply.[4,13]

A strict dilating regimen is necessary for prevention of neovaginal stenosis. A video demonstration and live instruction can help to ensure patients properly perform dilation. If primary vaginoplasty fails due to neovaginal stenosis, a conservative approach with aggressive dilation can be used in attempt to reform the neovaginal cavity. Soft

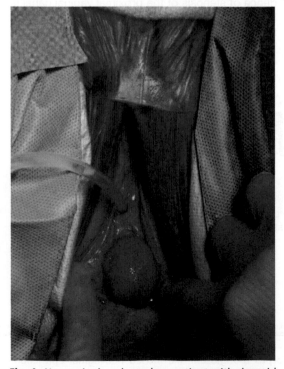

Fig. 4. Neovaginal prolapse in a patient with sigmoid neovagina.

silicone dilators may be used in place of the standard rigid dilators because they are better tolerated when the neovaginal caliber and length have been compromised as a result of scarring.[15] Adjunctive use of oil-based lubricants also can be helpful to soften the tissues lining the neovagina and may help with stretch at the time of dilation. When dilation is accompanied by significant pain, deep dilation in the operating room may be performed prior to attempting more aggressive dilation.

If these more conservative measures fail, multiple surgical approaches exist for reconstruction and may be required in up to 41% of cases.[6,13] Repair with buccal mucosal augmentation involves lateral relaxing incisions through the wall of the neovagina at the 3-o'clock and 9-o'clock positions followed by fixation of appropriately sized buccal mucosal grafts (BMGs) (**Fig. 5**).

A skin graft or an isolated bowel segment on its vascular pedicle can be used to increase depth of a neovagina.[9,17] Both approaches have good success and do not differ significantly in terms of complications.[13] Intestinal vaginoplasty with a sigmoid or ileal segment provides a neovagina with greater vaginal depth and the tissue is self-lubricating with less tendency to shrink, decreasing the need for lifelong dilation; however, it is a more invasive option involving intestinal surgery and bowel anastomosis.[13] A laparoscopic or robotic approach provides greater exposure and eliminates the need for an extensive perineal dissection, which is more challenging due to scarring. A full-thickness skin graft vaginoplasty using abdominal, inguinal, labial, or upper leg donor sites is performed by incising the preexisting neovagina and creating a dissection tunnel in the vesicorectal space to create a neovaginal cavity and fix the graft.[13] A rectal probe as well as a urinary catheter may be used to facilitate the dissection and decrease the risk of a rectal or urethral injury.

Neovaginal Fistulas

One of the most dreaded complications after vaginoplasty is the development of a rectovaginal fistula. Rectovaginal fistula can occur after a rectal injury, a postoperative abscess, an infection, a hematoma, or a dilation injury and, rarely, in cases of neovaginal malignancy.[10,15] The overall incidence of this complication is 2%, with a range between 0.8% to 17%.[4,6] There is a strong correlation between neovaginal fistulas and rectal injuries that are identified and repaired during the initial vaginoplasty surgery.[4,11] There also have been reports of urethroneovaginal fistulas, which may exist in isolation or arise secondary to another

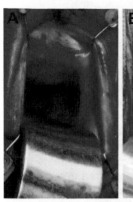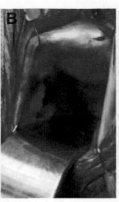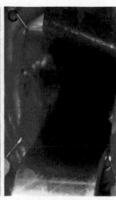

Fig. 5. Buccal mucosal augmentation for neovaginal stenosis. (*A*) Preoperative image depicting neovaginal stenosis. (*B*) Lateral neovaginal incisions. (*C*) BMG fixation.

complication, such as meatal stenosis (**Fig. 6**).[10] It is the authors' opinion, based on several observations, that urologists should exercise caution when performing procedures for the treatment of benign prostatic hyperplasia in patients with a history of vaginoplasty, because the prostatic capsule and the external urinary sphincter may be compromised during the initial surgical dissection. Similarly, dissection of the neovaginal space could be affected in patients with a history of prior prostate surgeries and increase the risk of fistula formation.

A small rectoneovaginal fistula may be managed conservatively with low residual diet, whereas surgical intervention is needed for more complex cases. Consultation and collaboration with colorectal surgery may be helpful for fistula repair. Surgical approaches include fistulectomy with primary closure in layers, local advancement flaps,

and interposition of pedicled flaps, such as a gracilis flap or an inferior gluteal artery fasciocutaneous flap. Another approach for large fistulas is the interposition of omentum and conversion to an intestinal vaginoplasty. Repairs may be performed transanally, transperineally, intraabdominally, or transneovaginally, depending on the integrity of the surrounding tissues, the size and location of the fistula, and surgeon preference.[10] Another important consideration is whether or not to perform a diverting ileostomy or colostomy, because it may improve outcomes of complex fistula repairs.[15]

Repair of a genitourinary fistula can be performed via a transvaginal or transabdominal approach. Repairs that involve tissue interposition strategies improve healing and the chances of a successful outcome.[15]

PHALLOPLASTY

Phalloplasty involves removal of the female genitalia and subsequent creation of male-appearing genitalia. For a majority (up to 98%) of transmen, voiding from a standing position is an important goal and many transmen undergo reconstructive surgery with the construction of a neourethra to achieve this goal.[25–28] For patients who prioritize sexual functioning, erogenous sensation and a phallus with sufficient length and girth for penetrative intercourse are important. The ideal phalloplasty has been described as a single-stage, reproducible procedure that allows for standing urination, tactile and erogenous sensation, sufficient girth to accommodate an erectile prosthesis, and an esthetically acceptable result.[2] Staged procedures often are necessary, however, to meet patient goals.[29]

Currently, several different techniques exist for phalloplasty. Broadly, these are categorized as free flaps and pedicled flaps. The most commonly used technique is the radial forearm free flap

Fig. 6. Prostato-neovaginal fistula in a patient with a prior transurethral resection of prostate. Foley catheter is seen through the fistula tracts.

phalloplasty because it provides the best cosmetic and functional results.[29–33] It involves tissue transfer from the forearm to the pubis with microsurgical vascular anastomoses. Pedicled flaps involve the transposition of tissue with an intact blood supply. The most common example is a pedicled anterolateral thigh flap phalloplasty.

Regardless of the flap, the neophallic urethra is created by connecting a urinary conduit within the neophallus to an elongated urethra. This results in 5 different segments of the neourethra that are classified from proximal to distal as (1) the native urethra, (2) the fixed perineal urethra (pars fixa), (3) the anastomotic urethra, (4) the phallic urethra (pars pendulans), and (5) the meatus.[26,34]

The placement of a penile prosthesis generally is a delayed procedure that occurs between 9 and 12 months after adequate healing has occurred.[3,35,36] Placement of a penile prosthesis is deferred if a neophallus is bulky enough on its own for penetrative intercourse.[35,36]

PHALLOPLASTY COMPLICATIONS

In general, phalloplasty is a more complex procedure than vaginoplasty and is associated with a higher rate of complications. Urologic complications, including urethrocutenaeous fistulas, persistent vaginal cavities, and urethral strictures, are the most commonly reported complications, which can present within a few weeks up to a few years after surgery.[32,37]

EVALUATION

Just as the history and physical are vital to the evaluation of a postvaginoplasty patient, they are the cornerstone to the evaluation of a postphalloplasty patient. Details of prior surgeries and any reconstructive efforts, which can be gathered from the patients or prior operative reports and clinical notes, are important. Specific complaints can help narrow down a differential diagnosis. For example, a patient who reports postvoid dribbling that persists long after a void is most likely to be diagnosed with a persistent vaginal cavity. During the physical examination, it is particularly important to evaluate the abdominal, flank, and genital regions. Evaluation of each may provide information regarding infection, urinary retention, fistula, or another abnormality. It cannot be overstated that blind calibration of the urethra should not be used to assess caliber of the urethra due to possibility of injury.

Beyond the history and physical, a urinalysis and culture, basic metabolic panel, complete blood cell count, and blood cultures may be useful. A uroflow and a bladder scan to obtain a postvoid residual can provide information regarding how well a patient is emptying his bladder. Infections should be appropriately treated and consideration should be given to possible urinary diversion via suprapubic access, which also allows for antegrade cystourethroscopy to facilitate eventual reconstruction.

RUG and VCUG combined with endoscopy using a cystoscope or pediatric cystoscope versus a ureteroscope are invaluable to delineate anatomy (**Fig. 7**). When the neourethra is tortuous, a guide wire ensures safe gradual advancement of a flexible scope. Additional imaging is dictated by the initial evaluation and may include ultrasound, CT scan, or MRI. Any fluid collection or abscess seen on imaging should be drained, and urine and cavity cultures should be sent to determine appropriate antibiotic treatment prior to urologic intervention.

URETHROCUTANEOUS FISTULA

Urethrocutaneous fistula is the most common complication after phalloplasty, with an incidence ranging from 15% to 70%.[32] Although fistulas may occur anywhere along the neourethra, the most common location is at the anastomotic sites between the phallic urethra and the fixed urethra and in the ventral suture line area between the fixed urethra and the native urethra (**Fig. 8**).[29,38] Decreased vascularity of the flap, poor quality of local tissue in the multilayer closure, and the discrepancy between the luminal diameters of the different urethral segments due to primary flap design or secondary to contraction during healing are thought to contribute to fistula formation.[29,38] In the presence of a stricture, proximal fistula formation is cited as 40%.[38]

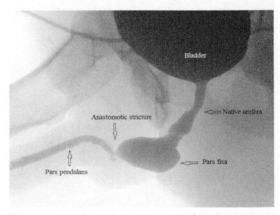

Fig. 7. RUG and simultaneous VCUG showing an anastomotic stricture between pars pendulans and pars fixa.

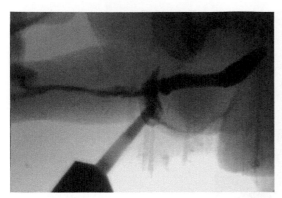

Fig. 8. Injection of contrast through an anastomotic urethrocutaneous fistula.

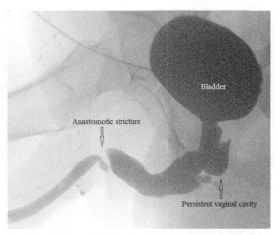

Fig. 9. RUG and simultaneous VCUG performed demonstrating an anastomotic stricture along with a persistent vaginal cavity posterior to the neourethra.

Observation is the initial course of management, because spontaneous closure of fistulous tracts may occur in up to 36% of patients within 2 months of diagnosis.[39] Fistulas that persist for greater than 3 months or are large with low potential for spontaneous closure can be corrected surgically.

Successful repair depends on complete excision of the fistula tract, the use of absorbable sutures, a tension-free multilayer closure with well-vascularized tissue, nonoverlapping suture lines, and low-pressure healing, which means elimination of distal obstruction (ie, stricture repair), maximal urinary drainage through a catheter (urethral and/or suprapubic), and prevention of detrusor overactivity.[37] A cystourethroscopy is first performed in retrograde or antegrade fashion, and external probing of the fistula tract with a guide wire or a lacrimal duct probe assists in identification of the fistula and delineation of the tract. Placement of concentric retraction sutures at the edges of the fistula tract can facilitate excision. After the tract is excised, the resulting opening can be closed in multiple nonoverlapping layers. A fasciocutaneous groin flap, a labial fat pad flap, or a musculofascial gracilis flap can be performed to decrease the risk of fistula recurrence. A catheter provides maximal urinary drainage for low-pressure healing. Repair of a concomitant neourethral stricture or persistent vaginal cavity also decreases the risk of fistula recurrence by allowing for low-pressure healing.[40]

PERSISTENT VAGINAL CAVITY

A persistent vaginal cavity may communicate with a neourethra and lead to prolonged postvoid dribbling, pelvic pain, or fullness and/or persistent urinary tract infections postphalloplasty. In patients who present for treatment of a neourethral stricture, this complication is present in approximately half of patients (**Fig. 9**).[37] It is hypothesized that pressurized urine due to neourethral stricture breaks through the suture lines of the fixed urethra into the previously obliterated vaginal cavity.[37] Inadequate vaginal de-epithelialization during colpocleisis or incomplete vaginectomy also makes patients more susceptible to this complication.[37] Presence of a persistent vaginal cavity should be investigated during reconstructive surgery, regardless of whether it is detected radiographically during the preoperative evaluation to ensure this complication is not missed.

Surgery involves complete excision and obliteration through an open perineal approach or a transabdominal robotic-assisted laparoscopic approach.[37,40] (**Fig. 10**). Subepithelial injection of lidocaine with epinephrine into the lining of the cavity is helpful in tissue hydrodissection and in reducing intraoperative bleeding. Placement of bilateral ureteral stents and a urethral catheter prior to the dissection can facilitate identification of these structures and possibly decrease the risk of injury.

URETHRAL STRICTURES

Urethral strictures occur with an incidence between 25% to 58%[35,38,41,42]; 41% of strictures occur in the anastomotic urethra between pars fixa and pars pendulans, 28% occur in the phallic urethra, 15% occur in the meatus, 13% occur in the fixed urethra, and 8% occur in multiple urethral segments, with most strictures presenting in association with fistulas.[34,38] A majority of strictures occur at anastomotic sites with poor blood flow due to ischemia.[29,41] Contracture of neourethral tissue during healing can also lead to stricture formation.[2]

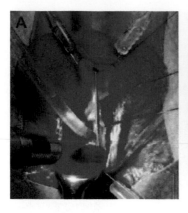
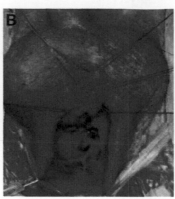

Fig. 10. Persistent vaginal cavity repair. (*A*) Intraoperative photograph of a remnant vaginal cavity repaired at the time of neourethral stricture repair (*B*) Obliterated vaginal cavity via redo colpocleisis.

Urethral strictures often require surgery but can be temporized with catheter dilation until the inflammation surrounding the tissue has abated.[35] Endoscopic management with dilation or direct visualization internal urethrotomy is a reasonable, less-invasive, first-line treatment option for short, single strictures.[43] These techniques are performed under direct endoscopic or radiographic guidance to ensure the proper location is dilated or incised. Placement of a Foley catheter for at least 2 weeks postoperatively allows for urinary drainage to promote healing.[43] Self-catheterization or self-calibration techniques can be used after catheter removal to help maintain urethral patency. Durable success after endoscopic management is low, with the rate of recurrence as high as 88% likely due to the lack of a corpus spongiosum and poor blood supply.[2,37,42]

Urethral reconstruction via urethroplasty is the best option for definitive management of strictures. Techniques after neophallus construction include meatotomy and excision and primary anastomosis, free graft urethroplasty, pedicled flap urethroplasty, and 2-stage urethroplasty.[34,35] In the largest study to date on outcomes after urethroplasty following phalloplasty, meatotomy and 2-staged urethroplasty had the lowest recurrence rates, at 25% and 30.3%, respectively.[34] Perineal urethrostomy is reserved for patients with multiple failed reconstructive attempts or those who choose to avoid extensive reconstruction.

Extended meatotomy is the standard approach for surgically correcting short stenotic segments at the meatus.[44] This technique is performed by incising the meatus with a simple ventral incision and then reapproximating the inner urethral mucosa and glanular tissue with sutures. Meatoplasty is performed for recurrent or longer meatal strictures. It includes numerous techniques that may incorporate flaps or grafts and can be performed in a single or staged procedure similar to more proximal urethral reconstruction.[44] The Asopa

urethroplasty is a 1-stage technique that involves ventral sagittal urethrotomy and dorsal graft placement without mobilization of the urethra.[45] A single-stage ventral onlay BMG is another distal urethroplasty technique.[46] A double-face BMG technique that involves opening the stenosed segment ventrally and raising glanular wings for placement of a ventral graft followed by a dorsal urethrotomy incision for placement of a dorsal graft is another option.[47] A more novel technique that involves a ventral transurethral wedge resection of the stenosed segment and transurethral delivery and spread fixation of appropriate BMG inlay into the resultant urethrotomy may be applied as well.[48] Augmented staged surgeries are important for patients with a completely obliterated meatus or those with prior failures (**Fig. 11**).

For a primary short urethral anastomotic stricture, a single-stage anastomotic technique without the use of additional flaps or grafts is an option. Excision and primary anastomosis or a nontransecting anastomotic urethroplasty, which is considered the gold standard approach for short strictures in cisgender male urethras, may be performed when a short anastomotic stricture is accompanied by reliable well-vascularized local tissue. This technique is performed by excising the stenosed urethral segment, spatulating the proximal and distal stumps in opposite, complementary directions, and then reapproximating the edges over an indwelling Foley catheter.[37] The overall success rate in this population is low, at 57%, which may be due to decreased tissue mobility, absence of corpus spongiosum, and reduced blood supply in transgender men with neophallic urethras.[28,34,42]

A dorsal inlay approach with BMG is a single-stage substitution technique that may be performed for longer or more complex strictures. The operation typically begins with a ventral urethrotomy followed by a vertical dorsal incision through the stenosed segment of the urethra and

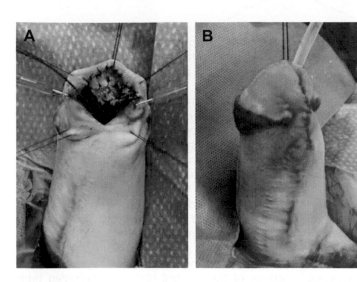

Fig. 11. Distal meatal reconstruction in a patient with prior extended meatotomy. (*A*) Buccal mucosa inlay placed dorsally prior to tubularization. (*B*) Postoperative image immediately after tubularization.

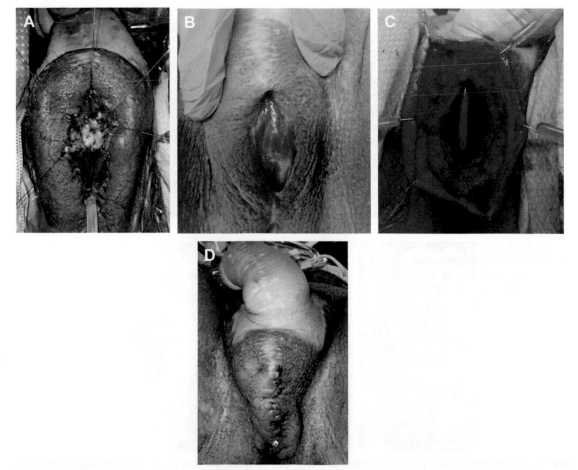

Fig. 12. Staged urethroplasty of anastomotic stricture. (*A*) Stage 1 repair with BMG placed at the site of anastomotic stricture to serve as a temporary perineal urethrostomy. (*B*) Matured urethral plate at 6 months postoperatively. (*C*) Intraoperative image during stage 2 urethroplasty showing lateral mobilization of urethral plate and tubularization over a Foley catheter. (*D*) Stage 2: immediate postoperative image.

advances 1 cm to 2 cm into the patent lumen proximally and distally. The graft is placed as a dorsal inlay to increase the size of the lumen and ensure patency prior to closure.[45] Dorsal placement may avoid the frequently unreliable vascularity and coverage of the ventral tissue; however, ventral repairs also have been described.[42,49] The double-face repair using simultaneous dorsal inlay and ventral onlay BMG is the authors' preferred urethroplasty method, which involves quilting each graft on an independent vascular bed.[50] Specifically, for the ventral graft, the authors utilize neoscrotal fat, similar to a Martius flap. Occasionally, a gracilis flap may be present in the perineum from the original neophallus construction.[37] Whenever available, gracilis can be carefully dissected, mobilized and reused as a vascular bed for the ventral BMG.[37] Incorporation of a fasciocutaneous

flap may be used to support a ventral onlay graft and improve its blood supply.[51]

A staged urethroplasty is the recommended option for long penile or recurrent neourethral strictures (**Figs. 12 and 13**). This technique begins with a ventral urethrotomy through the stenosed segment or, in cases of total neourethral obliteration, a complete ventral spatulation of the anterior urethral segment. The urethral plate either is then augmented with a graft or a new neourethral plate is created with a graft. The lateral edges of the urethral plate are then sutured to the borders of the skin incision and left to heal exposed. As the urethral plate matures over the next 3 months to 6 months, the patient voids through a temporary, more proximal urethrostomy. During the second stage, the lateral edges of the urethral plate are mobilized prior

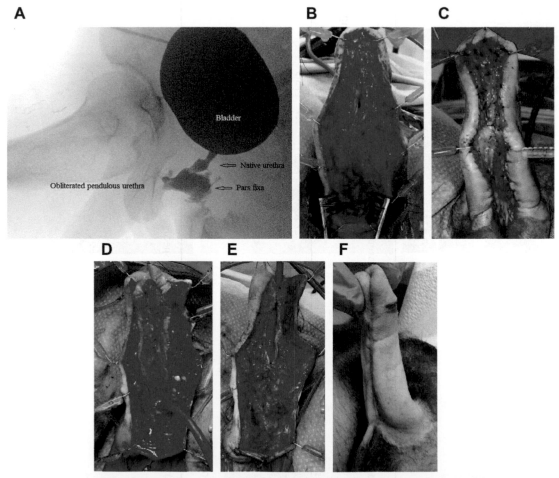

Fig. 13. Staged urethroplasty for panurethral stricture. (*A*) Preoperative RUG and VCUG showing a completely obliterated pars pendulans. (*B*) Intraoperative image showing absence of neourethra. (*C*) Stage 1: reharvested BMG fixation in multiple mosaic pieces in a patient with a prior bilateral BMG harvest. (*D*) Stage 2: mobilization of urethral plate 6 months later (note additional lingual mucosa inlay placed to widen the distal plate). (*E*) Stage 2: tubularization of the urethra over a Foley catheter. (*F*) Postoperative image at 8 months.

to tubularization of the neourethra over a catheter. Overall, this technique has been reported to have a success rate of up to 70%, which is the highest success rate among all types of neophallic urethroplasties.[34]

Perineal urethrostomy is an alternate option for patients who are not interested in reconstructive surgery or who have failed multiple reconstructive efforts. In other situations, it may be used as a temporary treatment until definitive reconstruction is pursued. This surgery results in a perineal urethra under the neoscrotum by opening the fixed urethra and approximating the lateral edges of the urethra to the perineum. It allows for unobstructed urine flow from the newly created urethra.

SUMMARY

Overall, reconstructive surgery is challenging after vaginoplasty and phalloplasty. Continued surgical advancements are critical for optimal treatment of patients with complications after surgery.

REFERENCES

1. Herman JL, Flores AR, Brown TNT, et al. Age of Individuals who Identify as Transgender in the United States. Los Angeles, CA: The Williams Institute; 2017.
2. Dy GW, Sun J, Granieri MA, et al. Reconstructive management pearls for the transgender patient. Curr Urol Rep 2018;19:36.
3. Pan S, Honig SC. Gender-affirming surgery: current concepts. Andrology and infertility. Curr Urol Rep 2018;19:62.
4. Dreher PC, Edwards D, Hager S, et al. Complications of the neovagina in male-to-female transgender surgery: a systematic review and meta-analysis with discussion of management. Clin Anat 2018;31(2):191–9.
5. Manrique OJ, Adabi K, Martinez-Jorge J, et al. Complications and patient-reported outcomes in male-to-female vaginoplasty-where we are today: a systematic review and meta-analysis. Ann Plast Surg 2018; 80(6):684–91.
6. Horbach SE, Bouman MB, Smit JM, et al. Outcome of vaginoplasty in male-to-female transgenders: a systematic review of surgical techniques. J Sex Med 2015;12:1499–512.
7. Gillies HD, Millard DR. The principles and art of plastic surgery. Boston, MA. Little, Brown & Company 1957;39(2): p 477.
8. Jacoby A, Maliha S, Granieri MA, et al. Robotic Davydov peritoneal flap vaginoplasty for augmentation of vaginal depth in feminizing vaginoplasty. J Urol 2019;201(6):1171–6.
9. Buncamper ME, van der Sluis WB, de Vries M, et al. Penile inversion vaginoplasty with or without additional full-thickness skin graft: to graft or not to graft? Plast Reconstr Surg 2017;139(3):649–56.
10. Van der Sluis WB, Bouman MB, Buncamper ME, et al. Clinical characteristics and management of neovaginal fistulas after vaginoplasty in transgender women. Obstet Gynecol 2016;127(6):1118–26.
11. Gaither TW, Awad MA, Osterberg EC, et al. Postoperative complications following primary penile inversion vaginoplasty among 330 male-to-female transgender patients. J Urol 2018;199:760–5.
12. Massie JP, Morrison SD, Van Maasdam J, et al. Predictors of patient satisfaction and postoperative complications in penile inversion vaginoplasty. Plast Reconstr Surg 2018;141(6):911–21.
13. Van der Sluis WB, Bouman MB, Buncamper ME, et al. Revision vaginoplasty: a comparison of surgical outcomes of laparoscopic intestinal versus perineal full-thickness skin graft vaginoplasty. Plast Reconstr Surg 2016;138(4):793–800.
14. Papadopulos NA, Zavlin D, Lelle JD, et al. Combined vaginoplasty technique for male-to-female sex reassignment surgery: operative approach and outcomes. J Plast Reconstr Aesthet Surg 2017;70:1483–92.
15. Ferrando CA. Vaginoplasty complications. Clin Plast Surg 2018;45(3):361–8.
16. Raigosa M, Avvedimento S, Yoon TS, et al. Male-to-female genital reassignment surgery: a retrospective review of surgical technique and complications in 60 patients. J Sex Med 2015;12(8):1837–45.
17. Suchak T, Hussey J, Takhar M, et al. Postoperative trans women in sexual health clinics: managing common problems after vaginoplasty. J Fam Plann Reprod Health Care 2015;41(4):245–7.
18. Goddard JC, Vickery RM, Qureshi A, et al. Feminizing genitoplasty in adult transsexuals: early and long term surgical results. BJU Int 2007;100:607–13.
19. Hoebeke P, Selvaggi G, Ceulemans P, et al. Impact of sex reassignment surgery on lower urinary tract function. Eur Urol 2005;47:398–402.
20. Krege S, Bex A, Lummen G, et al. Male to female transsexualism: a technique, results and long term follow up in 66 patients. BJU Int 2001;88:396–402.
21. Karim RB, Hage JJ, Bouman FG, et al. The importance of near total resection of the corpus spongiosum and total resection of the corpora cavernosa in the surgery of male to female transsexuals. Ann Plast Surg 1991;26(6):554–6.
22. Kuhn A, Santi A, Birkhauser M. Vaginal prolapse, pelvic floor function, and related symptoms 16 years after sex reassignment surgery in transsexuals. Fertil Steril 2011;95(7):2379–82.
23. Loverro G, Bettocchi C, Battaglia M, et al. Repair of vaginal prolapse following penoscrotal flap

vaginoplasty in a male-to-female transsexual. Gynecol Obstet Invest 2002;53:234–6.

24. Frederick RW, Leach GE. Abdominal sacral colpopexy for repair of neovaginal prolapse in male-to-female transsexuals. Urology 2004;64(3):580–1.

25. Hage JJ, Bout CA, Bloem JJ, et al. Phalloplasty in female-to-male transsexuals: what do our patients ask for? Ann Plast Surg 1993;30(4):323–6.

26. Hage JJ, Bloem JJ. Review of the literature on construction of a neourethra in female-to-male transsexuals. Ann Plast Surg 1993;30(3):278–86.

27. Dubin BJ, Sato RM, Laub DR. Results of phalloplasty. Plast Reconstr Surg 1979;64(2):163–70.

28. Puckett CL, Montie JE. Construction of male genitalia in the transsexual, using a tubed groin flap for the penis and a hydraulic inflation device. Plast Reconstr Surg 1978;61(4):523–30.

29. Blaschke E, Bales GT, Thomas S. Postoperative imaging of phalloplasties and their complications. AJR Am J Roentgenol 2014;203:323–8.

30. Chang TS, Hwang WY. Forearm flap in one-stage reconstruction of the penis. Plast Reconstr Surg 1984;74:251–8.

31. Song R, Gao Y, Song Y, et al. The forearm flap. Cin Plast Surg 1982;9:21–6.

32. Monstrey S, Hoebeke P, Selvaggi G, et al. Penile reconstruction: is the forearm flap really the standard technique? Plast Reconstr Surg 2009;124:510–8.

33. Garaffa G, Ralph DJ, Christoper N. Total urethral construction with the radial artery-based forearm free flap in the transsexual. BJU Int 2010;106:1206–10.

34. Lumen N, Monstrey S, Goessaert AS, et al. Urethroplasty for strictures after phallic reconstruction: a single-institution experience. Eur Urol 2011;60(1):150–8.

35. Morrison SD, Chen ML, Crane CN. An overview of female-to-male gender confirming surgery. Nat Rev Urol 2017;14(8):486–500.

36. Neuville P, Morel-Journel N, Maucourt-Boulch D, et al. Surgical outcomes of erectile implants after phalloplasty: retrospective analysis of 95 procedures. J Sex Med 2016;13:1758–64.

37. Nikolavsky D, Yamaguchi Y, Levine JP, et al. Urologic sequelae following phalloplasty in transgendered patients. Urol Clin North Am 2017;44:113–25.

38. Rohrmann D, Jakse G. Urethroplasty in female-to-male transsexuals. Eur Urol 2003;44(5):611–4.

39. Fang RH, Kao YS, Ma S, et al. Phalloplasty in female-to-male transsexuals using free radial osteocutaneous flap: a series of 22 cases. Br J Plast Surg 1999;52(3):217–22.

40. Groenman F, Nikkels C, Huirne J, et al. Robot-assisted laparoscopic colpectomy in female-to-male transgender patients; technique and outcomes of a prospective cohort study. Surg Endosc 2017;31(8):3363–9.

41. Monstrey SJ, Ceulemans P, Hoebeke P. Sex reassignment surgery in the female-to-male transsexual. Semin Plast Surg 2011;25(3):229–44.

42. Levine LA, Elterman L. Urethroplasty following total phallic reconstruction. J Urol 1998;160(2):378–82.

43. Lumen N, Oosterlinck W, Decaestecker K, et al. Endoscopic incision of short (<3 cm) urethral strictures after phallic reconstruction. J Endourol 2009;23(8):1329–32.

44. Daneshvar M, Hughes M, Nikolavsky D. Surgical management of fossa navicul016and distal urethral strictures. Curr Urol Rep 2018;19(6):43.

45. Asopa HS, Garg M, Singhal GG, et al. Dorsal free graft urethroplasty for urethral stricture by ventral sagittal urethrotomy approach. Urology 2001;58(5):657–9.

46. Chowdhury PS, Nayak P, Mallick S, et al. A single stage ventral onlay buccal mucosal graft urethroplasty for navicular fossa strictures. Indian J Urol 2014;30(1):17–22.

47. Goel A, Goel A, Dalela D, et al. Meatoplasty using double buccal mucosal graft technique. Int Urol Nephrol 2009;41(4):885–7.

48. Nikolavsky D, Abouelleil M, Daneshvar M. Transurethral ventral buccal mucosa graft inlay urethroplasty for reconstruction of fossa navicularis and distal urethral strictures: surgical technique and preliminary results. Int Urol Nephrol 2016;48(11):1823–9.

49. Pariser JJ, Cohn JA, Gottlieb LJ, et al. Buccal mucosal graft urethroplasty for the treatment of urethral stricture in the neophallus. Urology 2015;85(4):927–31.

50. Gelman J, Siegel JA. Ventral and dorsal buccal grafting for 1-stage repair of complex anterior urethral strictures. Urology 2014;83(6):1418–22.

51. Wilson SC, Stranix JT, Khurana K, et al. Fasciocutaneous flap reinforcement of ventral onlay buccal mucosa grafts enables neophallus revision urethroplasty. Ther Adv Urol 2016;8(6):331–7.

UNITED STATES POSTAL SERVICE®

Statement of Ownership, Management, and Circulation
(All Periodicals Publications Except Requester Publications)

1. Publication Title	2. Publication Number	3. Filing Date
UROLOGIC CLINICS OF NORTH AMERICA	000 – 711	9/18/2019

4. Issue Frequency	5. Number of Issues Published Annually	6. Annual Subscription Price
FEB, MAY, AUG, NOV	4	$387.00

7. Complete Mailing Address of Known Office of Publication (Not printer) (Street, city, county, state, and ZIP+4®)

ELSEVIER INC.
230 Park Avenue, Suite 800
New York, NY 10169

Contact Person: STEPHEN R. BUSHING
Telephone (Include area code): 215-239-3688

8. Complete Mailing Address of Headquarters or General Business Office of Publisher (Not printer)

ELSEVIER INC.
230 Park Avenue, Suite 800
New York, NY 10169

9. Full Names and Complete Mailing Addresses of Publisher, Editor, and Managing Editor (Do not leave blank)

Publisher (Name and complete mailing address)

TAYLOR BALL, ELSEVIER INC.
1600 JOHN F KENNEDY BLVD. SUITE 1800
PHILADELPHIA, PA 19103-2899

Editor (Name and complete mailing address)

KERRY HOLLAND, ELSEVIER INC.
1600 JOHN F KENNEDY BLVD. SUITE 1800
PHILADELPHIA, PA 19103-2899

Managing Editor (Name and complete mailing address)

PATRICK MANLEY, ELSEVIER INC.
1600 JOHN F KENNEDY BLVD. SUITE 1800
PHILADELPHIA, PA 19103-2899

10. Owner (Do not leave blank. If the publication is owned by a corporation, give the name and address of the corporation immediately followed by the names and addresses of all stockholders owning or holding 1 percent or more of the total amount of stock. If not owned by a corporation, give the names and addresses of the individual owners. If owned by a partnership or other unincorporated firm, give its name and address as well as those of each individual owner. If the publication is published by a nonprofit organization, give its name and address.)

Full Name	Complete Mailing Address
WHOLLY OWNED SUBSIDIARY OF REED/ELSEVIER, US HOLDINGS	1600 JOHN F KENNEDY BLVD. SUITE 1800 PHILADELPHIA, PA 19103-2899

11. Known Bondholders, Mortgagees, and Other Security Holders Owning or Holding 1 Percent or More of Total Amount of Bonds, Mortgages, or Other Securities. If none, check box ▶ ☐ None

Full Name	Complete Mailing Address
N/A	

12. Tax Status (For completion by nonprofit organizations authorized to mail at nonprofit rates) (Check one)
The purpose, function, and nonprofit status of this organization and the exempt status for federal income tax purposes:
☒ Has Not Changed During Preceding 12 Months
☐ Has Changed During Preceding 12 Months (Publisher must submit explanation of change with this statement)

PS Form 3526, July 2014 (Page 1 of 4 (see instructions page 4)) PSN: 7530-01-000-9931   PRIVACY NOTICE: See our privacy policy on www.usps.com.

---

13. Publication Title	14. Issue Date for Circulation Data Below
UROLOGIC CLINICS OF NORTH AMERICA	MAY 2019

15. Extent and Nature of Circulation			Average No. Copies Each Issue During Preceding 12 Months	No. Copies of Single Issue Published Nearest to Filing Date
a. Total Number of Copies (Net press run)			262	340
b. Paid Circulation (By Mail and Outside the Mail)	(1)	Mailed Outside-County Paid Subscriptions Stated on PS Form 3541 (Include paid distribution above nominal rate, advertiser's proof copies, and exchange copies)	118	165
	(2)	Mailed In-County Paid Subscriptions Stated on PS Form 3541 (Include paid distribution above nominal rate, advertiser's proof copies, and exchange copies)	0	0
	(3)	Paid Distribution Outside the Mails Including Sales Through Dealers and Carriers, Street Vendors, Counter Sales, and Other Paid Distribution Outside USPS®	90	129
	(4)	Paid Distribution by Other Classes of Mail Through the USPS (e.g. First-Class Mail®)	0	0
c. Total Paid Distribution (Sum of 15b (1), (2), (3), and (4))		▶	208	294
d. Free or Nominal Rate Distribution (By Mail and Outside the Mail)	(1)	Free or Nominal Rate Outside-County Copies included on PS Form 3541	43	29
	(2)	Free or Nominal Rate In-County Copies Included on PS Form 3541	0	0
	(3)	Free or Nominal Rate Copies Mailed at Other Classes Through the USPS (e.g. First-Class Mail)	0	0
	(4)	Free or Nominal Rate Distribution Outside the Mail (Carriers or other means)	0	0
e. Total Free or Nominal Rate Distribution (Sum of 15d (1), (2), (3) and (4))		▶	43	29
f. Total Distribution (Sum of 15c and 15e)		▶	251	323
g. Copies not Distributed (See Instructions to Publishers #4 (page 43))		▶	11	17
h. Total (Sum of 15f and g)		▶	262	340
i. Percent Paid (15c divided by 15f times 100)			82.87%	91.02%

* If you are claiming electronic copies, go to line 16 on page 3. If you are not claiming electronic copies, skip to line 17 on page 3.

16. Electronic Copy Circulation		Average No. Copies Each Issue During Preceding 12 Months	No. Copies of Single Issue Published Nearest to Filing Date
a. Paid Electronic Copies	▶		
b. Total Paid Print Copies (Line 15c) + Paid Electronic Copies (Line 16a)	▶		
c. Total Print Distribution (Line 15f) + Paid Electronic Copies (Line 16a)	▶		
d. Percent Paid (Both Print & Electronic Copies) (16b divided by 16c × 100)	▶		

☒ I certify that 50% of all my distributed copies (electronic and print) are paid above a nominal price.

17. Publication of Statement of Ownership

☒ If the publication is a general publication, publication of this statement is required. Will be printed in the NOVEMBER 2019 issue of this publication. ☐ Publication not required.

18. Signature and Title of Editor, Publisher, Business Manager, or Owner	Date
STEPHEN R. BUSHING - INVENTORY DISTRIBUTION CONTROL MANAGER	9/18/2019

I certify that all information furnished on this form is true and complete. I understand that anyone who furnishes false or misleading information on this form or who omits material or information requested on the form may be subject to criminal sanctions (including fines and imprisonment) and/or civil sanctions (including civil penalties).

PS Form 3526, July 2014 (Page 3 of 4)   PRIVACY NOTICE: See our privacy policy on www.usps.com

Moving?

Make sure your subscription moves with you!

To notify us of your new address, find your **Clinics Account Number** (located on your mailing label above your name), and contact customer service at:

Email: journalscustomerservice-usa@elsevier.com

800-654-2452 (subscribers in the U.S. & Canada)
314-447-8871 (subscribers outside of the U.S. & Canada)

Fax number: 314-447-8029

Elsevier Health Sciences Division
Subscription Customer Service
3251 Riverport Lane
Maryland Heights, MO 63043

*To ensure uninterrupted delivery of your subscription, please notify us at least 4 weeks in advance of move.